Board Review Series

Pharmacology
2nd edition

Board Review Series

Pharmacology
2nd edition

Gary C. Rosenfeld, Ph.D.
Associate Professor and Vice-Chairman
Director of Medical Education
Department of Pharmacology
University of Texas–Houston Medical School
Houston, Texas

Kathleen M. Rose, Ph.D.
Professor
Department of Pharmacology
University of Texas–Houston Medical School
Houston, Texas

David S. Loose-Mitchell, Ph.D.
Associate Professor
Department of Pharmacology
University of Texas–Houston Medical School
Houston, Texas

Contribution by
James B. Jones, Pharm. D.

M.D. candidate
University of Pennsylvania, School of Medicine
Philadelphia, Pennsylvania

Harwal Publishing

Philadelphia • Baltimore • Hong Kong • London • Munich • Sydney • Tokyo

A Waverly Company

Harwal

Library of Congress Cataloging-in-Publication Data

Rosenfeld, Gary C.
    Pharmacology / Gary C. Rosenfeld, Kathleen M. Rose, David Loose-Mitchell.
      —2nd ed.
      p.   cm—(Board review series)
    Rose's name appears first on the earlier edition.
    Includes index.
    ISBN 0-683-07361-3 (pbk. : alk paper)
    1. Pharmacology—Examinations, questions, etc. I. Rose, Kathleen M.
  II. Loose-Mitchell, David S.   III. Title. IV. Series.
    [DNLM: 1. Pharmacology—examination questions. QV 18 R 796 p 1993]
  RM301.13.R67 1993
615′.1′076—dc20
DNLM/DLC
for Library of Congress   93-18750
                                                               CIP

Accurate indications, adverse reactions, and dosage schedules for drugs are provided in this book, but it is possible that they may change. The reader is urged to review the package information data of the manufacturers of the medications mentioned.

10 9 8 7 6 5 4 3 2 1

Contents

Preface to the Second Edition

This concise review of medical pharmacology is designed for medical and dental students and others in the health care professions. It is intended primarily to help students prepare for licensing examinations such as the United States Medical Licensing Examination Step 1 (USMLE) or other similar examinations. This book presents the essentials of pharmacology in the form of condensed and succinct descriptions of relevant and current Board-driven information without the usual associated details. It is not meant to be a substitute for the comprehensive presentation of information and difficult concepts found in standard pharmacology texts.

Organization

The second edition begins with a chapter devoted to the general principles of drug action, followed by chapters concerned with drugs acting on the major body systems. Other chapters discuss autacoids, ergots, anti-inflammatory and immunosuppressive agents, drugs used to treat anemias and disorders of hemostasis, infectious diseases, cancer, and toxicology.

Each chapter includes a presentation of specific drugs with a discussion of their general properties, mechanism of action, pharmacologic effects, therapeutic uses, and adverse effects. Tables summarizing essential drug information are also included in several chapters.

Review questions and answers with explanations, all reflecting the new USMLE format, follow each chapter to help students assess their understanding of the information. Similarly, a Comprehensive Examination, with clinically oriented USMLE-type questions, has been added at the end of the book. This examination serves as a self-assessment tool for students to determine their fund of knowledge and to diagnose any weaknesses in pharmacology.

New to this edition

- Updated and current information
- Tables organizing essential information for quick recall
- 450 questions and explanations based on Board-driven information and reflecting current USMLE Step 1 format
- Comprehensive Examination including 100 clinically oriented questions and explanations

Gary C. Rosenfeld, Ph.D.
Kathleen M. Rose, Ph.D.
David S. Loose-Mitchell, Ph.D.

Acknowledgments

The authors acknowledge the organizational and secretarial skills of Ms. Marcia Waldbillig. The authors also are indebted to the redoubtable Ms. Susan Kelly, Managing Editor of the Board Review Series, for her seemingly unlimited patience and dedication to this project. Special thanks also to Ms. Mary Durkin for her inspired editing of the manuscript. Lastly, a thank you to our colleagues for their support and contributions to this book and to our medical students for being our harshest critics.

1

General Principles of Drug Action

I. Dose–Response Relationships

A. Drug effects

–are produced by altering the normal functions of cells and tissues in the body via one of four general mechanisms:

1. **Interaction with receptors,** naturally occurring target molecules (often proteins), which mediate the effects of endogenous physiologic substances such as neurotransmitters and hormones

2. **Alteration of the activity of enzymes**

3. **Antimetabolite action**

   –as a nonfunctional analog of a naturally occurring metabolite, interferes with normal metabolism.

4. **Nonspecific chemical or physical interactions**

   –are caused by antacids, osmotic agents, and chelators.

B. The graded dose–response curve

–expresses an individual's response to increasing doses of a given drug. The magnitude of a pharmacologic response is proportional to the number of receptors with which a drug effectively interacts (Figure 1.1).

–includes the following parameters:

1. **Magnitude of response**

   –is **graded;** that is, it continuously increases with the dose up to the maximal capacity of the system, and it is often depicted as a function of the log of the dose administered (to see the relationship over a wide range of doses).

2. **ED_{50}**

   –is the dose that produces the half-maximal response; the threshold dose is that which produces the first noticeable effect.

3. **Intrinsic activity**

   –reflects the ability of a drug to elicit a response.

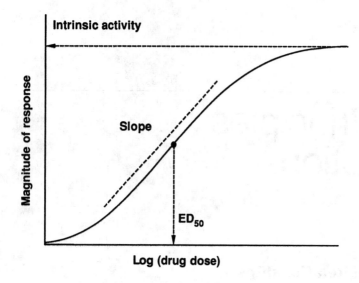

Figure 1.1. Graded dose–response curve.

a. Agonists
–are drugs capable of binding to, and activating, a receptor.
  (1) Full agonists occupy all receptors and have an intrinsic activity of 1.
  (2) Partial agonists can occupy all of the receptors but cannot elicit a maximal response. Such drugs have an intrinsic activity of less than 1 (Figure 1.2; drug C).

b. Antagonists
–bind to the receptor but do not initiate a response; that is, they block the action of an agonist or endogenous substance that works through the receptor.
  (1) Competitive antagonists combine with the same site on the receptor as the agonist but have little or no efficacy and an intrinsic activity of zero.
    –may be **reversible or irreversible**. Reversible—or equilibrium—competitive antagonists are not covalently bound, shift the dose–response curve for the agonist to the right, and increase the ED_{50};

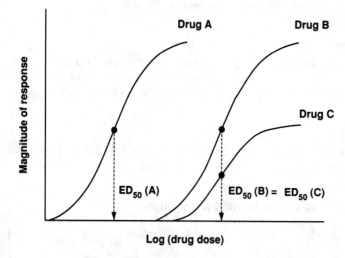

Figure 1.2. Graded dose–response curves for two agonists (A and B) and a partial agonist (C).

that is, more agonist is required to elicit a response in the presence of the antagonist (Figure 1.3). Because higher doses of agonist can overcome the inhibition, the maximal response can still be obtained.

   (2) Noncompetitive antagonists bind to the receptor at a site other than the agonist binding site (Figure 1.4) and either prevent the agonist from binding correctly or from activating the receptor. Consequently, the effective amount of receptor is reduced. Receptors unoccupied by antagonist retain the same affinity for agonist and the ED_{50} is unchanged.

4. Potency of a drug

–is a reflection of the relative amount of drug needed to produce a given response.
–can be demonstrated by comparing the ED_{50} values of two full agonists; the drug with the lower ED_{50} is more potent (see Figure 1.2; drug A is more potent than drug B).
–is partly determined by the **affinity** of a drug for its receptor.

5. Efficacy of a drug

–reflects its ability to elicit a maximal effect.

6. Slope

–is measured at the midportion of the dose–response curve.
–varies for different drugs and different responses. Steep dose–response curves indicate that a small change in dose produces a large change in response.

7. Variability

–reflects the differences between individuals in response to a given drug.

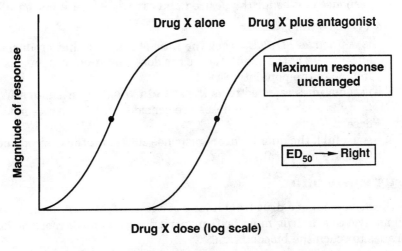

Figure 1.3. Graded dose–response curves illustrating the effects of competitive antagonists.

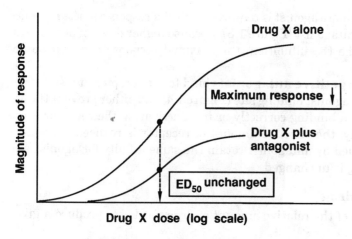

Figure 1.4. Graded dose–response curves illustrating the effects of non-competitive antagonists.

C. The quantal dose–response curve (Figure 1.5)

–relates the **dosage** of a drug to the **frequency** with which a designated response will occur within a population. The response may be an "all-or-none" phenomenon (e.g., individuals do or do not fall asleep after receiving a sedative) or some predetermined intensity of effect.

–is obtained via transformation of the data used for a frequency distribution plot to reflect the **cumulative frequency** of a response. In the context of the quantal dose–response curve, ED_{50} indicates the dose of drug that produces the response in half of the population. (Note that this differs from the meaning of ED_{50} in a graded dose–response curve.)

D. Therapeutic index and certain safety factor

1. Therapeutic index (TI)

–relates the desired therapeutic effect to undesired toxicity, using data provided by the quantal dose–response curve.

–is defined as TD_{50}/ED_{50} (i.e., the ratio of the dose that produces a toxic effect in half the population to the dose that produces the desired effect in half the population).

–should be used with caution in instances when the quantal dose–response curves for the desired and toxic effects are not parallel.

2. Certain safety factor

–is defined as TD_1/ED_{99} (i.e., the ratio of the dose that produces the toxic effect in 1% of the population to the dose that produces the desired effect in 99% of the population).

–is sometimes referred to as the **standard safety measure**. When mortality is a factor, lethal doses are considered; LD_{50} is the median lethal dose.

–is useful if the quantal dose–response curves for the desired and toxic effects are not parallel.

II. Drug Absorption

–is the movement of a drug from its site of administration into the bloodstream. In many cases, a drug must be transported across one or more biologic membranes to reach the bloodstream.

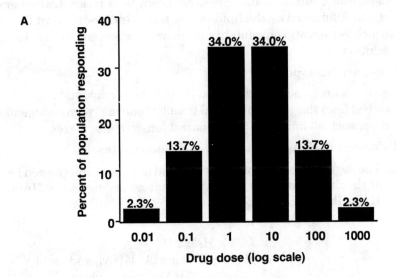

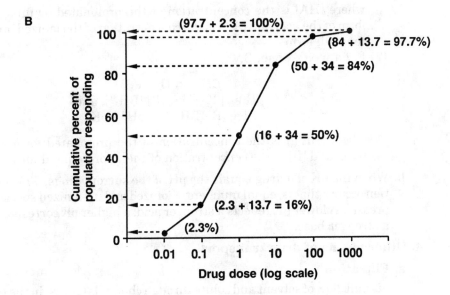

Figure 1.5. (*A*) Frequency distribution plot. Number of individuals (as percentage of the population) who require the indicated drug dose to exhibit an identical response. As illustrated, 2.3% of the population require 0.01 units to exhibit the response, 13.7% require 0.1 units, and so on. (*B*) Quantal dose–response curve. The cumulative number of individuals (as a percentage of the population) who will respond if the indicated dose of drug is administered to the entire population.

A. Drug transport across membranes

1. Diffusion of un-ionized drugs

−is the most common and most important mode of traversing biologic membranes; drugs diffuse passively down their concentration gradient.
−can be influenced by the lipid–water **partition coefficient** of the drug, which is the ratio of solubility in an organic solvent to that in aqueous solution.

2. Ion–pair transport

−occurs with some highly ionized (lipophobic) compounds, which are absorbed from the gastrointestinal tract by "pairing" with endogenous moieties, such as mucin, to form neutral ion–pair complexes.

3. Diffusion of drugs that are weak electrolytes

a. The degree of ionization of a weak acid or base is determined by the pK of the drug and pH of its environment according to the **Henderson-Hasselbalch equation**.

(1) For a **weak acid,** A,

$$HA \leftrightharpoons H^+ + A^-,$$
$$pH = pK + \log [A^-]/[HA], \text{ and}$$
$$\log [A^-]/[HA] = pH - pK$$

where [HA] is the concentration of the protonated or un-ionized form of the acid and [A$^-$] is the concentration of the ionized, unprotonated, form.

(2) For a **weak base,** B,

$$BH^+ \leftrightharpoons H^+ + B,$$
$$pH = pK + \log [B]/[BH^+], \text{ and}$$
$$\log [B]/[BH^+] = pH - pK$$

where [BH$^+$] is the concentration of the protonated form of the base, and [B] is the concentration of the unprotonated form.

b. When the pK of a drug equals the pH of the surroundings, 50% ionization occurs; that is, equal numbers of ionized and un-ionized species are present. A lower pK reflects a stronger acid; a higher pK corresponds to a stronger base.

4. Other means of drug transport

a. Filtration

−is bulk flow of solvent and solute through channels (pores) in the membrane.
−is seen with small molecules (usually with a molecular weight less than 100), which can pass through pores. Some substances of greater molecular weight, such as certain proteins, can be filtered through intercellular channels. Concentration gradients affect the rate of filtration.

b. Active transport

−is an energy-dependent process that can move drugs against a concentration gradient, as in **protein-mediated transport systems**.
−occurs in only one direction and is saturable.

 —is usually the mode of transport for drugs that resemble actively transported endogenous substances such as sugars, amino acids, and nucleosides. Examples of such transport include hepatic transport of digitalis glycosides and intestinal uptake of 5-fluorouracil.

c. Facilitated diffusion

 —is movement of a substance down a concentration gradient.

 —is carrier-mediated, specific, and saturable but does not require energy.

B. Routes of administration

1. Oral administration

 —is the most convenient, economical, and common route of administration and is generally safe for most drugs.

a. Sites of absorption

(1) Stomach

(a) **Lipid-soluble drugs** and **weak acids,** which are normally un-ionized at the low pH (1 to 2) of gastric contents, may be absorbed directly from the stomach.

(b) **Weak bases** and **strong acids** (pK 2 to 3) are not normally absorbed from this site, since they tend to be protonated at low pH.

(2) Small intestine

 —is the **primary site of absorption** because of the very large surface area across which drugs, including partially ionized weak acids and bases, may diffuse. Acids are normally absorbed more extensively from the small intestine than from the stomach, even though the intestine has a higher pH ($\sim$ 5).

b. Bioavailability of drugs

 —refers to the fraction of drug (administered by any route) that reaches the bloodstream unaltered.

(1) First-pass effect

 —influences drug absorption by metabolism in the liver or by biliary secretion.

 —after absorption from the stomach or small intestine, a drug must pass through the liver before reaching the general circulation and its target site. If the capacity of liver metabolic enzymes to inactivate the drug is great, only limited amounts of active drug will escape the process. Some drugs are metabolized so extensively as a result of hepatic metabolism during the first pass that it precludes their use.

(2) Other factors affecting bioavailability

 —the following may alter absorption from the stomach or small intestine:

(a) Stomach emptying time and passage of drug to the intestine may be influenced by **gastric contents,** intestinal motility, and blood flow.

(b) **Stomach acid** and inactivating enzymes may destroy certain drugs.

(c) **Interactions** with food, other drugs, and other constituents of the gastric milieu may influence absorption.

(d) **Inert ingredients** in oral preparations or the special formulation of those preparations may alter absorption.

2. Parenteral administration

–includes three major routes: **intravenous** (IV), **intramuscular** (IM), and **subcutaneous** (SC).

–generally results in more predictable bioavailability than oral administration.

a. With IV administration, the drug is injected directly into the **bloodstream**.

b. Many drugs can enter the **capillaries** directly after IM and SC administration.

c. Depot preparations for sustained release may be administered by IM or SC routes, but some preparations may cause irritation.

3. Other routes of administration

a. Inhalation

–results in **rapid absorption** due to the large surface area and rich blood supply of the alveoli.

–is frequently used for gaseous anesthetics but is generally not practical.

–may be useful for drugs that act on the airways, such as **epinephrine** used to treat bronchial asthma.

b. Sublingual administration

–is useful for drugs with **high first-pass metabolism**, such as **nitroglycerin,** since hepatic metabolism is bypassed.

c. Intrathecal administration

–is useful for drugs that do not readily cross the blood–brain barrier.

d. Rectal administration

–may be used to circumvent nausea and vomiting from oral administration.

–minimizes first-pass metabolism.

–may be limited by inconvenience or patient noncompliance.

e. Topical administration

–is used widely when a local effect is desired or to **minimize systemic effects,** especially in dermatology and ophthalmology. Preparations must be nonirritating.

–may sometimes produce systemic effects.

III. Drug Distribution

A. Binding of drugs by plasma proteins

1. General features of plasma protein binding

a. Drugs in the plasma may exist in the **free** form or may be **bound** to plasma proteins or other blood components such as red blood cells.

b. The extent of plasma protein binding is **highly variable** and ranges from virtually 0% to greater than 99% bound, depending on the specific drug. Binding is generally reversible.

c. Only the **free drug diffuses through capillary walls;** extensive binding retards the rate at which the drug reaches its site of action and may prolong duration of action.

    d. Some plasma proteins (e.g., serum albumin) bind many different drugs, and other proteins bind only one or a limited number.

2. Consequences of plasma protein binding

    a. Decreases in the following:

        (1) Distribution of drug from the plasma to tissue sites

        (2) Renal excretion as a result of reduced filtration

        (3) Metabolism as a result of diminished uptake by the liver or other metabolizing tissues

    b. Drug interactions

        –can be produced by **plasma protein binding** if several drugs (or drugs and endogenous compounds) compete for **binding sites on protein molecules**. Multiple drugs competing for the same binding site can result in higher free blood levels of one or more of the drugs, thereby possibly contributing to toxic effects.

B. Clinical distribution of drugs

    –is the process by which a drug leaves the bloodstream and enters the extracellular fluids and tissues. A drug must diffuse across cellular membranes if its site of action is intracellular. In this case, **lipid solubility** is important for effective distribution.

1. Importance of blood flow

    a. In most tissues, drugs can leave the circulation readily by diffusion across or between capillary endothelial cells. Thus, the **initial rate of distribution** of a drug is **heavily dependent on blood flow** to various organs.

    b. At **equilibrium,** or **steady state,** the amount of drug in an organ is related to the mass of the organ and its properties, as well as to the properties of the specific drug.

2. Volume of distribution (V_d)

    –is the **volume of total body fluid** into which a drug "appears" to distribute.

    –is determined by administering a known dose of drug (expressed in units of mass; e.g., milligrams) intravenously and measuring the initial plasma concentration (expressed in units of mass/volume; e.g., milligrams/liter, or mg/L):

$$V_d = \frac{\text{amount of drug administered (mg)}}{\text{initial plasma concentration (mg/L)}}$$

    –is expressed as units of volume (e.g., liters).

    a. Standard values

        –of volumes of fluid compartments in an average 70-kg adult: Plasma = 3 liters; extracellular fluid = 12 liters; and total body water = 41 liters.

    b. Features

        (1) V_d values for most drugs do not represent their actual distribution in bodily fluids. The use of V_d values is primarily conceptual; that is, drugs that distribute extensively have relatively large V_d values and vice versa.

(2) A very low V_d value may indicate extensive plasma protein binding of the drug. A very high value may indicate that the drug is extensively bound to tissue sites.

(3) Among other variables, V_d may be **influenced by age, sex, and weight**.

3. Redistribution of drugs

—infrequently, the action of a drug may be terminated by its **redistribution from the site of action to other organs**. For example, the action of the anesthetic **thiopental** is terminated largely by its redistribution from the brain (where it initially accumulates as a result of its high lipid solubility and the high blood flow to that organ) to more poorly perfused adipose tissue.

4. Barriers to drug distribution

a. Central nervous system (CNS)

(1) Because of the nature of the **blood–brain barrier,** ionized or polar drugs distribute poorly to the CNS since they must pass through rather than between endothelial cells.

(2) Inflammation, such as that which is a result of meningitis, may increase the ability of ionized, poorly soluble drugs to cross the blood–brain barrier.

b. Placenta

(1) Lipid-soluble drugs cross the placental barrier easier than polar drugs; drugs with molecular weight less than 600 pass the placental barrier better than larger molecules.

(2) The possibility that drugs administered to the mother may cross the placenta and reach the fetus is an important consideration in therapy.

c. Testis

—the blood–testis barrier may limit the effectiveness of chemotherapeutic agents in treating testicular neoplasms.

IV. Biotransformation (Metabolism) of Drugs

A. General properties

—biotransformation is a major mechanism for **drug elimination;** most drugs undergo biotransformation, or metabolism, after they enter the body.

—it usually terminates the pharmacologic action of the drug and increases removal of the drug from the body, although other consequences are possible.

1. Many drugs undergo several sequential biotransformation reactions. Biotransformation is catalyzed by **specific enzyme systems,** which may also catalyze the metabolism of endogenous substances such as steroid hormones.

2. The **liver** is the major site of biotransformation, although specific drugs may undergo biotransformation primarily or extensively in other tissues.

3. Biotransformation of drugs is **variable** and can be affected by many parameters, including **prior administration** of the drug in question or of other drugs; **physiologic status** (e.g., nutritional, hormonal); **age and**

developmental status; genetics; and **liver function** and the status of other metabolizing organs.

4. Possible **consequences** of biotransformation include production of **inactive metabolites** (most common), metabolites with increased or decreased potencies, metabolites with qualitatively different pharmacologic actions, toxic metabolites, or active metabolites from inactive prodrugs.

5. **Metabolites** are often **more polar** than the parent compounds, which may lead to a more rapid rate of clearance due to possible secretion by acid or base carriers in the kidney and also to decreased tubular reabsorption.

B. Classification of biotransformation reactions

   1. Nonsynthetic or phase I reactions

     –involve enzyme-catalyzed biotransformation of the drug without any conjugations.

     –include **oxidations, reductions,** and **hydrolysis reactions**.

     –frequently introduce a functional group (e.g., —OH) that serves as the active center for conjugation in a phase II reaction.

   2. Synthetic or phase II reactions

     –include **conjugation reactions,** which involve the enzyme-catalyzed combination of a drug (or drug metabolite) with an endogenous substance.

     –require a functional group—an **active center**—as the site of conjugation with the endogenous substance.

     –require energy indirectly for the synthesis of "activated carriers," the form of the endogenous substance used in the conjugation reaction (e.g., UDP-glucuronate).

C. Enzymes catalyzing biotransformation reactions

   –include cytochrome P-450, aldehyde and alcohol dehydrogenase, deaminases, esterases, amidases, and epoxide hydratases, which catalyze **phase I reactions;** and glucuronyl transferase (glucuronide conjugation), sulfotransferase (sulfate conjugation), transacylases (amino acid conjugation), acetylases, ethylases, methylases, and glutathione transferase, which catalyze **phase II reactions**.

   –are present in numerous tissues; some are present in plasma. Subcellular locations include cytosol, mitochondria, and endoplasmic reticulum. Only those enzymes located in the **endoplasmic reticulum** are inducible by drugs.

   1. Cytochrome P-450 monooxygenase (mixed function oxidase)

     a. General features

       –cytochrome P-450 monooxygenase plays a central role in drug biotransformation. A large family of cytochrome P-450s enzymes exist, each of which catalyzes the biotransformation of a unique spectrum of drugs, with some overlap in the substrate specificities. This enzyme system is that which is most frequently involved in **phase I reactions**.

       –catalyze numerous reactions including aromatic and aliphatic hydroxylations; dealkylations at nitrogen, sulfur, and oxygen atoms; heteroatom oxidations at nitrogen and sulfur atoms; and reductions at nitrogen atoms.

b. Mechanism of reaction

—in the overall reaction, the drug is oxidized and oxygen is reduced to water. Reducing equivalents are provided by **NADPH** (nicotinamide adenine dinucleotide phosphate), and generation of this cofactor is coupled to **cytochrome P-450 reductase**. The overall reaction for aromatic hydroxylation can be described as:

$$\text{Drug} + O_2 + \text{NADPH} + H^+ \rightarrow \text{Drug}-\text{OH} + \text{NADP}^+ + H_2O$$

c. Location

—cytochrome P-450 is primarily active in the **liver,** which has the greatest specific enzymatic activity and the highest total activity, but it is also found in **many tissues**. The enzyme's subcellular location is the **endoplasmic reticulum**. Lipid membrane location facilitates metabolism of lipid-soluble drugs.

d. Induction

—is brought about by **drugs** and **endogenous substances,** such as hormones. Any given drug preferentially induces one form of cytochrome P-450 or a particular set of P-450s.

—when caused by drugs, is pharmacologically important as a major source of **drug interactions**. A drug may induce its own metabolism (metabolic tolerance) and that of other drugs catalyzed by the induced P-450.

—can be caused by a wide variety of clinically useful drugs, such as **phenytoin, isoniazid, macrolide antibiotics, barbiturates, and carbamazepine**.

e. Inhibition

—can result in **reduced metabolism** of other drugs or endogenous substrates such as testosterone.

—can be caused by a number of commonly used drugs including **cimetidine, chloramphenicol, and disulfiram**.

2. Glucuronyl transferase

a. General features

—is the enzyme most commonly involved in **synthetic (phase II) reactions**.

—catalyzes the conjugation of glucuronic acid to a variety of active centers, including —OH, —COOH, —SH, and —NH$_2$.

b. Mechanism of reaction

(1) **UDP-glucuronic acid,** the active glucuronide donor, is formed from UTP and glucose 1-phosphate.

(2) **Glucuronyl transferase** then catalyzes the conjugation to the active center of the drug.

c. Location and induction

—is located in the **endoplasmic reticulum**.

—is **inducible by drugs** and is a possible site of drug interactions.

V. Excretion of Drugs

A. Routes of excretion

—may include urine, feces (e.g., unabsorbed drugs, drugs secreted in bile), saliva, sweat, tears, milk (with possible transfer to neonates), and lungs (e.g., alcohols and anesthetics). Any route may be important for a given drug, but the **kidney is the major site of excretion** for most drugs.

B. Clearance

—is a quantitative measure of the rate of removal of a drug from the body or specific body compartment.

1. Plasma clearance

—refers to the **volume of plasma** from which the drug is removed per unit time.

2. Total body clearance (CL)

—relates the volume of distribution (V_d) and the first-order **elimination rate constant (k)**; CL (mL/min) = k(min^{-1}) × V_d (mL).

3. Reabsorption

—may occur throughout the tubule.
—when **passive diffusion** is employed, only the un-ionized form of a drug is reabsorbed, depending on its lipid solubility.
—may be affected by **alterations of urinary pH,** which also affect elimination of weak acids or bases by affecting the degree of ionization. For example, acidification of the urine will result in a higher proportion of the un-ionized form of an acidic drug and will facilitate reabsorption.
—**ion trapping** may be used to increase excretion of drugs.
—some compounds (e.g., glucose) are actively reabsorbed.

4. Renal clearance of drugs

a. Measures the **volume of plasma** that is cleared of drug per unit time:
$$CL \text{ (mL/min)} = U \times V/P$$
where **U** = concentration of drug per milliliter of **urine, V = volume** of urine excreted per minute, and **P** = concentration of drug per milliliter of **plasma**.

(1) A drug excreted by **filtration alone** (e.g., inulin) will have a clearance equal to the GFR (125–130 mL/min).

(2) A drug excreted by **filtration and complete secretion** (e.g., *para*-aminohippuric acid) will have a clearance equal to renal plasma clearance (i.e., 650 mL/min).

(3) Clearance values between 130 and 650 mL/min suggest a drug is **filtered, secreted, and partially reabsorbed**.

b. A variety of factors influence renal clearance, including age, other drugs, and disease.

(1) In the presence of **renal failure,** the clearance of a drug may be reduced significantly, resulting in higher plasma levels. For those drugs with a narrow therapeutic index, dose adjustment may be required.

(2) Glomerulonephritis may result in a wasting of serum protein that would normally be available to bind drugs and thus may affect drug plasma concentration.

5. Hepatic clearance of drugs

a. General extraction by the liver

–occurs because of the liver's large size (1500 g) and high blood flow (1 mL/g/min). The **extraction ratio** is the amount of drug removed in the liver divided by the amount of drug entering the organ; a drug completely extracted by the liver would have an extraction ratio of 1. Highly extracted drugs can have an hepatic clearance approaching 1500 mL/min.

b. First-pass effect

(1) Drugs taken orally pass across membranes of the gastrointestinal tract into the portal vein and through the liver before entering the general circulation.

(2) Bioavailability of orally administered drugs is **decreased** by the fraction of drug removed by the first pass through the liver. For example, a drug with an hepatic extraction ratio of 1 would have 0% bioavailability; a drug such as lidocaine, with an extraction ratio of 0.7, would have 30% bioavailability.

(3) In the presence of hepatic disease, drugs with a high first-pass extraction may reach the systemic circulation in higher than normal amounts, and dose adjustment may be required.

VI. Pharmacokinetics

–describes **changes** in **plasma drug concentration** over time. Although it is ideal to determine the amount of drug reaching its site of action as a function of time after administration, it is usually impractical or not feasible. Therefore, the **plasma drug concentration is measured**. This provides useful information since the amount of drug in the tissues is generally related to plasma concentration.

A. Distribution and elimination

1. One-compartment model (Figure 1.6)

–the drug appears to distribute instantaneously after IV administration of a single dose. If the mechanisms for drug elimination, such as biotransformation by hepatic enzymes and renal secretion, are not saturated following the therapeutic dose, a semi-log plot of plasma concentration versus time will be **linear**.

–drug elimination is first order; that is, a constant fraction of drug is eliminated per unit time. For example, one-half of the drug is eliminated every 8 hours. Elimination of most drugs is a first-order process.

2. Two-compartment model (Figure 1.7)

–is a more common model for distribution and elimination of drugs. Initial rapid changes in the plasma concentration of a drug are observed due to a **distribution phase,** the time required for the drug to reach an equilibrium distribution between a central compartment, such as the plasma space, and a second compartment, such as the aggregate tissues and fluids to which the drug distributes.

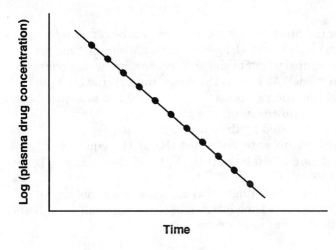

Figure 1.6. One-compartment model of drug distribution.

—after distribution, a linear decrease in the log drug concentration is observed if the **elimination phase** is first order.

3. First-order elimination

—accounts for elimination of most drugs.

—refers to the elimination of a constant fraction of drug per unit time; that is, the rate of elimination is a **linear function** of the plasma drug concentration.

—occurs when elimination systems are not saturated by the drug.

4. Zero-order elimination

—in this model, the plot of the log of the plasma concentration versus time will be concave upward, and a constant amount of drug will be eliminated per unit time (e.g., 10 mg drug will be eliminated every 8 hours). This is referred to as zero-order elimination, or **zero-order kinetics**. (Note that after an interval of time sufficient to reduce the drug level below the saturation point, first-order elimination occurs.)

—may occur when therapeutic doses of drugs exceed the capacity of elimination mechanisms.

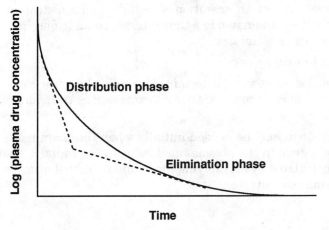

Figure 1.7. Two-compartment model of drug distribution.

B. Half-life ($t_{1/2}$)

- is the time it takes for the plasma drug concentration to be reduced by 50%.
- is determined from the log plasma–drug concentration versus time profile for drugs fitting a one-compartment model or from the elimination phase for the two-compartment model. As long as the dose administered does not exceed the capacity of elimination systems (i.e., dose does not saturate those systems), the $t_{1/2}$ will remain constant.
- applies only to drugs eliminated by **first-order kinetics**.
- is related to the **elimination rate constant (K)** by the equation $t_{1/2} = 0.693/K$ and to the **volume of distribution (V_d)** and **clearance (CL)** by the equation $t_{1/2} = 0.693\ V_d/CL$.
- for all doses in which first-order elimination occurs, approximately 94% of the drug will be eliminated in a time interval equal to four half-lives. This applies for therapeutic doses of most drugs.

C. Multidose kinetics

1. Repeat administration

- if a drug is administered repeatedly (e.g., one tablet every 8 hours), the average plasma concentration of the drug will increase until a mean **steady state** level is reached. The interval of time required to reach steady state is equal to four half-lives.
- results in elevation of plasma concentration of the drug above the mean steady state concentration, followed by a drop below that level. The actual concentration of the drug fluctuates around the mean steady state concentration.

2. Steady state

a. Some fluctuation in plasma concentration will occur even at steady state.

b. Levels will be at the high point of the steady state range shortly after a dose is administered, and at the low point immediately before administration of the next dose. Hence, steady state designates an **average plasma concentration** and the range of fluctuations above and below that level.

c. The magnitude of fluctuations can be controlled by the **dosing interval:** A shorter dosing interval decreases fluctuations, and a longer dosing interval increases them. On cessation of multidose administration, 94% of the drug will be eliminated in a time interval equal to four half-lives if first-order kinetics applies.

3. Maintenance and loading doses

a. The **maintenance dosage rate,** determined by multiplying the clearance by the desired plasma concentration, is expressed as the average dose per unit time.

b. A large **loading dose** may be needed initially when the therapeutic concentration of a drug in the plasma must be achieved rapidly. The loading dose is calculated by multiplying the volume of distribution by the desired plasma concentration.

Review Test

Directions: Each of the numbered items or incomplete statements in this section is followed by answers or by completions of the statement. Select the **one** lettered answer or completion that is **best** in each case.

1. The renal clearance of a drug is determined to be 60 mL/min. Which one of the following statements most likely explains this result?

(A) Extensive secretion
(B) Extensive reabsorption
(C) The drug is not bound to plasma proteins
(D) The drug is both filtered and secreted

2. Which of the following is characteristic of cytochrome P-450?

(A) Located in the lipophilic environment of mitochondrial membranes
(B) Catalyzes O-, S-, and N-methylation reactions
(C) Catalyzes aromatic and aliphatic hydroxylations
(D) Catalyzes conjugation reactions
(E) Activity is not inducible by drugs

3. A weak acid drug (A), with a $pK_a = 6$, is given orally. Assuming that the pH of the stomach equals 3 and the pH of the blood equals 7, which of the following statements is true?

(A) At equilibrium, there is roughly 1000 times more dissociated drug than undissociated drug in the stomach
(B) At equilibrium, the ratio of dissociated to undissociated drug in the blood is approximately 10
(C) At equilibrium, 10 times more undissociated drug is in the blood than in the dissociated drug.
(D) Drug concentrations on the blood side of the stomach barrier will never reach the concentration of drug in the stomach
(E) The drug will be more rapidly excreted if the urine is made acidic

4. Which of the following factors will determine the number of drug–receptor complexes formed?

(A) Efficacy of the drug
(B) Receptor affinity for the drug
(C) Therapeutic index of the drug
(D) Half-life of the drug
(E) Rate of renal secretion

5. Which of the following statements about phase II biotransformation reactions is true?

(A) They may introduce an active center for further conjugations
(B) They almost always yield water-soluble metabolites
(C) They are all inducible upon repeated drug administration
(D) They are often important in activating pro-drugs

6. Which one of the following results may occur from repeated administration of a drug?

(A) Increase in the drug's metabolism
(B) Increased metabolism of other drugs
(C) Induction of cytochrome P-450 or glucuronyl transferase
(D) Increased metabolism of endogenous compounds
(E) All of the above

7. Which of the following is an action of a noncompetitive antagonist?

(A) Alters the mechanism of action of an agonist
(B) Alters the potency of an agonist
(C) Shifts the dose–response curve of an agonist to the right
(D) Decreases the maximum response to an agonist
(E) Binds to the same site on the receptor as the agonist

8. Decreasing the pH of the intestinal contents is most likely to increase the rate of absorption from the intestine of a drug that is a

(A) weak base
(B) weak acid
(C) neutral organic compound
(D) quaternary (completely ionized) compound

17

9. Which of the following statements applies to a drug exhibiting a saturated elimination process?

(A) Upon multiple dosing, steady state plasma concentrations will be reached in approximately four to five biologic half-lives
(B) The fraction of drug eliminated per unit time is constant
(C) The biologic half-life ($t_{1/2}$) is affected by dose
(D) First-order kinetics are operable
(E) The rate of drug elimination is dependent on plasma drug concentration

10. Which of the following is NOT catalyzed by liver microsomal cytochrome P-450?

(A) Nitroreduction
(B) Sulfoxide formation
(C) Methylation
(D) *O*-Dealkylation
(E) Epoxidation

11. An acidic drug with a $pK_a = 4.0$ is placed in a solution that has a pH of 3.0. What is the ratio of un-ionized to ionized drug?

(A) 0.1
(B) 1.0
(C) 10
(D) 100
(E) 1000

12. Displacement of a drug from plasma protein binding sites would usually be expected to

(A) decrease tissue levels of the drug
(B) increase tissue levels of the drug
(C) decrease the volume of distribution
(D) decrease metabolism of the drug

13. Drug X is converted to a single inactive metabolite by a P-450–catalyzed biotransformation. Another drug, cimetidine, inactivates this particular P-450. If cimetidine and drug X are administered simultaneously, cimetidine will

(A) shift the dose–response curve of drug X to the right
(B) decrease the $t_{1/2}$ for plasma levels of drug X
(C) not affect the dose–response curve
(D) shift the dose–response curve of drug X and decrease the plasma $t_{1/2}$
(E) none of the above

14. The renal clearance of a drug is 10 mL/min. The drug has a molecular weight of 350 and is 20% bound to plasma proteins. It is most likely that renal excretion of this drug involves

(A) glomerular filtration
(B) active tubular secretion
(C) passive tubular reabsorption
(D) both glomerular filtration and active tubular secretion
(E) both glomerular filtration and passive tubular reabsorption

15. At equilibrium, the distribution ratio of a drug between two body compartments, A and B, is 100:1, respectively. The drug is a weak acid. In which compartment is the drug most highly ionized?

(A) A
(B) B
(C) It is equally ionized in both A and B

16. All of the following statements concerning a single form of cytochrome P-450 monooxygenase are true EXCEPT

(A) it may catalyze the biotransformation of many different drugs
(B) it catalyzes the biotransformation of a unique spectrum of drugs
(C) it may be preferentially induced (i.e., relative to other forms) by a given drug
(D) it may introduce the active center required for subsequent phase II biotransformation reactions
(E) it converts $NADP^+$ to NADPH

17. All of the following are possible consequences of phase I or nonsynthetic biotransformation EXCEPT

(A) production of a metabolite with increased pharmacologic activity
(B) combination of a drug with an endogenous substance
(C) introduction of an active center for amino acid conjugation
(D) production of a metabolite with qualitatively different pharmacologic activity
(E) production of a metabolite without pharmacologic activity

Questions 18 and 19

Questions 18 and 19 refer to the table below, which indicates the properties of drugs A–D, determined from quantal dose–response curves. Drugs A–D produce the same therapeutic effect via the same mechanism but each has a unique toxicity.

Drug	ED_{50} (mg)	Therapeutic Index	Certain Safety Factor
A	1	7	2.1
B	5	9	4.0
C	33	15	3.0
D	0.5	4	2.8

18. Which drug is the most potent?

(A) Drug A
(B) Drug B
(C) Drug C
(D) Drug D

19. When used at a maximally effective therapeutic dose (i.e., ED_{99}), which drug will produce the highest incidence of toxicity?

(A) Drug A
(B) Drug B
(C) Drug C
(D) Drug D

20. Administer a drug to a population of 100 patients and observe the following results for a therapeutic effect and for a toxic effect. What is the TI of the drug?

Dose (mg)	Therapeutic Effect*	Toxic Effect[†]
0.01	—	2
0.1	2	15
1.0	15	50
10.0	50	85
100.0	85	98

*Number of patients responding as cumulative total.
[†]Number of patients exhibiting toxic effect as cumulative total.

(A) 0.01
(B) 0.1
(C) 1.0
(D) 10
(E) 100

Directions: The group of items in this section consists of lettered options followed by a set of numbered items. For each item, select the **one** lettered option that is most closely associated with it. Each lettered option may be selected once, more than once, or not at all.

Questions 21–24

Match each route of administration with the description that best applies to it.

(A) Provides complete (100%) bioavailability of the drug
(B) Minimizes systemic effects
(C) May have limited use due to poor compliance
(D) Is frequently used for gaseous anesthetics
(E) Is useful for drugs that do not cross the blood–brain barrier

21. Rectal

22. Intrathecal

23. Intravenous

24. Topical

Answers and Explanations

1–B. Extensive reabsorption (or kidney disease) could lower the clearance rate. Normal glomerular filtration rate (GFR) is 125–130 mL/min. Extensive secretion would yield a higher clearance. If a drug were not bound to plasma proteins, clearance would be expected to be at least 130 mL/min.

2–C. Cytochrome P-450 catalyzes demethylation, not methylation or conjugation, reactions. The enzyme is located in the endoplasmic reticulum, not mitochondria. Drugs can induce cytochrome P-450 activity.

3–B. According to the Henderson-Hasselbalch equation, the pK equals the pH when the log of the ratio of ionized (dissociated) and protonated (undissociated) forms is 0 (i.e., their concentrations are equal and have a ratio of 1). When the pH of a solution (blood) is 7 and the pK of the acid is 6, at equilibrium, the log of the ratio of the concentrations of ionized form to protonated form is 1, (i.e., there is 10 times more ionized than protonated acid in the blood). When the pH of a solution (stomach) is 3 and the pK of the acid is 6, the log of the ratio of the concentrations of the ionized to protonated forms is −3 (i.e., the concentration of the ionized form is 1/1000 that of the protonated form, meaning there is 1000 times more protonated than ionized acid). Drug will accumulate in the compartment in which it is more highly charged (ion trapping)—in this case, the blood. Acidification of the urine will increase the protonation of an acid and increase reabsorption, thereby slowing renal excretion.

4–B. Receptor affinity for the drug will determine the number of drug–receptor complexes formed. Efficacy is the ability of the drug to activate the receptor after binding has occurred. Therapeutic index (TI) is related to safety of the drug. Half-life and secretion are properties of elimination that do not influence formation of drug–receptor complexes.

5–B. Phase II reactions typically yield water-soluble metabolites. Active centers are introduced during phase I, not phase II, biotransformation. Glucuronyl transferase is the only phase II enzyme inducible by drug administration. Prodrugs are often activated by phase I, not phase II, reactions; phase II reactions generally terminate drug action.

6–E. All of the choices are possible consequences of drug administration. Many enzymes involved in drug biotransformation also catalyze the metabolism of endogenous compounds such as steroids.

7–D. A noncompetitive antagonist decreases the magnitude of the response to an agonist but does not alter the agonist's potency (i.e., the ED_{50} remains unchanged). A competitive antagonist interacts at the agonist binding site.

8–B. An acid will become less ionized as the pH is decreased.

9–C. Biologic $t_{1/2}$ will be affected by dose in a drug when the elimination process is saturated. In that case, the drug will accumulate on repeated dosings, and elimination will be independent of plasma concentration. The amount (not fraction) of drug eliminated per unit time will be constant and zero-order elimination will be observed.

10–C. Methylation is a conjugation (i.e., phase II) reaction and so is not catalyzed by cytochrome P-450.

11–C. The ratio of un-ionized to ionized drug will be 10; this is obtained directly from the Henderson-Hasselbalch equation.

12–B. Displacement of a drug from plasma protein binding sites will tend to increase the amount available to distribute to tissue sites (including organs that metabolize this drug) and thus will increase the volume of distribution.

13–E. Inactivation of P-450 will shift the dose-response curve to the left and will increase plasma $t_{1/2}$ of the competing drug, drug X.

14–E. This drug will undergo filtration and passive reabsorption. Since the molecular weight of the drug is small, free drug will be filtered. Since 20% of the drug is bound to plasma proteins, 80% of it is free and available for filtration, which would be at a rate of 100 mL/min (i.e., 0.8×125 mL/min; 125 mL/min is the normal GFR). A clearance of 10 mL/min must indicate that most of the filtered drug is reabsorbed.

15–A. This is an example of ion trapping. The drug has accumulated in the compartment where it is most highly ionized.

16–E. NADPH supplies reducing equivalents for reduction of O_2 to H_2O.

17–B. Phase II reactions conjugate drugs with endogenous substances.

18–D. D is the most potent drug, because it has the lowest ED_{50}.

19–A. Drug A has the lowest certain safety factor and so will produce the highest incidence of toxicity at a maximally effective therapeutic dose. This is a more useful parameter than therapeutic index if the therapeutic and toxic dose-response curves are *not* parallel.

20–B. The TI of the drug would be 0.1, based on the following equation: $TI = TD_{50}/ED_{50} = 1/10 = 0.1$.

21–C. Patient discomfort may limit compliance.

22–E. This route of administration delivers drug directly into the cerebrospinal fluid.

23–A. This route of administration delivers drug directly to the bloodstream; bioavailability is defined as the amount of drug in the plasma.

24–B. With topical application, most of the drug is available only locally and systemic adverse effects are minimized.

2

Drugs Acting on the Autonomic Nervous System

I. The Peripheral Efferent Nervous System

A. Autonomic nervous system

—controls **involuntary activity**.

1. Parasympathetic nervous system

a. Long preganglionic axons originate from neurons in the **cranial and sacral areas** of the spinal cord and, with few exceptions, synapse on neurons in ganglia located close to or within the innervated organ.

b. Short postganglionic axons innervate **cardiac muscle, bronchial smooth muscle, and exocrine glands**.

2. Sympathetic nervous system

a. Short preganglionic axons originate from neurons in the **thoracic and lumbar areas** of the spinal cord and synapse on neurons in ganglia located outside of, but close to, the spinal cord. The **adrenal medulla,** anatomically considered a modified ganglion, is innervated by sympathetic preganglionic axons.

b. Long postganglionic axons innervate many of the same tissues and organs as the parasympathetic nervous system.

B. Somatic nervous system

—controls **voluntary activity**.

—contains long axons that originate in the spinal cord and directly innervate skeletal muscle.

C. Neurotransmitters of the autonomic and somatic nervous systems

1. Acetylcholine (ACh)

—is released by exocytosis from nerve terminals.

—transmits **nerve impulses** across synapses at the ganglia of the sympathetic and parasympathetic nervous system and across synapses in tissues innervated by the parasympathetic nervous system and the somatic nervous system.

—is synthesized in nerve terminals by the cytoplasmic enzyme **choline acetyltransferase,** which catalyzes the transfer of an acetate group from acetyl coenzyme A (**acetyl CoA**) to choline.

—is stored in nerve terminal vesicles that are released by nerve action potentials. On release, **ACh** is rapidly hydrolyzed and inactivated by tissue **acetylcholinesterase (AChE)** and also by nonspecific **butyrylcholinesterase** (pseudocholinesterase).

—because it is hydrolyzed nearly instantly by butyrylcholinesterase, it is not administered parenterally for therapeutic purposes.

2. Norepinephrine and epinephrine

—are **catecholamines,** possessing a catechol nucleus and an ethylamine side-chain.

a. Storage and release

(1) **Norepinephrine** is stored in vesicles that release their contents by exocytosis from nerve terminals at postganglionic nerve endings of the sympathetic nervous system (except at thermoregulatory sweat glands, where ACh is the neurotransmitter).

(2) A second pool of "protected" **norepinephrine** exists in the **neuronal cytoplasm** and is released by indirectly acting amines but not by nerve action potentials.

(3) **Norepinephrine,** and some epinephrine, is released from adrenergic nerve endings in the brain. In the periphery, **epinephrine,** along with some norepinephrine, is the major catecholamine released from adrenal medullary chromaffin cells into the general circulation.

b. Biosynthesis of catecholamines (Figure 2.1)

(1) In nerve endings, **tyrosine** is hydroxylated by tyrosine hydroxylase, the rate-limiting enzyme in the synthesis of catecholamines, to form **dihydroxyphenylalanine (dopa)** and is then decarboxylated by dopa decarboxylase to form dopamine. **Dopamine,** a neurotransmitter in the brain, interacts with dopamine receptors in renal and splanchnic vascular smooth muscle.

(2) Dopamine is hydroxylated in vesicles on the β carbon of the ethylamine side-chain by dopamine β-hydroxylase to form **norepinephrine**.

(3) In certain areas of the brain and in the adrenal medulla, **norepinephrine** is methylated on the amine group of the side-chain by phenylethanolamine-*N*-methyltransferase to form **epinephrine**.

c. Termination

(1) The action of **norepinephrine** is terminated primarily by active transport from the cytoplasm into the nerve terminal by a **carrier system**. There is also some simple diffusion away from the synapse.

(2) Norepinephrine is transported by a **second carrier system** into storage vesicles.

(3) **Norepinephrine and epinephrine** are oxidatively deaminated by mitochondrial **monoamine oxidase (MAO)** in nerve terminals and effector cells. **Effector cells** also contain **catechol-*O*-methyltransferase (COMT),** which metabolizes catecholamines.

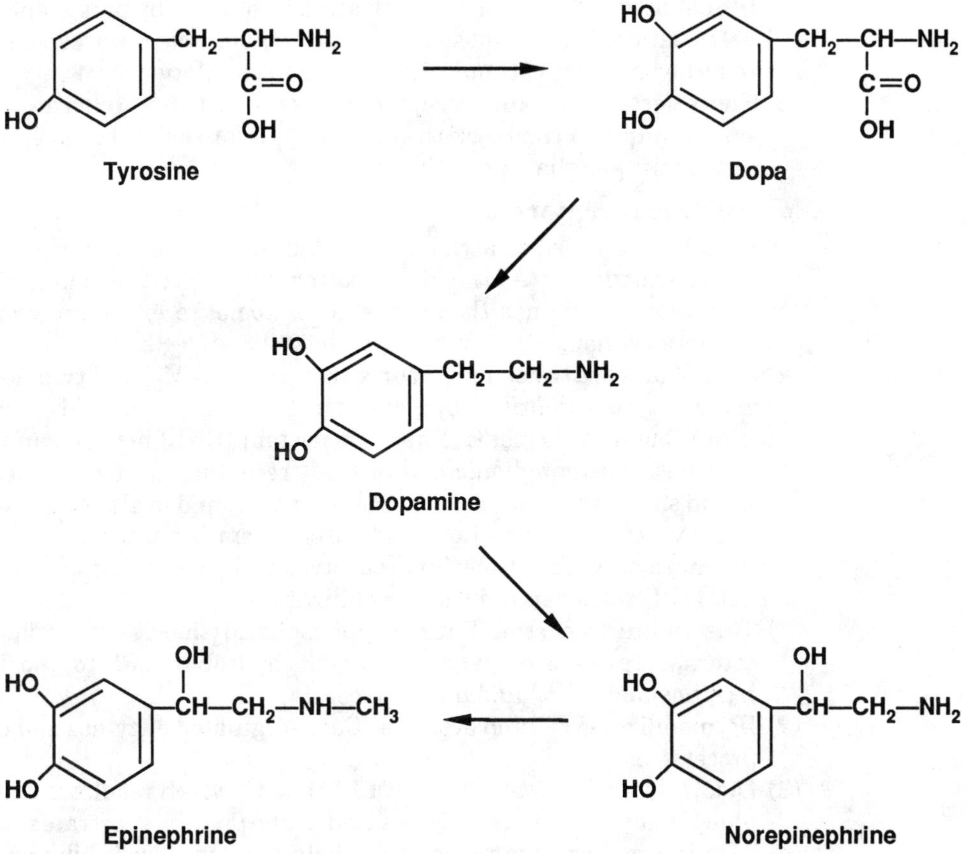

Figure 2.1. Biosynthesis of catecholamines.

D. Receptors of the nervous system

1. Cholinoceptors

a. Nicotinic receptors

  - are localized at neuromuscular junctions, autonomic ganglia, and certain areas in the brain.
  - consist of **five protein subunits** in skeletal muscle (α (2), β, γ, δ) and two in ganglia (α_2, β_2) that form ion channel pores in the cell membranes.
  - in skeletal muscle, ACh interacts with nicotinic receptors (one molecule ACh per α subunit) to open Na^+ channels. Na^+ current produces a membrane depolarization and a propagated action potential through the transverse tubules of skeletal muscle, resulting in the release of Ca^{2+} from the sarcoplasmic reticulum and, through a further series of chemical and mechanical events, muscle contraction. Hydrolysis of ACh by AChE results in **muscle cell repolarization**.
    (1) The continued presence of some nicotinic agonists at nicotinic receptors, or excessive cholinergic stimulation, can lead to a **phase I**

block, in which normal depolarization is followed by persistent depolarization. During phase I block, skeletal muscle is unresponsive to either neuronal stimulation or direct stimulation.

(2) The selective nicotinic receptor antagonists **tubocurarine and trimethaphan** can block the effect of ACh at skeletal muscle and autonomic ganglia, respectively.

b. Muscarinic receptors

–are localized on cardiac atrial muscle and cells of the sinoatrial (SA) and atrioventricular (AV) nodes, smooth muscle, exocrine glands, and vascular endothelium, although the latter do not receive parasympathetic innervation.

–consist of at least **three receptor subtypes** (M_1–M_3) and **two** additional **subtypes** identified by cloning techniques (m_4, m_5). M_1 receptors are found in the central nervous system (CNS) neurons and in sympathetic postganglionic neurons; M_2 receptors are found in cardiac and smooth muscle; and M_3 receptors are found in glandular cells and the vascular endothelium and vascular smooth muscle.

–ACh interacts with muscarinic receptors to increase phosphatidylinositol (PI) turnover and Ca^{2+} mobilization.

(1) This interaction stimulates polyphosphatidylinositol phosphodiesterase (**phospholipase C**), which hydrolyzes PI to inositol trisphosphate (IP_3) and diacylglycerol.

(2) IP_3 mobilizes Ca^{2+} and activates Ca^{2+}-regulated enzymes and cell processes.

(3) Diacylglycerol activates **protein kinase C,** which results in phosphorylation of cellular enzymes and other protein substrates.

(4) ACh interaction with muscarinic cholinoceptors also inhibits adenylate cyclase activity and activates K^+ flux across plasma membranes through K^+ channels.

2. Adrenoceptors

a. α-Adrenoceptors

–are generally excitatory, except in the gastrointestinal tract.

–contain two subtypes. α_1-**Receptors** are located in postjunctional effector cells; α_2-**receptors** are located primarily in prejunctional adrenergic nerve terminals and in postjunctional nerve terminals, platelets, smooth muscle, and adipocytes.

–mediate vasoconstriction, gastrointestinal relaxation, mydriasis, and inhibition of insulin release and lipolysis.

–are distinguished from β-adrenoceptors by their interaction (in descending order of potency) with the adrenergic agonists **epinephrine ≥ norepinephrine >> isoproterenol,** and by their interaction with relatively selective antagonists such as **phentolamine**.

(1) Prejunctional receptor activation inhibits neurotransmitter release.

(2) Although not well understood, activation of α-receptors results in an influx of extracellular Ca^{2+} through specific receptor-activated Ca^{2+} channels in the plasma membrane.

(3) α_1-Receptor activation in many cells also increases PI turnover and the production of IP_3 and diacylglycerol.

(4) α_2-Receptor activation, mediated by activation of an inhibitory guanine nucleotide–binding regulatory protein (G_i), inhibits adenylate cyclase activity and decreases intracellular cyclic AMP (**cAMP**) levels and the activity of cAMP-dependent protein kinases.

b. β-Adrenoceptors

—are generally inhibitory except in effects on the heart, lipolysis, and renin secretion.

(1) β_1-Receptor subtype

—mediates cardiac effects, lipolysis, and renin secretion in the kidney.

—is defined by its interaction (in descending order of potency) with the adrenergic agonists **isoproterenol** > **epinephrine** and **norepinephrine,** and by its interaction with relatively selective antagonists such as **atenolol**.

(2) β_2-Receptor subtype

—mediates vasodilation and intestinal and bronchial smooth muscle relaxation.

—is defined by its interaction (in descending order of potency) with the adrenergic agonists **isoproterenol** $\geq$ **epinephrine** >> **norepinephrine**.

(3) β-Receptor activation

—is mediated by a stimulatory guanine nucleotide–binding regulatory protein (G_s).

—stimulates adenylate cyclase activity and increases intracellular cAMP levels and the activity of cAMP-dependent protein kinases. Adrenoceptor-mediated changes in the activity of protein kinases (and also levels of intracellular Ca^{2+}) bring about changes in the activity of specific enzymes and structural and regulatory proteins, resulting in modification of cell and organ activity.

II. Parasympathomimetic Drugs

A. Direct-acting muscarinic cholinoceptor agonists (Figure 2.2)

1. Chemical structure

a. Bethanechol and **carbachol** are choline esters with a quaternary ammonium group. The β-methyl group of **bethanechol** substantially reduces its activity at nicotinic receptors.

b. Pilocarpine is a tertiary amine alkaloid.

2. Pharmacologic effects

a. Eye

—contract circular smooth muscle fibers of the ciliary muscle and iris to produce, respectively, spasm of accommodation and an increased outflow of aqueous humor into the canal of Schlemm with a **reduction in intraocular pressure**.

—contract the smooth muscle of the iris sphincter to cause **miosis**.

b. Cardiovascular system

—produce a negative chronotropic effect (reduced SA node activity).

—decrease conduction velocity through the AV node.

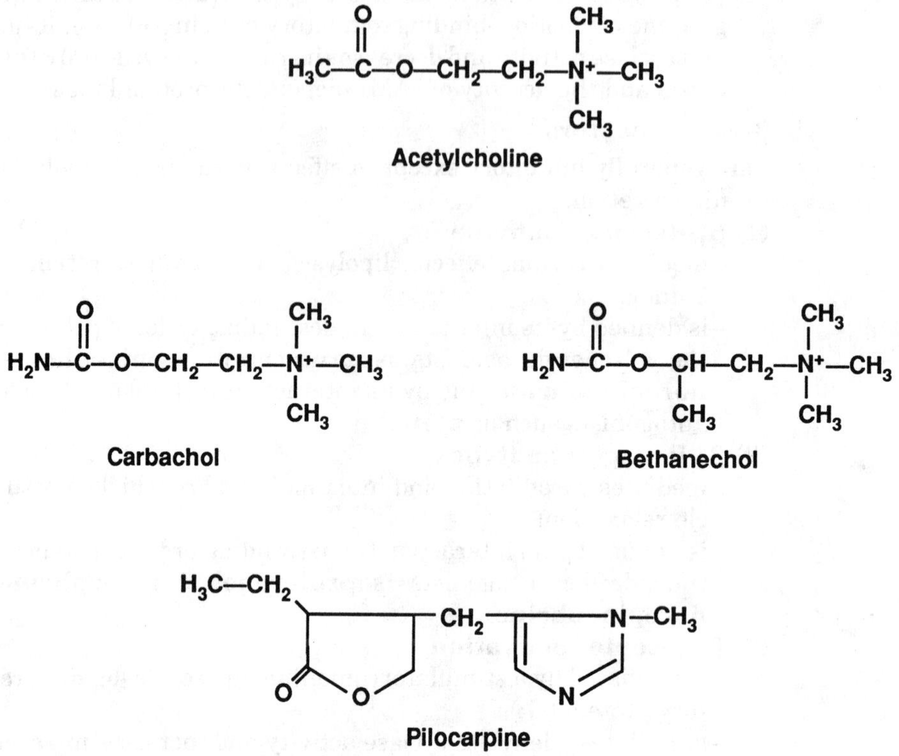

Acetylcholine

Carbachol

Bethanechol

Pilocarpine

Figure 2.2. Direct-acting cholinoceptor agonists.

—have no effect on force because there are no muscarinic receptors on, or parasympathetic innervation of, ventricles.

–produce **vasodilation**. Vascular smooth muscle has muscarinic receptors but no parasympathetic innervation. (Intravenous infusion of low doses of ACh causes a reflex sympathetic-stimulated increase in heart rate; higher doses directly inhibit heart rate.)

c. **Gastrointestinal tract**

–increase smooth muscle contractions, with increased peristaltic activity and motility.

–increase salivation and acid secretion.

d. **Urinary tract**

–increase contraction of the ureter and bladder smooth muscle.

–increase sphincter relaxation.

e. **Other effects**

–produce bronchoconstriction with increased resistance and increased bronchial secretions.

–increase secretion of tears from lacrimal glands and sweat gland secretion.

–produce tremor and ataxia.

3. Specific drugs and their therapeutic effects

a. Bethanechol [Urecholine]

- is used to stimulate smooth muscle motor activity to prevent **urine retention**.
- is used occasionally to stimulate gastrointestinal smooth muscle motor activity for **postoperative abdominal distention** and for **gastric atony** following bilateral vagotomy (in the absence of obstruction).
- is administered **orally** or **subcutaneously,** not by IV or IM route, because parenteral administration may cause cardiac arrest.
- has **low lipid solubility** and is poorly absorbed from the gastrointestinal tract. When given orally, gastrointestinal effects predominate, and there are relatively minor cardiovascular effects.
- has limited distribution to the CNS.
- is resistant to hydrolysis and thus has longer duration of action than ACh (2–3 hours).

b. Pilocarpine

- is used topically for **open-angle glaucoma,** either as eye drops or as sustained-release ocular insert [Ocusert]. Other drug classes used to treat open-angle glaucoma include indirectly acting parasympathomimetics, **epinephrine,** the β-adrenergic receptor antagonists **timolol** and **betaxolol,** and the carbonic anhydrase inhibitor **acetazolamide**.
- when used to treat **acute narrow-angle glaucoma** (a medical emergency), is given in combination with an indirectly acting muscarinic agonist such as **physostigmine**.
- is well absorbed from the gastrointestinal tract and enters the CNS.

c. Carbachol

- is used if pilocarpine is ineffective as a treatment for **open-angle glaucoma**.

4. Adverse effects and contraindications

- are extensions of pharmacologic activity: nausea, vomiting, diarrhea, sweating, salivation, bronchoconstriction, and vasodilation. Systemic effects are minimal for drugs applied topically to the eye.
- are contraindicated in the presence of peptic ulcer disease because they increase acid secretion, asthma because they produce bronchoconstriction, cardiac disease, and parkinsonian disease. Also, they are not recommended in hyperthyroidism because they predispose to arrhythmia nor when there is mechanical obstruction of the gastrointestinal or urinary tract.

B. Indirect-acting parasympathomimetic agents

1. Chemical structure

a. **Edrophonium** is an alcohol with a quaternary ammonium group.

b. **Neostigmine** and **physostigmine** are examples of carbamic acid esters of alcohols (carbamates) with either quaternary or tertiary ammonium groups.

c. Echothiophate and **isoflurophate** are examples of organic derivatives of phosphoric acid.

2. Mechanism of action and selected drugs

—inhibit AChE and **increase ACh levels** at both muscarinic and nicotinic cholinoceptors. AChE interacts with ACh at two sites: The **anionic site** binds N^+ of choline (ionic bond), and the **esteratic site** (serine residue) binds the acetyl ester. As ACh is hydrolyzed, the serine-OH side-chain is acetylated and free choline is released. Acetyl-serine is hydrolyzed to serine and acetate. The $t_{1/2}$ of acetyl-serine hydrolysis is 100–150 μsec.

a. Edrophonium [Tensilon]

—has a short duration of action (5–15 minutes).
—competitively inhibits ACh hydrolysis by AChE by the following processes:
(1) N^+ of edrophonium binds the anionic site.
(2) Phenolic hydroxyl of edrophonium interacts with histidine imidazolium N^+ of the esteratic site.

b. Neostigmine [Prostigmin], physostigmine [Eserine, Antilirium], and demecarium [Humorsol]

—like ACh, interact with AChE and undergo a **two-step hydrolysis**. However, the serine residue of the enzyme is covalently carbamylated rather than acetylated. Hydrolysis of the carbamyl-serine residue is much slower than that of acetyl-serine (30 minutes–6 hours).
—also have direct agonist action at skeletal muscle nicotinic cholinoceptors.
—differ in absorption as follows:
(1) Neostigmine is poorly absorbed from the gastrointestinal tract and has negligible distribution into the CNS.
(2) Physostigmine is well absorbed after oral administration and enters the CNS.

c. Echothiophate [Phospholine] and isoflurophate [Floropryl]

—result in phosphorylation of AChE rather than acetylation. With time, the strength of the bond increases ("aging"), and AChE becomes **irreversibly** inhibited. The enzyme can be reactivated within the first 30 minutes by **pralidoxime**. Hydrolysis of the covalent alkylphosphoryl-serine bond takes days.
—differ in absorption and distribution as follows:
(1) Echothiophate is poorly absorbed from the gastrointestinal tract and has negligible distribution into the CNS.
(2) Isoflurophate is highly lipid-soluble and is well absorbed across all membranes, including skin.

d. Pralidoxime [Protopam]

—is an **AChE reactivator**. Must be administered IV within minutes of exposure to an AChE inhibitor because it is effective only prior to "aging".

—acts as an **antidote for insecticide and nerve gas poisoning**. It binds the anionic site and undergoes a nucleophilic reaction with P = O group of alkylphosphorylated serine to cause hydrolysis of the phospho-serine bond that is at least 10^6 times faster than that occurring in water.

—is most effective at the neuromuscular junction, but is ineffective in the CNS and is ineffective against carbamylated AChE.

—produces few adverse effects in normal doses.

3. Pharmacologic effects

—are similar to those of direct-acting muscarinic cholinoceptor agonists.

—by increasing ACh at the neuromuscular junction, increase contraction strength of skeletal muscle. The effect is more pronounced if muscle contraction is already weak, as occurs in **myasthenia gravis**.

4. Therapeutic uses

  a. Glaucoma

   (1) Physostigmine is often concurrently used with **pilocarpine** for maximum effect.

   (2) Demecarium, echothiophate, and **isoflurophate** are long-acting AChE inhibitors that are used when other drugs are ineffective. Prolonged use may increase the possibility of cataracts.

  b. Gastrointestinal and urinary tract atony

   —can be treated with **neostigmine,** used much like **bethanechol**.

  c. Myasthenia gravis

   —is an **autoimmune disease** in which antibodies complex with nicotinic receptors at the neuromuscular junction to cause skeletal muscle weakness and fatigue. **Neostigmine,** or the related AChE inhibitors **pyridostigmine** [Mestinon, Regonol] or **ambenonium** [Mytelase], is used to increase ACh levels at the neuromuscular junction to activate fully the remaining receptors.

   —can be diagnosed using the **Tensilon test,** which can also assess the adequacy of treatment with AChE inhibitors. Small doses of **edrophonium** improve muscle strength in untreated myasthenics or in treated patients in whom AChE inhibition is inadequate. If there is no effect, or if muscle weakness increases, the dose of the AChE inhibitor is too high (excessive ACh stimulation at the neuromuscular junction results in depolarizing blockade).

  d. Atropine poisoning

   —**physostigmine** reverses the central, and to some extent, the peripheral effects of competitive muscarinic antagonists and is useful in treating cases of severe overdose with muscarinic antagonists such as **atropine or scopolamine**.

5. Adverse effects and toxicity

—are an extension of pharmacologic activity and arise from excessive cholinergic stimulation.

—include muscarinic effects similar to those of direct-acting cholinergic drugs and nicotinic effects: **muscle weakness, cramps, and fasciculations**.

—many lipid-soluble organophosphates are used as insecticides or nerve gases and may be absorbed in sufficient quantities from the skin or lungs to cause **cholinergic intoxication**. Treatment includes the following steps:

a. Maintain respiration.

b. Administer **atropine** parenterally to inhibit muscarinic effects.

c. Administer **pralidoxime** within minutes of exposure.

III. Muscarinic-Receptor Antagonists

A. Mechanism and chemical structure

—are competitive antagonists of ACh at muscarinic cholinoceptors.

1. **Atropine, scopolamine,** and **homatropine** are natural and semisynthetic tertiary amine alkaloids with ester linkages to tropic acid or mandelic acid (Figure 2.3).

2. **Cyclopentolate** [Cyclogyl], **dicyclomine** [Bentyl], and **tropicamide** [Mydriacyl] are synthetic tertiary amines.

3. **Methantheline** [Banthine] and **propantheline** [Pro-Banthine] are semisynthetic and synthetic quaternary amines.

4. Other drugs include **glycopyrrolate** [Robinul] and **ipratropium** [Atrovent].

B. Pharmacologic effects

1. Eye

—produce **cycloplegia** by blocking parasympathetic tone, leading to paralysis of the ciliary muscle with loss of accommodation.

—produce **mydriasis** by blocking parasympathetic tone to the iris circular (constrictor) muscle. Unopposed sympathetic stimulation of the radial muscle results in dilation of the pupil.

2. Cardiovascular system

—increase heart rate due to cholinergic blockade at the SA node.

—dilate blood vessels in facial blush area (**atropine flush**), which is not related to antagonist action.

3. Gastrointestinal tract

—decrease salivation.

—reduce peristalsis, resulting in prolonged gastric emptying and intestinal transit.

—reduce gastric acid secretion.

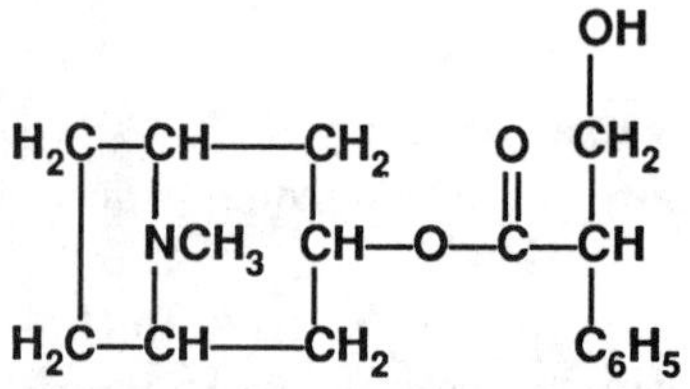

Figure 2.3. Atropine structure.

4. Other effects

- —produce some **bronchodilation** and decrease mucus secretion.
- —relax the ureters and bladder in the urinary tract and constrict the urinary sphincter.
- —tertiary amines can produce restlessness, headache, excitement, hallucinations, and delirium.
- —produce **anhidrosis** and dry skin due to inhibition of sympathetic cholinergic innervation of sweat glands.

C. Pharmacologic properties

- —except for quaternary ammonium drugs such as **methantheline and propantheline,** most are well absorbed across the gastrointestinal tract or mucosal surfaces and distribute throughout the body, including the brain. **Atropine and scopolamine** have relatively long durations of action.

D. Therapeutic uses

1. Eye

a. Shorter-acting muscarinic-receptor antagonists are administered topically as eye drops or as ointments for **refractive measurements** and for **ophthalmoscopic examination** of the retina and other structures of the eye (often in combination with **phenylephrine**).

b. Longer-acting muscarinic-receptor antagonists (such as **homatropine**) are generally preferred as adjuncts to **phenylephrine** (also glucocorticoids and antibiotics) to prevent synechia formation in **anterior uveitis and iritis**.

2. Cardiovascular system

- —are used occasionally for **acute myocardial infarction** with accompanying bradycardia and hypotension or arrhythmias.

3. Gastrointestinal tract

a. Large doses are used to treat **peptic ulcer** disease by reducing acid secretion, but often with accompanying typical adverse effects. To avoid adverse CNS effects, quaternary ammonium drugs are given. Muscarinic-receptor antagonist drug therapy has been supplanted to a large degree by histamine$_2$ (H$_2$)-receptor antagonists such as **cimetidine** and **ranitidine**.

b. Antispasmodic action helps treat **mild diarrhea;** these agents are often used in combination with an opioid such as **diphenoxylate**.

4. Urinary tract

- —are used for symptomatic treatment of **urinary urgency** in inflammatory bladder disorder.

5. Central nervous system

a. Antimuscarinic drugs are used as adjunct to **levodopa** therapy for **parkinsonian disease**.

b. **Scopolamine** (used orally, intravenously, or transdermally) prevents **motion sickness;** blocks muscarinic receptors in the vestibular system and in the CNS.

6. Other uses

a. Glycopyrrolate is used to suppress bronchiolar secretions during **surgical anesthesia. Scopolamine** or **atropine** administered intravenously are also given during spinal anesthesia to prevent bradycardia during surgery, or to prevent muscarinic effects of AChE inhibitors used to reverse muscle paralysis at the end of surgery. **Scopolamine** also has amnestic and sedative properties.

b. Tertiary agents such as **atropine** are used to block peripheral and CNS effects due to **cholinergic excess,** especially those caused by **poisoning** with AChE inhibitor–containing insecticides and muscarine-containing mushrooms.

E. Adverse effects and contraindications

—are extensions of pharmacologic activity and include mydriasis, cycloplegia, dry mouth, tachycardia, elevated temperature, dry skin, urine retention, agitation, hallucinations, and delirium. **Physostigmine** administered intravenously prevents or reverses peripheral and CNS effects resulting from poisoning with tertiary muscarinic antagonists. **Neostigmine** is used to treat poisoning with quaternary muscarinic antagonists.

1. Contraindications (relative)

—are contraindicated in glaucoma, particularly angle-closure glaucoma, and in urinary tract obstruction (e.g., prostatic hypertrophy). **Atropine** and other muscarinic-receptor antagonists are contraindicated in heart disease, because they may cause tachycardia and ventricular arrhythmias.

2. Drug interactions

—produce additive effects when administered with other drugs with muscarinic-receptor antagonist activity (e.g., tricyclic antidepressants).

IV. Ganglionic-Blocking Drugs

A. Mechanism and pharmacologic effects

—inhibit the effect of ACh at nicotinic receptors by acting competitively (**nondepolarizing blockade**) at both sympathetic and parasympathetic autonomic ganglia.

—**decrease blood pressure** by decreasing sympathetic tone to the vasculature; the extent of hypotensive action is dependent on the degree of sympathetic activity. Less effect is observed in patients in a completely recumbent position; if the patient stands or has his head elevated, there can be a precipitous fall in blood pressure (**postural hypotension**).

B. Specific drugs and their therapeutic uses

1. Trimethaphan [Arfonad]

—is a tertiary sulfur compound that is poorly absorbed after oral administration.

—is extremely **short-acting** (< 10 minutes); is usually administered by IV infusion to maintain antihypertensive action. It is actively secreted by the kidney.

−stimulates **histamine release** and may cause flushing, dizziness, and headache. This does not appear to contribute to the hypotensive effect.

2. Mecamylamine [Inversine]

−is a secondary amine that is absorbed well from the gastrointestinal tract and penetrates the CNS.

−has a duration of action of 4–12 hours and is eliminated by the kidney.

3. Therapeutic uses

−are used to treat the following conditions, but infrequently (**mecamylamine** is almost never used) because of the availability of more selective and less toxic agents:

a. Hypertensive emergencies

b. Acute dissecting aneurysm of the aorta

c. Autonomic hyperreflexia

d. Produce controlled hypotension and minimize bleeding during certain types of skin surgery

C. Adverse effects

−although relatively selective for nicotinic receptors, these agents inhibit all autonomic outflow, resulting in numerous adverse clinical effects.

1. Eye

−produce mydriasis and cycloplegia.

2. Cardiovascular system

−produce moderate tachycardia, decrease cardiac contractility, and cause a precipitous decrease in blood pressure.

3. Gastrointestinal tract

−produce constipation as a result of reduced gastrointestinal tone and motility.

−produce dry mouth by inhibiting salivary secretion.

4. Central nervous system

−may produce insomnia, confusion, depression, or seizures when higher doses are given.

5. Other effects

−include urine retention, inhibition of sweating with dry skin, and impotence.

V. Skeletal Muscle Relaxants

A. Classification

1. Neuromuscular junction-blocking drugs

−are structurally similar to ACh.

−except **vecuronium,** are quaternary ammonium compounds with poor lipid solubility (do not penetrate the CNS).

a. Depolarizing neuromuscular junction-blocking drugs have a linear structure (e.g., **succinylcholine** is two ACh molecules linked end to end).

b. Nondepolarizing neuromuscular junction-blocking drugs are arranged in a bulky, rigid conformation.

2. Spasmolytic drugs

—act to increase or mimic the activity of γ-aminobutyric acid (**GABA**) in the spinal cord and brain or to interfere with the release of calcium in skeletal muscle.

B. Nondepolarizing agents

1. Mechanism

—competitively **inhibit the effect of ACh** at the postjunctional membrane nicotinic receptor of the neuromuscular junction. There is some prejunctional inhibition of ACh release.

—prevent depolarization of the muscle and propagation of the action potential.

2. Pharmacologic properties

—are usually administered intravenously and are generally used for long-term paralysis. Paralysis and muscle relaxation occur within 2–5 minutes.

—have a duration of action that ranges from 20–90 minutes. Primarily a function of redistribution, this can be extended by supplemental fractional dosing and is increased by larger initial doses (although this also increases the likelihood of adverse effects).

3. Specific drugs

a. *d*-Tubocurarine (prototype)

—is seldom used at this time.

—releases histamine and has some ganglionic-blocking action.

—is partially metabolized by the liver and excreted unchanged by the kidney; duration of action may be prolonged by hepatic or renal disease. Average duration of action is 60 minutes.

b. Metocurine [Metubine]

—is a derivative of *d*-tubocurarine with the same properties but less histamine release and thus less hypotension and bronchoconstriction.

c. Atracurium [Tracrium]

—is structurally related to *d*-tubocurarine.

—has an intermediate duration of action (30 minutes).

—has minimal vagolytic or ganglionic activity and minimal histamine release.

—is inactivated by nonspecific esterases, an advantage for patients with liver or renal dysfunction.

d. Pancuronium [Pavulon]

—has **steroid nucleus** with two attached quaternary amine groups.

—has a duration of action similar to that of *d*-tubocurarine.

—produces no histamine release or blockade of ganglia.

—causes moderate increase in heart rate.

—is excreted by the kidney with only minimal hepatic metabolism.

e. Vecuronium [Norcuron]

—has an intermediate duration of action.

–has little vagolytic, histaminic, or ganglionic activity.

–is primarily metabolized by the liver.

f. Gallamine [Flaxedil]

–has vagolytic action and sympathomimetic action on the heart.

–has no histaminic or ganglionic activity.

–may cause marked **tachycardia**.

4. Therapeutic uses

–are used during surgery as **adjuncts to general anesthetics** to induce muscle paralysis and muscle relaxation. The order of muscle paralysis is small, rapidly contracting muscles (e.g., extrinsic muscles of the eye) before slower-contracting muscle groups (e.g., face and extremities), followed by intercostal muscles, and then the diaphragm. Recovery of muscle function is in reverse order, and respiration often must be assisted.

–are also used for **short surgical procedures** such as tracheal intubation and to control muscle contractions during **electroconvulsive therapy**.

–are occasionally used for the **diagnosis of myasthenia gravis**.

5. Adverse effects and contraindications

a. Cardiovascular system

–produce **hypotension** due to histamine release and ganglionic-blocking activity.

–produce **tachycardia** due to vagolytic and sympathomimetic activity, leading to potential arrhythmias. Should be used cautiously in patients with cardiovascular disease.

b. Respiratory system

–produce **prolonged apnea,** which is controlled with mechanical ventilation. AChE inhibitors such as **neostigmine** are administered for pharmacologic antagonism with **atropine** to prevent muscarinic effects.

–can produce **bronchospasm** due to histamine release. Agents that release histamine are contraindicated for asthmatics and patients with a history of anaphylactoid reactions.

6. Drug interactions

a. General inhalation anesthetics

–have neuromuscular blocking action of their own. Depending on the anesthetic, the dose of the neuromuscular junction-blocking drug may have to be reduced.

b. Aminoglycoside antibiotics and lincomycin, among others, inhibit presynaptic ACh release and potentiate the effect of nondepolarizing and depolarizing neuromuscular junction-blocking drugs.

C. Depolarizing agents

–include **succinylcholine** [Anectine, Quelicin, Sucostrin], the only depolarizing drug of clinical importance. It consists of two ACh molecules joined together.

1. Mechanism of action

—is a nicotinic receptor agonist that acts at the neuromuscular junction to produce a persistent stimulation and depolarization of the muscle, thus **preventing stimulation of contraction by ACh**. It maintains an open state of membrane ion channel.

—after a single IV injection and depolarization of the muscle, there are initial muscle contractions or fasciculations (first 30–60 seconds). Because **succinylcholine** is metabolized more slowly than ACh, the muscle cells remain depolarized (**phase I block**) and unresponsive to further stimulation, resulting in a flaccid paralysis (5–10 minutes).

—with continuous long-term exposure (45–60 minutes), the muscle cells repolarize. However, they cannot depolarize again while succinylcholine is present and, therefore, remain unresponsive to ACh (**phase II block**).

—AChE inhibition will enhance initial depolarization and phase I block by succinylcholine but provides inconsistent reversal of phase II block.

2. Pharmacologic properties

—has a rapid onset and short duration of action. Action is rapidly terminated (5–10 minutes) by hydrolysis by **plasma cholinesterase**.

a. Abnormally prolonged action causes **apnea** (1–4 hours) in a small percentage of patients (1:10,000) with genetically atypical or low levels of plasma cholinesterase. Mechanical ventilation is necessary.

b. Reduced plasma cholinesterase synthesis in end-stage hepatic disease or reduced activity following the use of irreversible AChE inhibitors may increase the duration of action.

3. Therapeutic use

—is primarily used to induce brief paralysis in short surgical procedures such as **tracheal intubation**.

4. Adverse effects and contraindications

a. Postoperative **muscle pain**

b. Hyperkalemia, resulting from loss of tissue potassium during depolarization.

    (1) Risk is enhanced in patients with burns, muscle trauma, or spinal cord transections.

    (2) It can be life-threatening, leading to **cardiac arrest** and circulatory collapse.

c. Malignant hyperthermia, a rare but often fatal complication in genetically susceptible patients, which results from rapid increase in muscle metabolism. This is more likely to occur when used with **halothane** and other potent inhalation general anesthetics.

    (1) It is characterized initially by unexplained **tachycardia or tachyarrhythmia,** followed later by **muscle rigidity** (75% of patients) and then by a rapid and profound **hyperthermia**.

    (2) Drug treatment is with **dantrolene**.

d. Increased intraocular pressure is caused by extraocular muscle contractions; may be contraindicated for penetrating eye injury.

e. Increased intragastric pressure, which may result in fasciculations of abdominal muscles and danger of aspiration.

f. Bradycardia or increased bronchial secretions from stimulation of muscarinic cholinoceptors or autonomic ganglia in the absence of atropine.

g. Tachycardia, in the presence of **atropine** or at high doses.

D. Spasmolytic drugs

1. Therapeutic uses

–**reduce the spasticity** associated with a variety of nervous system disorders (e.g., **cerebral palsy, multiple sclerosis,** and **stroke**) that result in hyperexcitability of alpha motoneurons in the spinal cord with abnormal skeletal muscle, bowel, and bladder function.

2. Selected drugs

a. Dantrolene [Dantrium]

–acts directly on muscle to reduce skeletal muscle contractions.

–interferes with Ca^{2+} release from the sarcoplasmic reticulum. Benefit may not be apparent for a week or more.

–is used to reduce spasticity in **stroke, spinal cord injury, cerebral palsy,** and **multiple sclerosis**.

–is also used to treat **malignant hyperthermia**.

b. Baclofen [Lioresal]

–is a $GABA_B$-receptor agonist that inhibits synaptic transmission in the spinal cord.

–is often used to reduce spasticity in **spinal cord injury** and **multiple sclerosis**.

c. Benzodiazepines (e.g., diazepam, clonazepam)

–act on the **spinal cord** and the **CNS** to facilitate GABA activity. Part of their spasmolytic action may be due to their antianxiety or sedative effects.

–are used for **spinal spasticity, multiple sclerosis,** and **flexor and extensor spasms**.

3. Adverse effects and contraindications

a. The major adverse effect of **dantrolene** is **muscle weakness,** which may limit therapy. Chronic use may result in **hepatotoxicity,** which may be fatal. Hepatic function should be monitored during treatment. Other effects include drowsiness, dizziness, diarrhea, seizures, and pericarditis. Contraindicated in patients with liver disease and respiratory muscle weakness.

b. Adverse effects of **baclofen** are generally mild and include fatigue, nausea, euphoria, confusion, depression, hypotension, and possible lowered seizure threshold.

VI. Sympathomimetic Drugs

A. Mechanism and chemical structure

–mimic effects of endogenous epinephrine and norepinephrine.

—act on **postjunctional adrenoceptors,** and also on prejunctional adreno-ceptors, to inhibit release of catecholamines from nerve endings (some also act within nerve endings to indirectly increase release of norepinephrine). Their actions can generally be predicted from the type and location of the receptors with which they interact, and whether or not they cross the blood–brain barrier to enter the CNS.

—are usually derived from the parent compound β-phenylethylamine. Chem-ical substitutions modify their relative selectivity and intrinsic activity at α- and β-receptors, and their metabolism.

1. **Noncatechols** (lacking hydroxyl groups on the benzene ring) are less po-lar than catechols, are better absorbed, and can cross the blood–brain bar-rier more readily. They are not metabolized by COMT.

2. Substitutions on the α carbon of the side-chain protect against metabolism by MAO and prolong drug action.

3. Substitutions on the side-chain nitrogen influence receptor specificity.

B. **Pharmacologic effects**

1. **Cardiovascular system**

   a. **β_1-Receptor agonists** increase the rate and force of myocardial con-traction and conduction velocity through the AV node and decrease the refractory period.

   b. **β_2-Receptor agonists** cause relaxation of vascular smooth muscle and may invoke a reflex increase in heart rate.

   c. **α_1-Receptor agonists** constrict smooth muscle of resistance blood vessels (e.g., in the skin and splanchnic beds), causing increased pe-ripheral resistance and venous return. In normotensive patients (less effect in those with hypotension), the increased blood pressure may in-voke a reflex baroreceptor vagal discharge and a slowing of the heart, with or without an accompanying change in cardiac output.

   d. **α_2-Receptor agonists** reduce blood pressure by a prejunctional action on neurons in the CNS.

2. **Eye**

   a. **β-receptor agonists** cause relaxation of the ciliary muscle with some decrease in accommodation.

   b. **α-receptor agonists** contract the radial muscle of the iris and dilate the pupil (mydriasis).

   c. **Epinephrine and β-receptor antagonists** decrease intraocular pressure.

3. **Respiratory system**

   —**β_2-receptor agonists** relax bronchial smooth muscle and decrease air-way resistance.

4. **Gastrointestinal tract**

   —**α- and β-receptor agonists** relax gastrointestinal smooth muscle. α-receptor agonists reduce the release of ACh by a prejunctional action; β-receptors are located directly on smooth muscle.

5. Metabolic and endocrine effects

    a. β-Receptor agonists increase liver and skeletal muscle glycogenolysis and increase lipolysis in fat cells.

    b. β-Receptor agonists increase and α-**receptor agonists** decrease insulin and renin secretion.

6. Genitourinary tract

    —**β₂-receptor agonists** relax uterine smooth muscle.

C. Specific drugs

—are selected depending on the **duration of drug action** and the **route of administration,** and also on the specific **effect on a particular tissue,** which in turn depends on the tissue population of adrenoceptor subtypes.

1. Epinephrine and norepinephrine

—are poorly absorbed from the gastrointestinal tract and do not enter the CNS to any appreciable extent. Absorption of **epinephrine** from subcutaneous sites is slow because of local vasoconstriction. Although rarely used, nebulized and inhaled solutions and topical preparations of epinephrine are available. **Epinephrine and norepinephrine** are most often administered **intravenously** (with caution to avoid cardiac arrhythmias or local tissue necrosis).

—are metabolized extensively by enzymes in the liver: **COMT** methylates the *meta*-hydroxyl group of the catechol and **MAO** removes the amine group of the side-chain. Metabolites are excreted by the kidney.

—are terminated by active uptake into sympathetic nerve terminals and subsequent active transport into storage vesicles. Actions are also partially terminated at neuroeffector junctions by metabolism by extraneuronal COMT and intraneuronal MAO.

a. Epinephrine

—activates β₁, β₂, and α-adrenoceptors. At low concentrations β-receptor effects predominate; at high concentrations α-receptor effects predominate.

—at **low doses, increases systolic pressure** as a result of positive inotropic and chronotropic effects on the heart (β₁-receptor activation) and **decreases total peripheral resistance** as a result of vasodilator activity in the vascular bed of skeletal muscle (β₂-receptor activation). In other vascular beds, has **vasoconstrictor activity** (α-receptor activation).

—the **net effect of a low dose** of epinephrine is **decreased total peripheral resistance** and **decreased diastolic pressure,** with no change in mean blood pressure, and therefore, no reflex slowing of the heart rate.

—at **high doses,** also will **activate α-receptors** in the vascular bed of skeletal muscle with vasoconstriction.

—at a **high dose,** the **increase in heart rate** may be offset somewhat by reflex vagal discharge to the SA node and bradycardia in response to increased total peripheral resistance and an increase in mean arterial pressure.

—increases coronary blood blow as a result of increased cardiac work load. May precipitate **angina** in patients with coronary insufficiency.

—increases drainage of aqueous humor and reduces pressure in **open-angle glaucoma**. Causes **mydriasis** by contraction of the radial muscle of the eye.

—relaxes bronchial smooth muscle (β_2-receptor activation) already constricted by other agents or in **bronchial asthma**.

b. Norepinephrine

—**activates β_1-receptors** (equipotent to epinephrine) and **α-receptors** (slightly less potent than epinephrine, but has little activity at β_2-receptors).

—**increases total peripheral resistance and diastolic blood pressure** to a greater extent than epinephrine because of its vasoconstrictor activity and lack of effect on β_2-receptors in the skeletal muscle vascular bed.

—increases systolic blood pressure and mean arterial pressure.

—has a direct stimulant effect on heart rate but this is overcome by reflex baroreceptor-mediated vagal bradycardia.

—is rarely used therapeutically.

2. Dopamine [Dopastat, Intropin]

—activates peripheral β_1-receptors to increase heart rate and contractility.

—**activates** specific **prejunctional and postjunctional dopamine receptors** in the renal, coronary, and splanchnic vessels to reduce arterial resistance and increase blood flow. Prejunctionally, **dopamine** inhibits norepinephrine release.

—at **low doses** has a positive inotropic effect and increases systolic pressure with little effect on diastolic pressure or mean blood pressure.

—at **higher doses** activates α-receptors and causes vasoconstriction with a reflex decrease in heart rate.

3. β-Adrenoceptor agonists

a. Dobutamine [Dobutrex]

—is a **synthetic catecholamine** that is related to **dopamine**.

—has relatively selective effect on β_1-receptors (no effect on dopamine receptors).

—increases cardiac output (less tachycardia than **isoproterenol**) and lowers peripheral resistance. Larger doses may increase heart rate and blood pressure.

—is administered by **IV infusion** because of short $t_{1/2}$ (2 minutes).

b. Metaproterenol [Metaprel, Alupent], terbutaline [Brethine, Bricanyl], ritodrine [Yutopar], albuterol [Proventil, Ventolin], and bitolterol [Tornalate]

—are more selective β_2-receptor agonists that **relax bronchial smooth muscle** with fewer cardiac effects and longer duration of action than epinephrine. **Ritodrine** and **terbutaline** are used to suppress premature labor.

c. Isoproterenol [Isuprel]

—**activates β-receptors** with little activity on α-receptors. It is infrequently used due to availability of selective β_2-adrenoceptor agonists.

−dilates **bronchial smooth muscle**.

−increases **heart rate** and **contractility** and causes **vasodilation** with decreased total peripheral resistance and decreased diastolic blood pressure.

−is administered orally, parenterally, sublingually, or as an aerosol.

−is erratically absorbed after oral administration and is **metabolized by COMT**.

4. α-Adrenoceptor agonists

a. Phenylephrine, methoxamine [Vasoxyl], and metaraminol [Aramine]

−produce effects primarily by **direct α-receptor stimulation** that results in vasoconstriction and increased total peripheral resistance. **Metaraminol** also has **indirect activity;** it is taken up and released at sympathetic nerve endings, where it acts as a false neurotransmitter. It also releases **epinephrine**.

−are less potent but have longer durations of action than norepinephrine because they are not metabolized by COMT.

b. Xylometazoline [Otrivin], oxymetazoline [Afrin], and phenylpropanolamine

−have selective action at α-receptors.

−at **high doses,** may cause clonidine-like effect by action in the CNS.

c. Clonidine [Catapres], methyldopa [Aldomet], and guanabenz [Wytensin]

−**activate α$_2$-receptors** in the vasomotor center of the medulla to reduce sympathetic tone.

−**reduce blood pressure** with a decrease in total peripheral resistance and minimal long-term effects on cardiac output and heart rate.

−**methyldopa** is a prodrug that is metabolized to the active agent α-methylnorepinephrine in nerve endings, where it replaces norepinephrine and acts as a potent false neurotransmitter. At higher, nontherapeutic doses, it activates peripheral α-receptors to cause vasoconstriction.

5. Other adrenoceptor agonists

a. Ephedrine

−releases norepinephrine from nerve terminals and has some direct action on adrenoceptors.

−has effects similar to **epinephrine,** but is less potent; has a longer duration of action because it is resistant to metabolism by COMT and MAO.

−is effective orally and, unlike catecholamines, penetrates the brain and can produce mild CNS stimulation.

−after continued use, **tachyphylaxis** may develop.

b. Amphetamine [Dexedrine], methamphetamine [Desoxyn], phenmetrazine [Preludin], methylphenidate [Ritalin], and hydroxyamphetamine [Paredrine]

−produce effects similar to **ephedrine,** with direct and indirect activity. Minor metabolite, *p*-OH amphetamine, is taken up by adrenergic nerve endings and metabolized to the false neurotransmitter *p*-OH norephedrine.

−**dextroamphetamine** has more CNS stimulatory activity than the levo-isomer, which has more cardiovascular activity.

−are well absorbed and, except for **hydroxyamphetamine,** enter the CNS readily and have marked stimulant activity.

D. Therapeutic uses

1. Overview

a. α_1-**Adrenoceptor agonists** are used to treat hypotension and paroxysmal atrial tachycardia, to induce mydriasis, and to induce vasoconstriction (with local anesthetics).

b. α_2-**Adrenoceptor agonists** are used to treat hypertension.

c. β_1-**Adrenoceptor agonists** are used to treat cardiac arrest or decompensation.

d. β_2-**Adrenoceptor agonists** are used to treat bronchospasm, asthma, and emphysema.

2. Cardiovascular system

a. Sympathomimetic drugs are used for **short-term hypotensive emergencies** when there is inadequate perfusion of the heart and brain. Direct-acting α-receptor agonists such as **norepinephrine, phenylephrine,** and **methoxamine** are used if vasoconstriction is desired.

b. Use of sympathomimetic agents in **shock** is controversial. Further vasoconstriction may be harmful.

(1) Low to moderate doses of **dopamine** or **dobutamine** in **cardiogenic or septic shock** may be useful because they increase cardiac output with minimal vasoconstrictive effect on the peripheral vasculature.

(2) Epinephrine is used to reverse hypotension and angioedema associated with **anaphylactic shock, during spinal anesthesia** to maintain blood pressure (**phenylephrine** is also used for this purpose), and topically to reduce **superficial bleeding**.

c. Dobutamine is used to treat **congestive heart failure**.

d. Isoproterenol and **epinephrine** may be used for temporary emergency treatment of cardiac arrest and heart block (**Stokes-Adams syndrome**) because they increase ventricular automaticity and rate and increase AV conduction.

e. Epinephrine is commonly used in combination with **local anesthetics** (1:200,000) to reduce blood flow. α-Receptor agonist activity causes local vasoconstriction, which prolongs local anesthetic action and allows the use of lower doses.

3. Respiratory system

a. For symptomatic relief of **hay fever** and **rhinitis** of the common cold, **phenylephrine** and other short- and longer-acting agents, including

phenylpropanolamine, oxymetazoline, xylometazoline, tet-rahydrozoline, and **pseudoephedrine,** are available, many as over-the-counter (OTC) medications. Chronic use may result in ischemia and rebound hyperemia with development of chronic rhinitis and congestion.

b. When treating **asthma,** preferred drugs (e.g., **metaproterenol, ter-butaline, albuterol,** and **bitolterol**) have greater β_2-receptor stimulatory activity. **Epinephrine** is also used for management of acute bronchospasm.

c. Epinephrine is administered subcutaneously to treat bronchospasm, congestion, angioedema, and cardiovascular collapse of **anaphylaxis.**

4. Eye

a. Phenylephrine facilitates **examination of the retina** because of its mydriatic effect. It is also used for **minor allergic hyperemia of the conjunctiva.**

b. Used in **chronic open-angle glaucoma, epinephrine** and α-receptor agonists lower intraocular pressure by increasing aqueous outflow (and formation).

5. CNS

a. Amphetamine or related analogs are used for somewhat controversial treatment of **narcolepsy** (sleep disorder) for their arousal effects and their ability to increase the attention span; as occasional adjunct therapy for **obesity** because of their anorexiant effects; and to treat **attention-deficit hyperactivity disorder** in children.

b. Hydroxyamphetamine is used for the **diagnosis of Horner's syndrome.**

6. Other uses

–**ritodrine** and **terbutaline** are used to suppress premature labor by relaxing the uterus.

E. Adverse effects and toxicity

–are generally extensions of pharmacologic activity.

1. Overdose may result in **severe hypertension** with possible cerebral hemorrhage, pulmonary edema, arrhythmias, and ventricular fibrillation. Milder effects include headache, dizziness, and palpitations. Increased cardiac work load may result in angina or myocardial infarction in patients with coronary insufficiency. **Muscle tremor** may result, particularly with β_2-selective agonists.

2. Drug abuse may occur with amphetamine and amphetamine-like drugs.

3. Drug interactions

a. Tricyclic antidepressants and **guanethidine** block catecholamine reuptake and may potentiate the effects of norepinephrine and epinephrine.

b. Some **halogenated anesthetic agents** and **digitalis** may sensitize the heart to β-receptor stimulants, resulting in ventricular arrhythmias.

VII. Adrenergic Receptor Antagonists

—interact with either α- or β-receptors to prevent or reverse the actions of endogenously released norepinephrine or epinephrine or exogenously administered sympathomimetic agents.

A. α-Adrenoceptor antagonists

1. **Pharmacologic effects** are predominantly cardiovascular and include lowered peripheral vascular resistance and blood pressure. These agents prevent pressor effects of α-receptor agonists.

   —convert pressor response of agonists with combined α- and β-receptor agonist activity to a depressor response; this is referred to as epinephrine reversal.

2. **Specific drugs**

   a. **Phentolamine [Regitine]**

      —is the prototype of competitive antagonists that are equiactive at both α$_1$- and α$_2$-receptors. It is infrequently used at this time.
      —**reduces peripheral resistance** and **decreases blood pressure** partly as a result of nonadrenergic action on vascular smooth muscle.
      —is **administered intravenously** because absorption after oral administration is erratic.
      —has a **rapid onset of action** and is metabolized in the liver.
      —**tolazoline [Priscoline],** a somewhat more selective α-receptor antagonist, is less potent than phentolamine but is absorbed better from the gastrointestinal tract.

   b. **Prazosin [Minipress]**

      —is the prototype of competitive antagonists selective for α$_1$-receptors. Others include **terazosin** [Hytrin] and **doxazosin** [Cardura].
      —reduces peripheral resistance and blood pressure.
      —is administered orally. Has a **slow onset** (2–4 hours) and **long duration of action** (10 hours) and is extensively metabolized by the liver (50% during first pass).

   c. **Labetalol [Normodyne and Trandate]**

      —is a **competitive antagonist** (partial agonist) that is relatively selective for α$_1$-receptors and also blocks β-receptors.
      —reduces heart rate and myocardial contractility, decreases total peripheral resistance, and lowers blood pressure.
      —is administered **orally** or **intravenously** and undergoes extensive first-pass metabolism.

   d. **Phenoxybenzamine [Dibenzyline]**

      —is a noncompetitive, irreversible α$_1$-receptor antagonist that is mostly of historical interest.
      —binds covalently, resulting in long-lasting (15–50 hours) blockade.

3. **Therapeutic uses** (Table 2.1)

   a. **Overview**

      (1) **α$_1$-Adrenoceptor antagonists** are used to treat **hypertension**.
      (2) **α$_2$-Adrenoceptor antagonists** have no important therapeutic use.

Table 2.1. Therapeutic Uses of Adrenoceptor Antagonists

Drug	Receptor	Features	Major Uses
Propranolol [Inderal, others]	β_1 and β_2	Prototype	Hypertension; angina pectoris; pheochromocytoma; cardiac arrhythmias; migraine headache; hypertrophic subaortic stenosis
Timolol [Blocadren, Timoptic]			Hypertension; glaucoma
Metipranolol [OptiPranolol]			Glaucoma
Levobunolol [Betagan]			Glaucoma
Nadolol [Corgard]		Long duration of action (15–25 hr)	Hypertension; angina pectoris
Pindolol [Visken]		Partial agonist*	Hypertension
Penbutolol [Levatol]		Partial agonist*	Mild to moderate hypertension
Carteolol [Cartrol]		Partial agonist*	Hypertension
Metoprolol [Lopressor]	$\beta_1 > \beta_2$	Prototype	Hypertension; angina pectoris
Atenolol [Tenormin]			Hypertension, angina pectoris
Esmolol [Brevibloc]		Ultrashort acting	Supraventricular tachycardia
Betaxolol [Betoptic, Kerlone]			Glaucoma; hypertension
Acebutolol [Sectral]		Partial agonist*	Hypertension; ventricular arrhythmias
Labetalol [Normodyne, Trandate]	α_1 and β_1 and β_2	Partial agonist*; rapid blood pressure reduction	Mild to severe hypertension; hypertensive emergencies
Phentolamine [Regitine]	α_1 and α_2	Short duration of action (1–2 hr)	Hypertension of pheochromocytoma
Phenoxybenzamine [Dibenzyline]		Long duration of action (15–50 hr)	Hypertension of pheochromocytoma
Prazosin [Minipress]	α_1	Minimal reflex tachycardia	Mild to moderate hypertension (often with a diuretic or a β-adrenoceptor antagonist); severe congestive heart failure (with a cardiac glycoside and a diuretic)
Terazosin [Hytrin]			Mild to moderate hypertension
Doxazosin [Cardura]			Mild to moderate hypertension

Drugs listed in **boldface type** are considered prototype drugs.
*Lower blood pressure without significant reduction in cardiac output or resting heart rate; also do not elevate triglyceride levels or decrease high-density lipoprotein cholesterol.

b. Pheochromocytoma

—is a **tumor** of the **adrenal medulla** that secretes excessive catecholamines. Symptoms include hypertension, tachycardia, and arrhythmias.

(1) **Phentolamine** and **phenoxybenzamine** are used to treat the tumor in the preoperative stage; they also are used for long-term management of inoperable tumors.

(2) β-Receptor antagonists are often used to prevent cardiac effects of excessive catecholamines after α-receptor blockade is established.

    c. Adrenoceptor antagonists are occasionally used to **reverse hypertensive crisis** due to sudden increase in α-receptor stimulation caused by, for example, overdose with sympathomimetic agonists or pheochromocytoma.

    d. Prazosin and **labetalol** are used to treat essential hypertension.

    e. Other uses

        –include reversible **peripheral vasospasm** (e.g., Raynaud's syndrome) and **urinary obstruction** (e.g., prostatic hypertrophy) in patients who are poor candidates for surgery; treatment has limited success.

4. Adverse effects

    a. Adverse effects of **phentolamine** include **postural hypotension, reflex tachycardia, arrhythmias, angina,** and **diarrhea.**

    b. Prazosin, terazosin, and **doxazosin** produce **postural hypotension** and **bradycardia** on initial administration, and no significant tachycardia.

    c. Adverse effects of **labetalol** include **postural hypotension** and **gastrointestinal disturbances.** Bradycardia occurs with overdose. Labetalol produces fewer adverse effects on the bronchi and cardiovascular system than selective β-receptor antagonists.

B. β-Adrenoceptor antagonists

1. Pharmacologic effects

    a. Cardiovascular system

        –**lower blood pressure,** possibly due to their combined effects on the heart, the renin–angiotensin system, and the CNS.

        –reduce sympathetic-stimulated increases in heart rate and contractility and cardiac output.

        –lengthen AV conduction time and refractoriness and suppress automaticity.

        –in some cases, inhibit β_2-receptor–mediated vasodilation. Initially, they may increase peripheral resistance.

        –reduce renin release.

    b. Respiratory system

        –**increase airway resistance** as a result of β_2-receptor blockade, an effect that is more pronounced in asthmatics.

    c. Eye

        –in some cases, decrease production of aqueous humor and **reduce intraocular pressure** by an unknown mechanism.

    d. Endocrine and metabolic

        –inhibit **lipolysis.**

        –inhibit **glycogenolysis** in the liver (may increase the hypoglycemic effect of insulin).

2. Specific drugs

a. Overview

–include **propranolol,** the prototype drug, and others. Experience with most drugs other than propranolol is limited.

–have an **antihypertensive effect** that is slow to develop (mechanism is unclear).

–are absorbed well after oral administration. Except for **pindolol** (90%), all have low bioavailability (30%–50%) because of extensive first-pass metabolism; marked interpatient variability is seen. Most have a $t_{1/2}$ of 2–5 hours.

b. Propranolol [Inderal] (Figure 2.4)

–is a competitive antagonist at β_1- and β_2-receptors (Pan-beta).

–is employed in **long-term treatment of hypertension** but it is not useful for hypertensive crisis.

–is used to treat **supraventricular and ventricular arrhythmias** and is administered intravenously for emergency treatment of arrhythmias.

–is 90% bound to plasma proteins.

–is cleared by hepatic metabolism and therefore has prolonged action in the presence of liver disease.

–is also available in sustained-release preparation.

c. Metoprolol [Lopressor], betaxolol [Betoptic], atenolol [Tenormin], acebutolol [Sectral], and esmolol [Brevibloc]

–are somewhat selective β_1-receptor antagonists that may offer some advantage in asthmatic patients.

(1) Atenolol has little local anesthetic activity; it enters the CNS poorly.

(2) Acebutolol has partial agonist activity.

(3) Betaxolol is used topically for **chronic open-angle glaucoma**.

(4) Esmolol is ultrashort-acting ($t_{1/2}$ = 10 minutes) due to esterase metabolism; it is administered by **IV infusion**.

d. Nadolol [Corgard]

–has a longer duration of action than other antagonists (15–25 hours).

e. Timolol [Blocadren] and levobunolol [Betagan]

–are nonselective antagonists that have excellent **ocular effects** when applied topically for **glaucoma**. **Metipranolol** [OptiPranolol] is also used to treat **glaucoma**.

–have no local anesthetic activity.

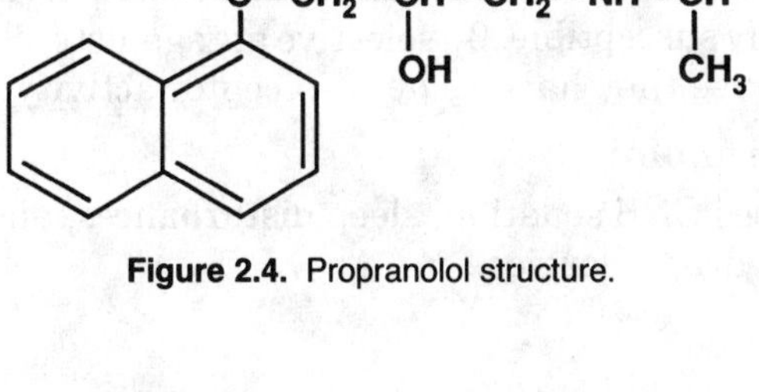

Figure 2.4. Propranolol structure.

f. Pindolol [Visken, carteolol [Cartrol], and penbutolol [Levatol]

–are **nonselective antagonists** with partial agonist activity.

3. Therapeutic uses (see Table 2.1)

a. Cardiovascular system

–are used to treat **hypertension,** often in combination with a diuretic or vasodilator. β_1-Adrenoceptor antagonists are used to treat hypertension. Drugs with β_1- and β_2-adrenoceptor antagonist activity are used for hypertension, angina, and arrhythmias.

–provide prophylaxis for **supraventricular and ventricular arrhythmias**.

–provide prophylaxis for **angina pectoris**. Long-term use may prolong survival after acute myocardial infarction.

–**propranolol** relieves angina, palpitations, dyspnea, and syncope in **obstructive cardiomyopathy**. This effect is thought to be related to slowing of ventricular ejection and decreased resistance to outflow.

b. Eye

–topical application of **timolol, betaxolol,** and **levobunolol** reduces intraocular pressure in **glaucoma**. Sufficient **timolol** can be absorbed after topical application to increase airway resistance and decrease heart rate and contractility.

c. Other uses

(1) **Propranolol** is used to control clinical symptoms of sympathetic overactivity in **hyperthyroidism** by an unknown mechanism. It may also inhibit conversion of thyroxine to triiodothyronine.

(2) **Propranolol** may be beneficial in prophylaxis of **migraine**.

(3) β-Adrenoceptor antagonists such as **propranolol** relieve **anxiety** by inhibiting overactivity of the sympathetic nervous system.

4. Adverse effects and contraindications

a. All agents

–can cause **heart failure** or heart block; should be administered with extreme caution in patients with preexisting compromised cardiac function.

–may augment insulin action in diabetics and mask tachycardia associated with hypoglycemia.

–may mask signs of developing hyperthyroidism.

–after abrupt withdrawal, adrenoceptor "supersensitivity" and increased risk of angina and arrhythmias may occur.

b. β_2-Adrenoceptor antagonists

–may cause **bronchoconstriction** and so are contraindicated for asthmatics. Patients with chronic obstructive lung disease are particularly susceptible. β_1-selective antagonists should be used cautiously, because they have some β_2-receptor activity.

c. Propranolol

–causes CNS sedation, sleep disturbances, and depression, as well as rare drug allergies.

Review Test

Directions: Each of the numbered items or incomplete statements in this section is followed by answers or by completions of the statement. Select the **one** lettered answer or completion that is **best** in each case.

1. Competitive antagonist at the neuromuscular junction nicotinic cholinoceptors include which one of the following drugs?

(A) Dantrolene
(B) Atracurium
(C) Mecamylamine
(D) Isoflurophate
(E) Succinylcholine

2. In which one of the following ways does metoprolol differ from propranolol?

(A) Metoprolol is used for the management of hypertension
(B) Metoprolol has some selectivity for β_2-adrenoceptors
(C) Metoprolol is less likely to reduce cardiac output
(D) Metoprolol is less likely to precipitate bronchoconstriction
(E) Metoprolol inhibits release of renin from the kidney

3. Administration of a moderately high dose of epinephrine to a patient results in a severe decrease in blood pressure. Which of the following drugs might the patient have previously taken that could account for this unexpected effect?

(A) Cocaine
(B) Atropine
(C) Guanethidine
(D) Prazosin

4. A drug that stimulates β_1- and β_2-adrenoceptors can be expected to cause

(A) a decrease in heart rate
(B) a decrease in total peripheral resistance
(C) a constriction of airway smooth muscle
(D) a decrease in renin release

5. All of the following drugs produce either direct or indirect parasympathomimetic effects EXCEPT

(A) bethanechol
(B) neostigmine
(C) nicotine
(D) atropine
(E) pilocarpine

6. Which one of the following drugs can be used to reduce intraocular pressure in the treatment of glaucoma?

(A) Pilocarpine
(B) Acetazolamide
(C) Neostigmine
(D) Timolol
(E) All of the above

7. Hereditary deficiency of which of the following enzymes can lead to prolonged effects of succinylcholine?

(A) Glucose-6-phosphate dehydrogenase
(B) Plasma cholinesterase
(C) Heme oxygenase
(D) Cytochrome oxidase
(E) Liver transaminase

8. Dantrolene is the drug of choice to treat malignant hyperthermia caused by succinylcholine because

(A) dantrolene blocks Ca^{2+} release from sarcoplasmic reticulum
(B) dantrolene induces contraction of skeletal muscle
(C) dantrolene increases the rate of succinylcholine metabolism
(D) succinylcholine binding to nicotinic receptors is antagonized by dantrolene
(E) dantrolene acts centrally to reduce fever

9. Which one of the following drugs is least likely to enter the CNS?

(A) Guanethidine
(B) Methyldopa
(C) Clonidine
(D) Propranolol
(E) Ephedrine

10. Clonidine and methyldopa act as agonists at α_2-adrenoceptors to cause

(A) a sustained increase in mean arterial pressure
(B) an increase in intestinal motility
(C) a CNS-mediated decrease in sympathetic nerve activity
(D) an increase in myocardial contractility
(E) bronchoconstriction

11. Which of the following drugs is the shortest-acting acetylcholinesterase inhibitor?

(A) Neostigmine
(B) Physostigmine
(C) Edrophonium
(D) Echothiophate
(E) Trimethaphan

12. Drug X causes an increase in blood pressure and a decrease in heart rate when administered intravenously. If an antagonist at ganglionic nicotinic receptors is administered first, drug X causes an increase in blood pressure and an increase in heart rate. Drug X most likely is

(A) propranolol
(B) norepinephrine
(C) isoproterenol
(D) terbutaline
(E) curare

13. Poisoning with a carbamate insecticide is best managed by administration of which one of the following agents?

(A) Physostigmine
(B) Bethanechol
(C) Propranolol
(D) Pilocarpine
(E) Atropine

14. Receptor actions of acetylcholine are mimicked by nicotine at which one of the following sites?

(A) Adrenal medullary chromaffin cells
(B) Urinary bladder smooth muscle cells
(C) Iris circular (constrictor) muscle
(D) Heart sinoatrial pacemaker cells

15. Which one of the following drugs would decrease release of norepinephrine from adrenergic nerves?

(A) Prazosin
(B) Propranolol
(C) Phenylephrine
(D) Clonidine

16. Muscarinic cholinoceptor agonists may induce vasodilation largely by causing release of endothelial

(A) histamine
(B) norepinephrine
(C) acetylcholine
(D) nitric oxide

17. Which one of the following agents would be most likely to induce bronchial dilation?

(A) Norepinephrine
(B) Phenylephrine
(C) Clonidine
(D) Metaproterenol

18. Which one of the following agents, when applied topically to the eye, would induce both mydriasis and cycloplegia?

(A) Phenylephrine
(B) Carbachol
(C) Prazosin
(D) Atropine

19. The reflex change in heart rate associated with administration of metaproterenol could be blocked by administration of which one of the following agents?

(A) Atropine
(B) Propranolol
(C) Prazosin
(D) Physostigmine

20. Which one of the following drugs generally should NOT be administered to a patient with asthma?

(A) Atropine
(B) Propranolol
(C) Epinephrine
(D) Isoproterenol

21. Neostigmine would be expected to reverse which one of the following conditions?

(A) Paralysis of skeletal muscle induced by a competitive (nondepolarizing) muscle relaxant
(B) Paralysis of skeletal muscle induced by a depolarizing muscle relaxant
(C) Cardiac slowing induced by stimulation of the vagus nerve
(D) Pupillary miosis induced by bright light

22. The pressor effect of epinephrine can be converted to a depressor effect by prior administration of

(A) prazosin
(B) propranolol
(C) atropine
(D) reserpine

23. The direct cardiac effects of dobutamine would be blocked by which one of the following agents?

(A) Prazosin
(B) Metoprolol
(C) Clonidine
(D) Isoproterenol

24. Topical application of timolol to the eye would be expected to induce which of the following?

(A) miosis
(B) mydriasis
(C) decreased formation of aqueous humor
(D) increased outflow of aqueous humor

25. Phenylephrine is applied to the nasal mucosa in order to

(A) block histamine receptors
(B) block β-adrenergic receptors
(C) induce vasodilation
(D) induce vasoconstriction

Directions: The group of items in this section consists of lettered options followed by a set of numbered items. For each item, select the **one** lettered option that is most closely associated with it. Each lettered option may be selected once, more than once, or not at all.

Questions 26–30

Match the action below with the receptor that is most closely associated with it.

(A) α_1-Adrenoceptors
(B) β_1-Adrenoceptors
(C) α_2-Adrenoceptors
(D) β_2-Adrenoceptors
(E) Muscarinic cholinoceptors

26. Norepinephrine acts directly on these receptors to increase heart rate

27. Epinephrine acts at these receptors to contract arteriolar smooth muscle

28. Acetylcholine act at these receptors to increase gastric acid secretion and intestinal motility

29. Terbutaline acts on these receptors to relax bronchial smooth muscle

30. Stimulation of these receptors in the CNS leads to a sustained decrease in mean arterial pressure

Answers and Explanations

1–B. Atracurium is a nondepolarizing neuromuscular blocking agent that competitively inhibits the effect of acetylcholine at neuromuscular junction nicotinic cholinoceptors. Dantrolene interferes with the release of calcium from the sarcoplasmic reticulum. Mecamylamine is a nicotinic cholinoceptor ganglionic-blocking agent. Isoflurophate is a cholinesterase inhibitor. Succinylcholine is a depolarizing cholinoceptor agonist at the motor end-plate.

2–D. Metoprolol is more selective at β_1-adrenoceptors, which are more abundant in the heart than in the lungs.

3–D. Prazosin blocks postsynaptic α_1-adrenoceptors and inhibits epinephrine-mediated vasoconstriction.

4–B. β_2-Adrenoceptor agonists relax vascular smooth muscle and reduce blood pressure. Heart rate is stimulated reflexively (β_2 activation) and directly (β_1 activation). Bronchial smooth muscle is relaxed (β_2 activation) and renin release is increased (β_1 activation).

5–D. Atropine is a muscarinic cholinoceptor antagonist.

6–E. All of these agents can be used to treat glaucoma. Pilocarpine is a muscarinic cholinoceptor agonist. Acetazolamide inhibits carbonic anhydrase. Neostigmine is a cholinesterase inhibitor. Timolol is a β-receptor antagonist.

7–B. Plasma cholinesterase is responsible for the rapid inactivation of succinylcholine.

8–A. In patients with malignant hyperthermia, a rare hereditary disorder, an impaired sarcoplasmic reticulum is unable to sequester calcium. The sudden release of calcium results in extensive muscle contraction that can be reduced with dantrolene.

9–A. Unlike methyldopa, clonidine, propranolol, and ephedrine, guanethidine's action is limited to the periphery (a highly basic nitrogen makes it too polar to enter the CNS).

10–C. Both clonidine and methyldopa are useful antihypertensive agents.

11–C. Edrophonium has a short duration of action (5–15 min), and is used in the diagnosis of myasthenia gravis.

12–B. In the absence of a nicotinic receptor antagonist, norepinephrine may result in a reflex baroreceptor-mediated increase in vagal activity. The presence of such an agent unmasks the direct stimulant effect of norepinephrine on heart rate.

13–E. Atropine blocks the effects of increased acetylcholine resulting from cholinesterase inhibition. Physostigmine indirectly, and bethanechol and pilocarpine directly, activate cholinoceptors. Propranolol is a β-adrenoceptor antagonist.

14–A. Nicotinic cholinoceptors are found in adrenal medullary chromaffin cells. At the other sites, acetylcholine activates muscarinic cholinoceptors.

15–D. Clonidine decreases release of norepinephrine by activation of prejunctional α_2-adrenoceptors. Prazosin inhibits postjunctional α_1-adrenoceptors (norepinephrine release could be decreased indirectly by negative feedback). Phenylephrine is a relatively pure α-adrenoceptor agonist. Propranolol is a β-adrenoceptor antagonist.

16–D. Release of nitric oxide activates guanylate cyclase, increasing guanosine 3',5'-monophosphate (cyclic GMP) and sequestering calcium. This leads to relaxation of vascular smooth muscle.

17–D. Metaproterenol, a selective β_2-adrenoceptor agonist, is most likely to cause bronchial dilation.

18–D. Atropine produces both mydriasis and cycloplegia (the inability to accommodate for near vision). Phenylephrine causes mydriasis without cycloplegia. Carbachol causes pupillary constriction. Prazosin is an α-adrenoceptor antagonist.

19–B. Metaproterenol, a relatively selective β_2-adrenoceptor agonist, will cause vasodilation and reflex sympathetic activation of the heart, which can be blocked with propranolol.

20–B. Blockade of bronchial β_2-adrenoceptors by propranolol can exacerbate asthma.

21–A. Acetylcholine accumulation due to neostigmine inhibition of cholinesterase will reverse the action of the competitive neuromuscular blocking agents.

22–A. Prazosin blocks the α_1-adrenoceptor vasoconstrictor effect (increase in blood pressure) of epinephrine, which reveals its β_2-adrenoceptor vasodilator action (decrease in blood pressure or, "epinephrine reversal").

23–B. The β_1-adrenoceptor antagonist metoprolol blocks the β_1-adrenoceptor activity of dobutamine.

24–C. β-Adrenoceptor blocking agents such as timolol reduce aqueous humor formation.

25–D. Phenylephrine activates α-adrenoceptors, producing vasoconstriction.

26–B. Norepinephrine acts directly on β_1-adrenoceptors to increase heart rate.

27–A. Epinephrine acts at α_1-adrenoceptors to contract arteriolar smooth muscle.

28–E. Acetylcholine acts at muscarinic cholinoceptors to increase gastric acid secretion and intestinal motility.

29–D. Terbutaline acts on β_2-adrenoceptors to relax bronchial smooth muscle.

30–C. Stimulation of α_2-adrenoceptors in the CNS leads to a sustained decrease in mean arterial pressure.

3

Drugs Acting on the Renal and Cardiovascular Systems

I. Agents that Alter Kidney Function

A. Diuretics

—**increase urine flow** through effects on the kidney. Most agents affect **water balance** indirectly by altering electrolyte reabsorption or secretion. Osmotic agents affect water balance directly.

—produce **diuresis** associated with increased Na^+ excretion. This results in concomitant loss of water and reduction of extracellular volume.

—are generally used for management of **congestive heart failure (CHF)** and abnormalities in body fluids (e.g., edema and glaucoma) and for reducing plasma volume in **hypertensive patients**.

—can cause electrolyte imbalances such as **hypokalemia, hyponatremia, and hypochloremic alkalosis**.

1. Thiazide diuretics

a. Mechanism

—these agents **inhibit active reabsorption of NaCl** in the ascending loop of Henle and in the early distal part of the nephron (distal convoluted tubule), which results in net excretion of Na^+ and accompanying volume of water.

—also **increase absorption of Ca^{2+}**.

—can be derivatives of sulfonamides (sulfonamide diuretics). Many also **inhibit carbonic anhydrase,** resulting in diminished HCO_3^- reabsorption by the proximal tubule.

b. Prototype drugs

—include **chlorothiazide** [Diuril, others] and **hydrochlorothiazide** [Esidrix, HydroDIURIL, Oretic, others]. Other agents include **chlorthalidone** [Hygroton, others], **benzthiazide** [Exna, others], and **cyclothiazide** [Anhydron], among many others.

—**increase excretion** of Cl^-, Na^+, K^+ and, at high doses, HCO_3^- They **reduce excretion** (increase absorption) **of Ca^{2+}**.

—are **absorbed from the gastrointestinal tract** and produce diuresis within 1–2 hours.

–are **secreted into the lumen** of the proximal tubule by organic acid carrier with some secretion via the hepatic–biliary route. They exert effects only after reaching the lumen.

c. **Related drugs**

–include **indapamide** [Lozol, Lozide] and **metolazone** [Zaroxolyn, Diulo], **indoline** and **quinazoline** diuretics, respectively, that have properties generally similar to those of the thiazide diuretics. Unlike thiazides, these agents may be effective in the presence of some renal impairment.

d. **Therapeutic uses**

–thiazide diuretics are the preferred class of diuretic for treatment of **hypertension** when renal function is normal; they are often used in combination with other antihypertensive agents to enhance their blood pressure-lowering effects.

–reduce formation of new calcium stones in **idiopathic hypercalciuria**.

–may be useful in patients with **diabetes insipidus** not responsive to antidiuretic hormone (ADH).

–are often used in combination with a potassium-sparing diuretic to manage mild cardiac **edema,** cirrhotic or nephrotic edema, and edema produced by hormone imbalances.

–should be approached cautiously in the presence of renal or hepatic diseases, such as cirrhosis.

–should be used only as an ancillary treatment in nephrotic syndrome.

e. **Adverse effects and contraindications**

–produce electrolyte imbalances such as **hypokalemia, hyponatremia,** and **hypochloremic alkalosis;** are often exhibited by central nervous system (CNS) disturbances, including dizziness, confusion, and irritability; muscle weakness; cardiac arrhythmias; and by increased sensitivity to digitalis-like drugs. Diets high in K^+ are recommended; K^+ supplementation may be required.

–often **elevate serum urate,** presumably as a result of competition for the organic acid secretory carrier (which also eliminates uric acid). Gout-like symptoms may appear.

–can cause **hyperglycemia,** especially in patients with diabetes, and **hypersensitivity reactions**.

2. **Loop diuretics**

a. **Mechanism**

–inhibit active NaCl reabsorption in the thick ascending limb of the loop of Henle. Because of high capacity for NaCl reabsorption in this segment, agents active at this site markedly increase water and electrolyte excretion and are referred to as **high-ceiling diuretics**. These drugs are often effective in producing diuresis in patients responding maximally to other types of diuretics.

b. **Prototype drugs**

–include **furosemide** [Lasix] and its derivatives **piretanide and bumetanide** [Bumex], as well as **ethacrynic acid** [Edecrin] and other phenoxyacetic acid derivatives.

   –reduce reabsorption of Cl^- and Na^+; increase K^+, Mg^{2+}, and Ca^{2+} excretion.
   –are **absorbed by the gastrointestinal tract**. They are administered either orally or parenterally. Diuresis occurs within 5 minutes after intravenous (IV) administration and within 30 minutes after oral administration.
   –are **eliminated by filtration** and by **tubular secretion** (may cause increases in serum uric acid); some elimination occurs via the hepatic–biliary route.

   c. Therapeutic uses
   –are used in the treatment of **CHF** by reducing **acute pulmonary edema** and edema refractory to other agents. They are synergistic with thiazide diuretics when coadministered.
   –are used to treat **hypertension,** especially in individuals with diminished renal function.
   –are also used to treat **acute hypercalcemia** and **halide poisoning**.

   d. Adverse effects and contraindications
   –produce **hypotension** and **volume depletion,** as well as **hypokalemia** due to enhanced secretion of K^+ and **alkalosis** due to enhanced H^+ secretion. Mg^{2+} wasting can also occur; therapy is often instituted gradually to minimize electrolyte imbalances and volume depletion.
   –can cause dose-related **ototoxicity,** more often in individuals with renal impairment. These effects are more pronounced with ethacrynic acid than furosemide. These agents should be administered cautiously in the presence of renal disease or with use of other ototoxic agents such as **aminoglycosides**.
   –can cause **hypersensitivity** reactions. **Ethacrynic acid** produces **gastrointestinal disturbances**.

3. Potassium-sparing diuretics

   a. Mechanism
   –**interfere with K^+ secretion and N^+ reabsorption** in the distal part of the nephron (collecting tubule). These are not potent diuretics when used alone; major use is in combination with other diuretics.

   b. Selected drugs
   (1) Structural analogs of aldosterone
   –include agents such as **spironolactone** [Aldactone], the active metabolite of which is **canrenone**.
   –**inhibit the action of aldosterone** by competitively binding to the cytoplasmic receptor and preventing subsequent cellular events that regulate K^+ and H^+ secretion and Na^+ reabsorption.
   –are active only when endogenous mineralocorticoid is present; effects are reduced when hormone levels are elevated.
   –are **absorbed** from the **gastrointestinal tract** and **metabolized** in the **liver;** therapeutic effects are achieved only after several days.
   –are generally used in combination with a thiazide or loop diuretic to treat **hypertension, CHF, and refractory edema**.

—are also used to induce diuresis in clinical situations associated with hyperaldosteronism, such as in **adrenal hyperplasia** and in the presence of **aldosterone-producing adenomas** when surgery is not feasible.

—can cause **hyperkalemia, hyperchloremic metabolic acidosis,** and **gynecomastia**.

—can cause menstrual abnormalities in females.

—are **contraindicated in renal insufficiency,** especially in diabetic patients. They must be used cautiously in the presence of liver disease.

—are contraindicated in the presence of other potassium-sparing diuretics and should be used with extreme **caution in individuals taking** an angiotensin-converting enzyme inhibitor (**ACE inhibitor**).

(2) Amiloride [Midamor] and triamterene [Dyrenium]

—decrease membrane permeability and inhibit electrogenic absorption of Na^+ and excretion of K^+ in the cortical collecting tubule, independent of the presence of mineralocorticoids.

—produce diuretic effects within 2–4 hours after oral administration. **Triamterene** is metabolized in the liver. Both drugs are secreted in the proximal tubule.

—are used to manage **CHF, cirrhosis,** and **edema** caused by secondary hyperaldosteronism. These agents are available in combination products containing thiazide or loop diuretics; for example, **triamterene/hydrochlorothiazide** [Dyazide]. **Amiloride** in combination with thiazide diuretics—such as **amiloride/hydrochlorothiazide** [Moduretic]—is used to treat hypertension.

—produce **hyperkalemia,** the most serious adverse effect. Dietary potassium should be reduced. Minor adverse effects include nausea and vomiting.

—are contraindicated in the presence of diminished renal function.

4. Carbonic anhydrase inhibitors

a. Mechanism

—inhibit carbonic anhydrase in all parts of the body. In the kidney, the effects are predominantly in the proximal tubule.

—reduce HCO_3^- reabsorption and concomitant Na^+ uptake. They also inhibit excretion of H^+ (and coupled Na^+ uptake).

b. Prototype drugs

—include **acetazolamide** [Diamox] and **dichlorphenamide** [Daranide, Oratrol].

—are **sulfonamide derivatives,** forerunners of thiazide diuretics. (Thiazides separate natriuresis from carbonic anhydrase inhibition.)

—are **absorbed** from the **gastrointestinal tract** and **secreted** by the **proximal tubule**. Urine pH changes are observed within 30 minutes.

c. Therapeutic uses

—are most useful in the treatment of **glaucoma** (decrease the rate of HCO_3^- formation in aqueous humor and consequently reduce ocular pressure).

—are sometimes used as adjuvants for the treatment of **seizure disorder** but development of tolerance limits use.

—may be used to produce desired alkalinization of urine to enhance renal secretion of uric acid and cysteine.

—may reduce symptoms of **acute mountain sickness** in mountain climbers.

—are rarely used as diuretics.

d. Adverse reactions and contraindications

—include **metabolic acidosis** due to reduction in bicarbonate stores. Alkalinity of urine decreases solubility of calcium salts and increases the propensity for renal calculi formation. Potassium wasting may be severe.

—following large doses, commonly produce drowsiness and paresthesias.

—are **contraindicated in hepatic cirrhosis**.

5. Agents influencing water excretion

a. Osmotic agents

—include **mannitol** [Osmitrol], **glycerin,** and **isosorbide**.

—are easily filtered, poorly reabsorbable solutes that alter the diffusion of water relative to sodium by "binding" water. Net reabsorption of Na^+ is reduced.

(1) Mannitol

—is administered intravenously.

—is used in **prophylaxis of acute renal failure** resulting from physical trauma or surgery. Even when filtration is reduced, sufficient mannitol usually enters the tubule to promote urine output.

—may also be useful for **reducing cerebral edema and intraocular pressure**.

—because osmotic forces that reduce intracellular volume ultimately expand extracellular volume, serious adverse effects may occur in patients with CHF. Minor adverse effects include headache and nausea.

(2) Glycerin and isosorbide

—are administered orally.

—are used primarily for **ophthalmic procedures**. Topical anhydrous glycerin is useful for **corneal edema**.

b. Agents that influence the action of ADH (vasopressin)

—ADH increases the permeability of the luminal surface of the medullary collecting duct to water. Under conditions of dehydration, ADH levels increase to conserve body water. Agents that **elevate** or mimic ADH are **antidiuretic;** agents that **lower** or antagonize ADH action are **diuretic**.

(1) Vasopressin [Pitressin] or analogs

—are useful in the management of ADH-sensitive **diabetes insipidus. Desmopressin** [DDAVP], one of the most useful analogs, is used to treat **nocturnal enuresis**.

—produce serious **cardiac-related adverse effects,** and they should be used with caution in individuals with coronary artery disease.

**(2) Chlorpropamide [Diabinese], acetaminophen, indometha-
cin, and clofibrate [Atromid-S]**

(a) Chlorpropamide, acetaminophen, and indomethacin enhance the action of ADH, at least partially by reducing production of prostaglandins in the kidney.

(b) Clofibrate increases the release of ADH centrally.

(c) These agents are also useful as antidiuretics in diabetic patients.

(3) ADH antagonists

−include **demeclocycline and lithium carbonate**.

−may be useful in the treatment of **inappropriate secretion of
ADH** in individuals refractory to water restriction.

6. Other diuretics

a. Xanthine diuretics act by increasing cardiac output and promoting a
higher glomerular filtration rate. They are seldom used as diuretics, but
diuresis occurs under other clinical applications (e.g., bronchodilatation).

b. Acidifying salts such as **ammonium chloride** lower pH and increase
lumen concentrations of Cl^- and Na^+. They are sometimes used in
combination with high-ceiling diuretics to counteract alkalosis.

B. Nondiuretic inhibitors of tubular transport

−influence transport of organic anions, including the endogenous anion uric
acid, and cations. Transport takes place in the proximal tubule; organic compounds enter a cell by Na^+-facilitated diffusion and are excreted from the cell
into the lumen by a specific organic ion transporter. *Para*-aminohippurate,
not used clinically, is a classic compound used to study these phenomena.

1. Uricosuric agents

a. Mechanism

−**increase excretion of uric acid.** Paradoxically, because of the balance between uptake into a cell, excretion from the cell, and reabsorption from the lumen, low doses of these agents often decrease excretion, whereas high doses increase excretion. These drugs are often
used in the **treatment of gout**.

b. Selected drugs

(1) Probenecid [Benemid]

−inhibits secretion of organic acids. It was developed to **decrease
secretion of penicillin** (an organic acid) and thus prolong elimination of this antibiotic. Other drugs whose secretion is inhibited
by probenecid include **indomethacin** and **methotrexate**.

−also **decreases reabsorption of uric acid** with a net increase in
secretion (thus may be useful in gout).

−inhibits the transport of organic acids from the subarachnoid
space to the plasma.

−is **absorbed from the gastrointestinal tract** and **secreted by
the proximal tubule**.

−is used to **prevent gout** in individuals with normal renal function
and as an adjuvant to penicillin therapy when prolonged serum
levels following a single dose are required or to enhance antibiotic
concentrations in the CNS.

−produces hypersensitivity reactions and gastric irritation as the
most common adverse effects.

(2) Sulfinpyrazone [Anturane]

–is a strong organic acid that inhibits reabsorption of uric acid. May also inhibit secretion of drugs transported by an organic acid carrier.

–is **absorbed from the gastrointestinal tract** and **secreted by the proximal tubule**.

–is used in the treatment of **gout,** often in **combination with colchicine** or a nonsteroidal anti-inflammatory drug.

–is contraindicated in the presence of peptic ulcer disease.

(3) Allopurinol [Zyloprim]

–is not a true uricosuric agent. It **inhibits xanthine oxidase,** which is involved in the synthesis of uric acid.

–is metabolized by xanthine oxidase to produce **alloxanthine,** which has long-lasting inhibitory effects on the enzyme; net result is **decreased production of uric acid**.

–is used in the treatment of **gout**.

C. Drugs that act on the renin–angiotensin system

1. Principles of the renin–angiotensin system

a. Several parameters regulate **release of renin** from the kidney cortex: Reduced arterial pressure, decreased sodium delivery to the cortex, increased sodium at the distal tubule, and stimulation of sympathetic activity all increase renin release.

b. Renin cleaves the protein α_2-globulin and **releases angiotensin I**. This decapeptide is converted enzymatically (mostly in the lung) to an octapeptide, **angiotensin II,** or the heptapeptide **angiotensin III**. Angiotensin II is a vasoconstricting agent and causes sodium retention via release of **aldosterone**. In the adrenal gland, angiotensin II is converted to angiotensin III, which is less active as a vasoconstricting agent than angiotensin II.

c. Both angiotensin II and angiotensin III stimulate the **release of aldosterone**.

2. ACE inhibitors

a. Mechanism

–**inhibit** the production of angiotensin II from angiotensin I.

–**counteract** elevated peripheral vascular resistance and sodium and water retention resulting from angiotensin II and aldosterone.

–also **prevent inactivation of bradykinin,** which is a potent vasodilator. Net effect is **reduced blood pressure**.

b. Therapeutic uses

–are very useful in the treatment of **CHF** and **hypertension**. They have the advantage of minimal electrolyte disturbances and fewer adverse effects than other agents used to treat hypertension.

c. Selected drugs

(1) Captopril [Capoten]

–is **absorbed from the gastrointestinal tract,** and is metabolized to disulfide conjugates. It does not enter the CNS.

–is used in the treatment of **mild to moderate hypertension**. Diuretics enhance the effects.

−produces **adverse effects** that include rashes, taste disturbances, pruritus, weight loss, and anorexia. It rarely produces
bone marrow suppression and proteinuria. Dose reduction may be
required in patients with impaired renal function.

(2) Enalapril [Vasotec]

−is a prodrug that is deesterified in the liver to produce **enala-
prilat,** which inhibits ACE.

−is used to treat **mild to severe hypertension,** especially in the
presence of CHF. Diuretics enhance its activity.

(3) Lisinopril [Zestril, Prinivil]

−is an ACE inhibitor that permits once-a-day dosing. Bioavailability is not affected by food.

II. Drugs that Lower Plasma Lipids

A. Overview

1. Dietary or pharmacologic reduction of elevated plasma cholesterol
levels can reduce the risk of atherosclerosis and subsequent cardiovascular disease. Exact factors linking elevated cholesterol levels to heart disease are not yet known.

2. The association between cardiovascular disease and elevated plasma triglycerides is less clear. However, **elevated triglycerides** can produce
life-threatening pancreatitis.

3. Hyperlipoproteinemias

a. Cholesterol is a nonpolar, poorly water-soluble substance, transported in the plasma in particles that have a hydrophobic core of cholesteryl esters and triglycerides surrounded by a coat of phospholipids,
free cholesterol (nonesterified), and one or more apoproteins. These lipoprotein particles vary in the ratio of triglyceride to cholesteryl ester
as well as in the type of apoprotein.

b. Diseases of plasma lipid can be manifest as an elevation in triglycerides
or as an elevation in cholesterol. In several of the complex or combined
hyperlipoproteinemias, both **triglycerides and cholesterol can be
elevated**.

4. Lipoprotein metabolism

a. Chylomicrons, rich in triglyceride with a lesser cholesterol component, are formed in the intestine and transported by the lymphatics to
the circulation. **Free fatty acids** are released from chylomicrons by
hydrolysis of triglyceride by lipoprotein lipase, an enzyme associated
with the endothelial cell. This catabolism provides fatty acids to muscle
and adipose cells and produces the relatively cholesterol-rich chylomicron remnant.

b. Chylomicron remnants are bound by cell-surface receptors in the
liver—probably both the **low-density lipoprotein (LDL) receptor**
and a unique remnant receptor—and deliver the chylomicron cholesterol to the hepatocytes. This cholesterol is used directly as a constituent of bile (or metabolized to bile acids) or for membrane biosynthesis,

or is reesterified by acyl coenzyme A (acyl CoA) cholesterol acetyltransferase and stored or repackaged into **very-low-density lipoprotein (VLDL) particles** and transported from the liver.

c. The triglyceride component of VLDL is hydrolyzed by lipoprotein lipase, eventually converting the VLDL particle to the cholesterol-rich **intermediate-density lipoprotein (IDL) particle**.

d. About 50% of the IDL particles are recirculated back to the liver and are bound by the LDL receptor, where the lipids are reutilized for VLDL synthesis; the remaining 50% are more fully metabolized by lipoprotein lipase to LDL. **LDL particles** constitute about 60% of total plasma cholesterol. These particles are slowly removed from the plasma, with a half-life ($t_{1/2}$) of about 1.5 days. LDL transports cholesterol to the peripheral circulation, where the particle is bound by cell-surface LDL receptors and internalized, and the cholesterol utilized or stored as a cholesteryl ester.

e. High concentrations of **high-density lipoprotein (HDL) particles** are correlated with a decreased incidence of cardiovascular disease. One role of these particles is removal of plasma cholesterol released from dead cells and produced by membrane turnover. In addition, these particles mediate **reverse cholesterol transport** from peripheral cells back to the liver.

f. About 50% of all cholesterol metabolism occurs in the liver, and about 50% of the LDL receptors are within the liver. Alterations of hepatic cholesterol metabolism can markedly affect the levels of cholesterol in the peripheral circulation.

B. Drugs useful in treating hyperlipidemias

1. Nicotinic acid (niacin) [Nicobid, Nicolar]

a. Mechanism

—can exert cholesterol- and triglyceride-lowering effects at high concentrations (nicotinamide cannot do this). This is distinct from the role of this molecule as a vitamin, where nicotinic acid is converted to nicotinamide and used for biosynthesis of the cofactors NAD and NADP.

—**reduces plasma VLDL** by inhibiting VLDL synthesis (20%–80% over 1–4 days); it markedly decreases plasma triglyceride levels. As the substrate VLDL concentration is reduced, the concentrations of IDL and LDL also fall, thereby reducing plasma cholesterol levels.

—the precise mechanism of inhibition of VLDL synthesis is unclear: **Lipolysis in adipocytes is inhibited,** reducing the major source of fatty acids for hepatic triglyceride biosynthesis; **VLDL catabolism is increased** by an elevation in the activity of lipoprotein lipase; and a slight **decrease in hepatic cholesterol synthesis** is observed.

—in much smaller doses, can also be used as a vitamin supplement in the treatment of **pellagra**.

b. Adverse effects

—nicotinic acid commonly produces **flushing and an itching or burning feeling in the skin,** which may reduce compliance. This is mediated by prostaglandin release and can be diminished by taking aspirin 30 minutes before taking nicotinic acid.

–produces **hepatic effects,** including increased transaminase activities; **hyperglycemia; gastrointestinal disturbances and peptic ulcer; renal effects** that include elevated plasma uric acid; and **macular edema.**

2. Fibric acid analogs

a. Clofibrate [Atromid-S]

–is an ethyl ester of chlorophenoxyisobutryic acid (CPIB).

(1) Mechanism

–**increases the peripheral catabolism of VLDL and chylomicrons** by increasing the activity of lipoprotein lipase. Results in a reduction in the plasma concentration of VLDL, most notably in triglycerides.

–**reduces hepatic synthesis of cholesterol,** probably as a result of altered VLDL metabolism.

(2) Pharmacologic properties

–has good oral absorption, with $t_{1/2}$ approximately 15 hours.

–is metabolized to the active metabolite CPIB, which is extensively bound to plasma albumin.

–is excreted by the kidney, mostly as a glucuronide.

(3) Therapeutic uses

–is used to treat **hyperlipidemia** of several etiologies, especially hypertriglyceridemia due to dysbetalipoproteinemia, a defect in apolipoprotein E, which impairs clearance of chylomicron remnants and VLDL.

–is ineffective in primary chylomicronemia (caused by a deficiency in lipoprotein lipase) and has little effect on reducing plasma cholesterol levels.

–has antidiuretic action in individuals with mild or moderate **diabetes insipidus**.

(4) Adverse effects and contraindications

–produces cholelithiasis and cholecystitis, gastrointestinal intolerance and nausea, and myalgia.

–frequently causes leukopenia, rash, and drowsiness, as well as decreased libido in a small percentage of men.

–can **displace** other albumin-bound drugs, most notably the **sulfonylureas and warfarin**.

–must be used cautiously in individuals with impaired renal or hepatic function.

b. Gemfibrozil [Lopid]

–is an analog of **clofibrate** that is more effective in some circumstances.

(1) Mechanism

–**decreases plasma concentration of VLDL** by decreasing lipolysis in fat tissue, which reduces free fatty acid substrates for hepatic triglyceride biosynthesis. It has little effect on total plasma cholesterol levels: It increases plasma HDL and slightly (10%) reduces LDL.

(2) Pharmacologic properties

–is completely absorbed after oral administration; $t_{1/2}$ is approximately 1½ hours.

—undergoes considerable enterohepatic circulation and is excreted by the kidney.

(3) Therapeutic uses

—are identical to those for clofibrate; may be more active in **reducing triglycerides** than clofibrate.

(4) Adverse effects

—are similar to those of clofibrate; skin rashes and cholelithiasis may occur.

3. Probucol [Lorelco]

—is a *bis*-phenol in a sulfur linkage and is highly **hydrophobic.**

a. Mechanism

—**reduces plasma cholesterol** (10%–15%).

—has antioxidant properties, which may reduce the atherogenic nature of plasma lipids by reducing uptake by macrophages.

—**increases bile acid excretion.**

—produces some inhibition of the early steps of cholesterol biosynthesis. HDL and LDL concentrations are reduced, but there is no effect on serum triglyceride levels.

b. Pharmacologic properties

—approximately 10% of an oral dose is absorbed; it partitions into adipose tissue and may remain there for several months.

—is excreted into the feces by the biliary route.

c. Therapeutic use

—is limited to patients who are refractory or hypersensitive to other cholesterol-lowering drugs.

d. Adverse effects

—include nausea, diarrhea, and flatulence; eosinophilia; and increased hematocrit. Fatal arrhythmias have been reported in experimental animals; prolongation of Q–T interval has been reported in humans.

4. Bile acid sequestrants

—include **cholestyramine** [Questran] and **colestipol** [Colestid].

a. Structure and mechanism

(1) Cholestyramine is a large copolymer of styrene and divinylbenzene that has ion-exchange capacity provided by trimethylbenzylammonium groups. The average molecular weight of the polymer is over 10^6. Chloride is the anion that is exchangeable.

(2) Colestipol is an ion-exchange resin that is a copolymer of diethyl pentamine and epichlorohydrin.

(3) Both of these resins are **hydrophilic** but are not absorbed across the intestine.

(4) In the intestine, the resins exchange chloride for bile salts and prevent enterohepatic reutilization of bile acids. In addition, they impair absorption of dietary cholesterol by the following mechanisms:

(a) Increase hepatic uptake of LDL and **reduce plasma LDL levels.** This is mediated by an increase in LDL receptors.

(b) Increase VLDL synthesis and release for a variable length of time; the elevation in VLDL synthesis is most prolonged in patients with preexisting hypertriglyceridemia.

b. Therapeutic uses

–are effective in **reducing plasma cholesterol** (by 15%–20%) in patients with some normal LDL receptors. This excludes patients who completely lack functional LDL receptors because of a genetic defect (homozygous familial hypercholesterolemia).

c. Adverse effects

–are generally quite safe, because they are not absorbed in the intestine.

–produce **gastrointestinal disturbances** (constipation, nausea, and discomfort), which may reduce compliance.

–**interfere with absorption of anionic drugs** (e.g., **digitalis, warfarin**).

5. Inhibitors of cholesterol biosynthesis

–include **lovastatin** (mevinolin) [Mevacor], **simvastatin** [Zocor], and **pravastatin** [Pravachol].

a. Mechanism

–function as competitive inhibitors of 3-hydroxy-3-methylglutaryl-coenzyme A reductase (HMG-CoA reductase), the rate-limiting enzyme in cholesterol biosynthesis. Reduced cholesterol synthesis results in a compensatory increase in hepatic uptake of plasma cholesterol mediated by an increase in the number of LDL receptors.

–reduce total cholesterol by as much as 33%; LDL and HDL cholesterols are reduced by 41% and 12%, respectively. LDL/HDL ratio is reduced by 46%.

b. Therapeutic uses

–are effective in reducing cholesterol levels in **familial and nonfamilial hypercholesterolemias**.

c. Adverse effects

–include myositis and hepatotoxicity and elevations in aminotransferases.

6. Other agents

a. Neomycin [Mycifradin]

–is an **aminoglycoside antibiotic** that is poorly absorbed from the gastrointestinal tract.

–appears to inhibit the absorption of bile acids and dietary cholesterol.

–is similar in action to the bile acid sequestrants and has no effect on triglycerides.

–may be useful in conjunction with other lipid-lowering agents, but adverse effects limit use as a primary cholesterol-lowering agent.

–produces adverse effects that include nausea, diarrhea, and abdominal cramps, and superinfection (overgrowth of resistant bacteria) in the intestine and colon.

b. β-Sitosterol [Cytellin]

–is a **poorly absorbed plant sterol** similar in structure to cholesterol. Large doses of β-sitosterol appear to inhibit intestinal absorption of cholesterol.

−may be useful in patients with unusual sensitivity to dietary cholesterol.

−is not known to produce adverse effects, even at high concentrations.

c. Thyroxine and D-thyroxine

(1) L-**Thyroxine,** the naturally occurring form of the thyroid hormone,
can reduce plasma cholesterol.

(2) The D-isomer, **dextrothyroxine** [Choloxin], retains the cholesterol-lowering capacity of thyroxine with some reduction in the hy-
permetabolic actions of the hormone. This is mediated through increased biliary cholesterol excretion, increased metabolism of
cholesterol to bile acids, and increased LDL receptors.

(3) Although the metabolic effects of D-**thyroxine** are reduced compared to the L-isomer, significant calorigenic activity remains. This
potentiates adrenergic action on the heart, leading to exacerbation
of angina and arrhythmias.

III. Agents Used to Treat Congestive Heart Failure (CHF)

A. Overview

1. CHF

−results when the output of the heart is insufficient to supply adequate
levels of oxygen for the body. **Impaired contractility** and **circulatory
congestion** are both components of failure. Compensatory elevation in
angiotensin II production results in sodium retention and vasoconstriction, which may contribute to cardiac hypertrophy.

2. Therapeutic agents

a. Increase cardiac contractility

b. Reduce preload (left ventricular filling pressure) and aortic impedance
(systemic vascular resistance)

c. Normalize heart rate and rhythm

B. Cardiac glycosides

−are the principal drugs for treatment of **CHF** and certain **arrhythmias**
(atrial fibrillation and flutter and paroxysmal atrial tachycardias).

1. Structure

−are **cardenolides** that contain a lactone ring and a steroid (aglycone)
moiety attached to sugar molecules. Most common agents are **digoxin
and digitoxin,** the major active ingredients found in digitalis plants,
collectively referred to as **digitalis.** (**Oubain** is another plant glycoside
that currently is not often used.)

2. Mechanism

−**inhibit Na$^+$,K$^+$-ATPase,** resulting in increased intracellular Na$^+$ and
decreased intracellular K$^+$. Increased Na$^+$ reduces normal exchange of
intracellular Ca^{2+} for extracellular Na$^+$ and yields elevated intracellular Ca^{2+}.

−with each action potential, there is a greater release of Ca^{2+} to activate
the contractile process. Net result is **positive inotropic effect.**

3. Cardiac effects

—increase the speed of shortening and the force of contraction in both the normal and failing heart.

a. Under normal cardiac conditions, **digitalis treatment** results in an increase in systemic vascular resistance and constriction of smooth muscles in veins (cardiac output may decrease).

b. In the failing heart, capacity to develop force during systole is compromised and increased end-diastolic volume is required to achieve the same amount of work. **Heart rate, ventricular volume, and pressure are elevated** while **stroke volume** is **diminished**. There is a compensating increase in sympathetic activity and decrease in vagal activity as well as an increase in blood volume.

  (1) Under these conditions, cardiac glycosides **increase stroke volume** and **enhance cardiac output**. Concomitantly, blood volume, venous pressure, and end-diastolic volume decrease.

  (2) The congested heart becomes smaller; efficiency of contraction is increased (restored toward normal). **Improved circulation** reduces sympathetic activity and permits further improvement in cardiac function as a result of decreased systemic arterial resistance and venous tone.

  (3) Improved renal blood flow augments elimination of Na^+ and water.

4. Pharmacologic properties and selected drugs

—distribute to most body tissues and **accumulate in cardiac tissue**. Concentration in the heart is twice that in skeletal muscle and at least 15 times higher than in plasma.

—must **individualize dose**. Initial loading (digitalizing) dose is often selected from prior estimates and adjusted for the patient's condition. **Maintenance dose** is based on daily loss of the drug.

—dosing levels for **treatment of CHF** generally are lower than for decreasing the ventricular response in atrial fibrillation.

a. Digoxin [Lanoxin]

  —has a somewhat variable oral absorption; can be given **orally or intravenously**. Peak effect after IV dose occurs in 1.5–2 hours; $t_{1/2}$ is approximately 1.5 days. Maintenance dose is approximately 35% of the loading dose.

  —produces therapeutic effect (and disappearance of toxic effects) more rapidly than digitoxin. However, because of a relatively rapid clearance, lack of compliance may influence therapeutic effects.

  —is **eliminated by renal route;** $t_{1/2}$ is prolonged in individuals with impaired renal function. Dosage can be adjusted based on creatinine clearance.

b. Digitoxin [Crystodigin, Purodigin]

  —is completely **absorbed** from the **gastrointestinal tract;** $t_{1/2}$ is approximately 5–6 days. Maintenance dose is approximately 10% of the loading dose. Long elimination $t_{1/2}$ is a disadvantage when toxicity is manifest but an advantage when compliance is problematic.

−is **metabolized in the liver** and **excreted** via **biliary route**. Impaired renal function does not alter $t_{1/2}$.

−should be administered cautiously in the presence of hepatic dysfunction.

5. **Adverse effects and toxicity**

  a. **Narrow therapeutic index**

    −can cause **fatal adverse effects**.

    −**induce** virtually every type of **arrhythmia**.

    −**affect** all **excitable tissues;** the most common site outside the heart is the **gastrointestinal tract** (anorexia, nausea, vomiting, and diarrhea can occur), resulting either from direct action or through stimulation of the chemoreceptor trigger zone.

    −**disorientation and visual disturbances** may occur.

    −gynecomastia and galactorrhea are rarely observed.

  b. **Toxicity** is treated primarily by discontinuing the drug.

    (1) **Potassium** may help in alleviating arrhythmias.

    (2) Antiarrhythmic agents such as **phenytoin and lidocaine** may be helpful.

    (3) **Antidigoxin antibodies** (digoxin immune FAB) [Digibind] or hemoperfusion may be useful in serious toxicity.

  c. **Drug interactions**

    −drugs that bind digitalis compounds, such as **cholestyramine and neomycin,** may interfere with therapy. Drugs that enhance hepatic metabolizing enzymes, such as **phenobarbital,** may lower concentrations of the active drug (especially **digitoxin**).

    −risk of toxicity is increased by the following:

    (1) **Hypokalemia**

      −K^+ interferes with binding of cardiac glycosides to Na^+,K^+-ATPase. Thus, hypokalemia enhances their effects and greatly increases the risk of toxicity; may be seen with **thiazide** or other potassium-lowering diuretics.

      −reduces therapeutic effects.

    (2) **Hypercalcemia and calcium-channel blocking agents** (e.g., verapamil)

      −cause toxicity by adding to drug effects on Ca^{2+} stores. Hypocalcemia renders digitalis less effective.

    (3) **Quinidine**

      −displaces digoxin from tissue binding sites. The $t_{1/2}$ of **digoxin** is prolonged because of decreased renal elimination.

C. **ACE inhibitors**

−are becoming increasingly important in the treatment of CHF.

−are most often used when treatment with digitalis has failed. As single agents, they are unique in improving mortality. A combination of **captopril and digitalis** may be more effective than either agent alone.

−**increase cardiac output and induce systemic arteriolar dilatation** (reduce afterload).

−cause **venodilatation and induce natriuresis,** thereby reducing preload.

−are especially useful for **long-term therapy**.

D. Other inotropic agents

1. Amrinone lactate [Inocor] and milrinone [Corotrope]

−are bipyridine derivatives related to the anticholinergic agent **biperiden.**

−**reduce left ventricular filling pressure** and **vascular resistance** and **enhance cardiac output.**

−**inhibit cardiac phosphodiesterase.**

−may act by increasing cyclic AMP (cAMP), which leads to elevated intra-cellular CA^{2+} levels and excitation-contraction.

−are used in patients who do not respond to digitalis and are most effective in individuals with elevated left ventricular filling pressure.

−produce considerable **toxicity on extended administration;** are administered intravenously only for short-term therapy. The most common **adverse effect** is **hypotension.** Fever and gastrointestinal disturbances occur occasionally.

−fewer and **less severe adverse effects** are seen with **milrinone** as compared to amrinone.

2. Dobutamine hydrochloride [Dobutrex]

−is a **synthetic catecholamine derivative** that **increases contractility;** it acts primarily on myocardial β_1-adrenoceptors with lesser effects on β_2- and α-adrenoceptors.

−moderate doses do not increase heart rate.

−does not activate dopamine receptors.

−is administered only by IV route.

−is employed in short-term therapy in individuals with **severe chronic cardiac failure** and for inotropic support after **cardiac surgery.** It does not substantially increase peripheral resistance and thus is not useful in cardiac shock with severe hypotension.

−combined infusion therapy with **nitroprusside** or **nitroglycerin** may improve cardiac performance in outpatients with **advanced heart failure.**

−produces tachycardia and hypertension, but is less arrhythmogenic than **isoproterenol.**

E. Diuretics

−reduce left ventricular filling pressure and decrease left ventricular volume and myocardial wall tension (lower oxygen demand).

−are often used as sole therapy in **mild CHF;** they also are employed for **acute pulmonary edema.**

F. Vasodilators

1. Cardiac effects

−reduce aortic impedance or increase venous capacitance. Net effect is **vasodilation.** In response to failures of pump function, sympathetic tone increases during resting state and ultimately reduces cardiac output and excessive venoconstriction. Thus, vasodilators can be effective in CHF and are particularly useful when heart failure is associated with hypertension, congestive cardiomyopathy, mitral or aortic insufficiency, or ischemia.

2. Therapeutic use

—are used to treat **severe, decompensated CHF** refractory to diuretics and digitalis.

a. Agents used in **short-term therapy** include **nitroprusside,** which has a direct balanced effect on arterial and venous beds, and **nitroglycerin,** which has more effect on venous beds than on arterial beds. Nitroglycerin is not as effective as nitroprusside in enhancing cardiac output.

b. Agents used in **long-term therapy** include the direct-acting vasodilators **isosorbide** and **hydralazine,** and **prazosin,** an adrenergic blocking agent that produces arterial and minor venous dilation.

IV. Antiarrhythmic Drugs

A. Causes of arrhythmias

—include improper impulse generation, conduction, or both. They manifest as abnormalities of rate, regularity, or disturbance in normal sequence of activation of atria and ventricles.

1. Altered automaticity

—can arise from the following:

a. Sinus node (sinus tachycardia and bradycardia)

—**increased vagal activity** can impair nodal pacemaker cells by elevating K^+ conductance, leading to hyperpolarization. **Increased sympathetic activity** increases the rate of phase 4 depolarization. Intrinsic disease yields faulty pacemaker activity (**sick sinus syndrome**).

b. Ectopic foci

—are areas within the conduction system that may, in the diseased state, develop high rates of intrinsic activity and function as pacemakers.

c. Triggered automaticity

—results from delayed after-polarizations that reach threshold and are capable of initiating an impulse.

2. Abnormal impulse conduction in conduction pathways

a. Heart blocks may produce **bradyarrhythmias**.

b. Reentry circus conduction may produce **tachyarrhythmias**.

B. Goal of therapy

—aims to restore normal pacemaker activity and modify impaired conduction that leads to arrhythmias.

—is achieved by sodium or calcium-channel blockade, prolongation of effective refractory period, or blockade of sympathetic effects on the heart. Many antiarrhythmic drugs affect depolarized tissue to a greater extent than they affect normally polarized tissue.

C. Treatment of tachyarrhythmias: Class I drugs

1. Mechanism

—depress fast inward movement of sodium, thereby reducing rate of phase 0 depolarization, prolonging effective refractory period, increasing threshold of excitability, and reducing phase 4 depolarization. They also have local anesthetic properties.

a. Class IA drugs prolong refractory period and slow conduction.

b. Class IB agents shorten duration of refractory period.

c. Class IC drugs slow conduction.

2. Class IA

a. Quinidine [Quinidex, Duraquin, Cardioquin]

(1) Effects and pharmacologic properties

—at therapeutic levels direct **electrophysiologic effects** predominate, including depression of the pacemaker rate and depressed conduction and excitability. At low doses, **anticholinergic** (vagolytic) **effects** predominate and may increase conduction velocity in the atrioventricular (AV) node and accelerate heart rate.

—is administered **orally** and is rapidly absorbed from the **gastrointestinal tract**.

—is **hydroxylated in the liver** and has a $t_{1/2}$ approximately 5–12 hours, which is longer in hepatic or renal disease and heart failure.

(2) Therapeutic uses

—is used for **supraventricular and ventricular ectopia** and is employed to **maintain sinus rhythm** after conversion of atrial flutter or fibrillation by **digoxin, propranolol,** or **verapamil**.

—is used to **prevent frequent premature ventricular complexes and ventricular tachycardia**. Paradoxical tachycardia may be seen.

—as the dextrorotary isomer of **quinine,** also exhibits antimalarial, antipyretic, and oxytocic actions.

(3) Adverse effects

—depresses all muscles, which can lead to skeletal muscle weakness, especially in individuals with myasthenia gravis.

—can produce severe hypotension and shock after rapid infusion.

—can produce **cinchonism** (ringing of ears and dizziness) and diarrhea.

—may induce thrombocytopenia, most probably as a result of platelet-destroying antibodies developed in response to circulating protein–quinidine complexes.

—can cause ventricular arrhythmias. **Quinidine syncope** (dizziness and fainting) may occur as a result of ventricular tachycardia. It is associated with a prolonged Q–T interval.

(4) Drug interactions

—increases digoxin plasma levels and the risk of **digitalis toxicity**.

—has $t_{1/2}$ reduced by agents that induce drug-metabolizing enzymes (**phenobarbital, phenytoin**).

–may enhance activity of **coumarin** anticoagulants and other drugs metabolized by hepatic microsomal enzymes.

–cardiotoxic effects are exacerbated by hyperkalemia.

b. Procainamide [Pronestyl, Procan]

–has action similar to quinidine but is safer to use intravenously and produces fewer adverse gastrointestinal effects.

–is acetylated in the liver to *N*-acetylprocainamide [NAPA] at a genetically determined rate. "Slow acetylators" have earlier onset and greater prevalence of drug-induced lupus-like syndrome than "fast acetylators." NAPA is also active as an antiarrhythmic.

–is eliminated by the kidney; $t_{1/2}$ is approximately 3–4 hours. Dose reduction is required in renal failure.

–has **high incidence of adverse effects with chronic use**. It is more likely than quinidine to produce severe or irreversible heart failure.

–often causes drug-induced **lupus-like syndrome** (symptoms resembling systemic lupus erythematosus).

c. Disopyramide [Norpace]

–has action similar to quinidine.

–is approved for treatment of **ventricular arrhythmias;** it is generally reserved for cases refractory or intolerant to quinidine or procainamide.

–produces **pronounced antimuscarinic effects,** including dry mouth, blurred vision, constipation, urine retention, and, rarely, acute angle-closure glaucoma. It may worsen heart block and adversely affect sinus node function.

3. Class IB

a. Lidocaine [Xylocaine]

–is the most widely used agent for **suppression and prevention of ventricular ectopic activity associated with myocardial infarction (MI):** It does not slow conduction and thus has little effect on atrial function.

–acts exclusively on the **sodium channel** (both activated and inactivated).

–undergoes large first-pass effect; is administered **intravenously or intramuscularly;** $t_{1/2}$ is approximately 1.5–2 hours.

–is administered in a loading dose followed by infusion. The dose must be adjusted in CHF or hepatic disease.

–has low level of cardiotoxicity; most common **adverse effects are neurologic**. In contrast to quinidine and procainamide, it has little effect on the autonomic nervous system (ANS).

b. Mexiletine [Mexitil] and tocainide [Tonocard]

–are agents similar in action to lidocaine and can be administered orally.

(1) Mexiletine is used primarily for **chronic treatment of ventricular arrhythmias associated with previous MI**.

(2) Tocainide is used for treatment of **ventricular tachyarrhythmias**.

  c. **Phenytoin and moricizine [Ethmozine]**
     (1) **Phenytoin,** an anticonvulsant drug, is useful in treating **digitalis-induced tachyarrhythmias**.
     (2) **Moricizine,** a phenothiazine, suppresses abnormal automaticity. It is approved for **life-threatening ventricular arrhythmias** and may be useful in treating asymptomatic or mild ventricular arrhythmias.

  4. **Other class I agents**

     a. **Class IC: Flecainide [Tambocor], encainide [Enkaid] and lorcainide**
        —are **orally** active, and are used for **ventricular tachyarrhythmias**.
        —are limited by propensity to **cause proarrhythmic actions;** cautious use is recommended in patients with sinus node dysfunction and CHF.

     b. **Propafenone [Rhythmol]**
        —has a spectrum of action similar to that of quinidine.
        —possesses some β-**adrenoceptor antagonist** activity.
        —is effective in a variety of **atrial and ventricular tachyarrhythmias**.
        —may cause bradycardia, CHF, or new arrhythmias.

     c. **Aprindine [Fibocil]**
        —**reverses** both **supraventricular and ventricular arrhythmias**.

  D. **Treatment of tachyarrhythmias: Class II drugs**

  1. **Mechanism**
     —are β-**adrenoceptor antagonists,** including **propranolol,** which act by reducing sympathetic stimulation. They inhibit phase 4 depolarization, depress automaticity, prolong AV conduction, and decrease heart rate (except for agents that have sympathomimetic activity) and contractility.

  2. **Major drugs** (see Table 2.1)

     a. **Propranolol** [Inderal, generic], a nonselective β-adrenoceptor antagonist, and the more selective $β_1$-adrenoceptor antagonists **acebutolol** [Sectral] and **esmolol** [Brevibloc] are used to treat ventricular arrhythmias. **Esmolol** is ultra–short-acting and is used to titrate block during surgery.

     b. **Propranolol, metoprolol** [Lopressor], **nadolol** [Corgard], and **timolol** [Blocadren] are frequently used to prevent MI.

  3. **Therapeutic uses**
     —are used to treat **tachyarrhythmias** caused by increased sympathetic activity. They also are employed for a variety of other arrhythmias, atrial flutter, and atrial fibrillation.
     —**prevent reflex tachycardia** produced by vasodilating agents. They sometimes are used for **digitalis toxicity**.

  4. **Adverse effects**
     —include **arteriolar vasoconstriction** and **bronchospasm**. Bradycardia and myocardial depression may occur. **Atropine** or **isoproterenol** may be used to alleviate bradycardia.

E. Treatment of tachyarrhythmias: Class III drugs

–prolong action potential duration and effective refractory period.

1. Bretylium [Bretylol]

–**inhibits neuronal release of catecholamines** and also has some direct antiarrhythmic action. It has properties of class II drugs.

–**prolongs ventricular action potential** but not atrial action potential.

–is used intravenously for **severe refractory ventricular tachyarrhythmias** and also for prophylaxis and treatment of **ventricular fibrillation**.

–may cause initial burst of norepinephrine release and may precipitate ventricular arrhythmias. The effect is exacerbated in the presence of vasopressors or digitalis. The major adverse effect is **hypotension,** which can be alleviated by administration of **dopamine or norepinephrine**.

2. Amiodarone [Cordarone]

–is structurally related to thyroxine and **increases refractoriness**. It also depresses sinus node automaticity and slows conduction.

–plasma concentration is not well correlated with the effects of the drug. Although electrophysiologic effects may be seen within hours after parenteral administration, effects on abnormal rhythms may not be seen for several days. Antiarrhythmic effects may last for weeks or months after the drug is discontinued.

–is used for **severe refractory supraventricular and ventricular tachyarrhythmias,** and it also possesses antianginal effects.

–produces **adverse effects** (especially **gastrointestinal-related**) in almost all patients. Other adverse effects include photosensitivity, "gray man syndrome," corneal microdeposits, and thyroid disorders (due to iodine in drug preparation).

F. Treatment of tachyarrhythmias: Class IV drugs

1. Mechanism

–selectively block slow-calcium channel; prolong nodal conduction and effective refractory period.

2. Verapamil [Calan, Isoptin]

–is a papaverine-derivative that blocks both **activated and inactivated slow-calcium channels**. Tissues that depend on slow-calcium channels are most affected.

–is **metabolized** by the **liver;** dose reduction is necessary in the presence of hepatic disease. Oral dosage is only partially (20%) available, and larger doses are required when administered intravenously.

–is useful in **reentrant supraventricular tachycardia,** and can also reduce ventricular rate in **atrial flutter and fibrillation**.

–has **negative inotropic action** that limits its use in damaged hearts; can lead to AV block when given in large doses or in patients with partial blockage. It can precipitate sinus arrest in diseased patients and causes peripheral vasodilation.

–**adverse cardiac effects** may be exacerbated in individuals taking β-**adrenoceptor antagonists;** this can be reversed by atropine, β-adrenoceptor agonists, or calcium.

G. Treatment of tachyarrhythmias: Class V drugs

1. Adenosine has cardiac effects similar to **verapamil** and is often preferred to the calcium-channel blocking agent for treatment of **reentrant supraventricular tachycardia**. Adenosine acts through specific purinergic (P_1) receptors rather than directly on calcium channels.

2. Digoxin can control ventricular response in **atrial flutter or fibrillation**.

H. Treatment of bradyarrhythmias

1. Atropine

–**blocks the effects of acetylcholine.** It elevates sinus rate and AV nodal and sinoatrial (SA) conduction velocity, and decreases refractory period.

–is used to treat bradyarrhythmias that accompany **MI**.

–produces adverse effects that include dry mouth, mydriasis, and cycloplegia; may induce arrhythmias.

2. Isoproterenol [Isuprel]

–**stimulates β-adrenoceptors** and increases heart rate and contractility.

–is used to **maintain adequate heart rate** and output in patients with AV block.

–may cause tachycardia, anginal attacks, headaches, dizziness, flushing and tremors.

V. Antianginal Agents

A. Goal of therapy

–is to restore the balance between oxygen supply and demand in the ischemic region of myocardium.

B. Types of angina

1. Classic angina (angina of exercise)

–occurs when oxygen demand increases and diseased coronary arteries cannot meet the demand.

2. Vasospastic (Prinzmetal's, or variant) angina

–results from reversible coronary vasospasm that decreases oxygen supply and occurs at rest. Some individuals have **mixed angina,** in which both exercise-induced and resting attacks may occur.

C. Nitrates and nitrites

1. Structure and mechanism

–are polyol esters of **nitric acid** (nitrates) or **nitrous acid** (nitrites) that relax vascular smooth muscle.

–activate guanylate cyclase and increase cyclic guanine nucleotides.

–dilate all vessels. Peripheral venodilation decreases cardiac preload and myocardial wall tension and thus lowers oxygen demand by decreasing the work of the heart.

–ameliorate symptoms of **classic angina** predominantly through improvement of hemodynamics. **Variant angina** is relieved through effects on coronary circulation.

–form nitrosothiol at smooth muscle by reaction with glutathione. Tolerance occurs upon glutathione depletion.

2. Bioavailability and selected drugs

—have **large first-pass effect** due to high-capacity organic nitrate reductase in liver, which inactivates drugs. Nitrates have $t_{1/2}$ of less than 10 minutes.

a. Nitroglycerin

—is preferably administered sublingually for rapid delivery and short duration. Sustained-delivery systems [Transderm-Nitro, Nitrodisc] are available and are used to maintain blood levels. Aerosol, topical, intravenous, and oral preparations are also available.

b. Amyl nitrite

—is a **volatile liquid** that is **inhaled**. An unpleasant odor and extensive cutaneous vasodilation render it less desirable than **nitroglycerin**.

c. Isosorbide dinitrate [Isordil, Sorbitrate]

—has active initial metabolites.

—is administered **orally** or **sublingually;** has better oral bioavailability and longer half-life (up to 1 hour) than **nitroglycerin**. Timed-release oral preparations are available.

d. Erythrityl tetranitrate [Cardilate]

—is similar to **nitroglycerin** and is administered **sublingually**.

3. Therapeutic uses

a. Sublingual **nitroglycerin** is most often used for severe, recurrent **Prinzmetal's angina**.

b. Continuous infusion or slowly absorbed preparations of nitroglycerin (including the now-favored transdermal patch) or derivatives with longer half-lives have been used for **unstable angina** and for **CHF in the presence of MI**.

4. Adverse effects

—produce **vasodilation,** which can lead to orthostatic hypotension, reflex tachycardia, throbbing headache (may be dose-limiting), and blushing. Continuous exposure may lead to tolerance.

—can produce **thiocyanate**. Large doses produce **methemoglobinemia**.

D. β-Adrenoceptor antagonists

—decrease heart rate, blood pressure, and contractility, resulting in **decreased myocardial oxygen requirements**. Combined therapy with nitrates is often preferred in the treatment of angina pectoris because of decreased adverse effects of both agents.

—are contraindicated in the presence of CHF and asthma.

E. Calcium-channel blocking agents

1. Mechanism

—produce blockade of slow-calcium channel, which decreases contractile force and oxygen requirements. Agents cause **coronary vasodilation and relief of spasm;** also dilate vasculature and decrease cardiac afterload.

2. Pharmacologic properties

—can be administered orally. When administered intravenously, they are effective within minutes.

−therapeutic use in angina is generally reserved for instances when nitrates are ineffective or when β-adrenoceptor antagonists are contraindicated.

−**serum lipids should not be increased.**

−produce **hypotension**.

3. Selected drugs

a. Verapamil [Calan, Isoptin]

−produces slowed conduction through AV node (predominant effect); may be an unwanted effect in some situations (especially in the treatment of hypertension).

−may produce AV block when used in combination with β-adrenoceptor antagonists. Toxic effects include myocardial depression, heart failure, and edema.

b. Nifedipine [Adalat, Procardia] and nicardipine [Cardene]

−**lower vascular resistance;** also decrease afterload and lower blood pressure.

−have pronounced **vasodilating effects** that can produce headaches, reflex tachycardia, and fluid retention.

c. Diltiazem [Cardizem]

−is intermediate in properties between **verapamil** and **nifedipine**.

−is used to treat **variant (Prinzmetal's) angina,** either naturally occurring or drug-induced.

d. Bepridil [Vascor]

−blocks both slow calcium and fast sodium channels and both voltage-dependent and receptor-mediated calcium channels.

−is used only in individuals in whom other agents have failed or have elicited intolerable adverse effects.

−may cause **ventricular arrhythmias**.

F. Prostaglandins and related agents

1. Principles of the prostaglandin (PG) system

−modulates vascular tone and platelet aggregation. **PGI_2** (prostacyclin, epoprostenol) is produced by blood vessels, dilates vascular beds, and inhibits platelet aggregation. Note that **thromboxane A_2 (TxA_2)** is released by platelets and causes vasoconstriction and platelet aggregation.

2. Dipyridamole [Persantine]

−is a coronary vasodilator that interferes with uptake of the vasodilator **adenosine**. Potentiates effect of **PGI_2** and dilates resistance vessels.

−may be used for **prophylaxis of angina pectoris** but efficacy is not proven.

−produces adverse effects that include worsening of angina, dizziness, and headache.

VI. Antihypertensive Drugs

A. Principles of blood pressure regulation

1. Blood pressure is regulated by the following:

a. Cardiac output

      b. Peripheral vascular resistance

      c. Volume of intravascular fluid (controlled at the kidney)

    2. Baroreflexes adjust moment-to-moment blood pressure.

      a. Carotid baroreceptors respond to stretch, and their activation inhibits sympathetic discharge.

      b. Reduction in renal perfusion pressure results in increased reabsorption of salt and water. Decreased renal pressure stimulates **renin production** and leads to enhanced levels of **angiotensin II**. This agent in turn causes resistance vessels to constrict and stimulates aldosterone synthesis, which ultimately increases the absorption of sodium by the kidney.

B. Goal of therapy

    —is to **reduce elevated blood pressure,** which would ultimately lead to end-organ damage.

    —is achieved through the use of various drug classes, and **treatment** often involves a **combination of agents** (Table 3.1).

C. Diuretics

    —increase sodium excretion and lower blood volume.

1. Thiazide diuretics

    —are effective in lowering blood pressure 10–15 mm Hg.

    —when administered alone, can provide relief for **mild or moderate hypertension**.

    —are used in combination with sympatholytic agents or vasodilators in **severe hypertension**.

2. Loop diuretics

    —are used in combination with sympatholytic agents and vasodilators.

3. Potassium-sparing diuretics

    —are used to avoid potassium depletion, especially when administered with cardiac glycosides.

D. Adrenoceptor antagonists

1. β-Adrenoceptor antagonists (see Table 2.1)

a. Propranolol [Inderal]

    —antagonizes **catecholamine action** at both β_1- and β_2-receptors. It produces sustained reduction in peripheral vascular resistance.

    —**blockade of cardiac β_1-adrenoceptors** reduces heart rate and contractility. β_2-adrenoceptor blockade increases airway resistance and decreases catecholamine-induced glycogenolysis and peripheral vasodilation.

    —**blockade of β-adrenoceptors** in the CNS decreases sympathetic activity.

    —also decreases renin release.

    —is used in **mild to moderate hypertension**.

b. Nadolol [Corgard], timolol [Blocadren], carteolol [Cartrol], pindolol [Visken], and penbutolol [Levatol]

Table 3.1. Some Antihypertensive Drugs

Class	Drug	Adverse Effects	Therapeutic Use
Diuretics			
Thiazide and thiazide-related agents	Chlorothiazide, hydrochlorothiazide, benzthiazide, cyclothiazide, chlorthalidone, metolazone, indapamide	Hypokalemia, hyperuricemia, hypersensitivity reactions, hyperglycemia	Alone to treat moderate hypertension; in combination with other classes of drugs to treat severe hypertension
Loop	Furosemide, bumetanide, ethacrynic acid	Hypotension, volume depletion, hypokalemia, hypomagnesemia, hyperuricemia, hyperglycemia, hypercalcemia	In the presence of azotemia
Potassium-sparing agents	Triamterene, spironolactone, amiloride	Hyperkalemia	Managing primary aldosteronism; may be beneficial in presence of hyperuricemia, hypokalemia, or glucose intolerance
Peripheral sympatholytics			
β-Adrenoceptor antagonists	Nonselective (β_1 and β_2): propranolol, timolol, nadolol, pindolol, penbutolol, carteolol; β_1-selective: acebutolol, atenolol, metoprolol	Most adverse effects are mild, rarely requiring withdrawal of drug: fatigue, depression, reduced exercise tolerance, bradycardia, CHF, bronchoconstriction in presence of asthma, gastrointestinal disturbances, masked hypoglycemia, increased triglycerides, decreased low-density lipoprotein cholesterol	All grades of hypertension; may be combined with a diuretic for additive effects, or with a diuretic plus an α-adrenoceptor antagonist for resistant hypertension; β_1-selective agents are advantageous for diabetic patients (less likely to cause hypotension during hypoglycemia and to delay recovery from hypoglycemia)
α_1- and β-Adrenoceptor antagonist	Labetalol	Similar to propranolol; more likely to cause orthostatic hypotension and sexual dysfunction	Intravenously for hypertensive emergencies due to rapid reduction in pressure

α-Adrenoceptor antagonists	Prazosin, terazosin, doxazosin	First-dose syncope, dizziness, palpitations, fluid retention, anticholinergic effects	As single agents in mild to moderate hypertension; may be useful with a diuretic and a β-adrenoceptor antagonist
Angiotensin-converting enzyme inhibitors	Captopril, enalapril, lisinopril, ramipril	Rash, dysgeusia, cough; individuals with high plasma renin activity may experience excessive hypotension	Mild to severe hypertension
Calcium-channel blockers	Verapamil, diltiazem, nicardipine, nifedipine, isradipine, felodipine	Peripheral edema	Broad range of hypertensive patients; cautious use in presence of heart failure
Central sympatholytics	Methyldopa, clonidine, guanabenz	Dry mouth, sedation, lethargy	Chronic hypertension
Adrenergic neuronal blocking drugs	Guanethidine, guanadrel	Orthostatic hypotension; severe hypertension in presence of pheochromocytoma	Severe refractory hypertension
	Reserpine	Gastrointestinal disturbances, mental depression	Mild-to-moderate hypertension
Vasodilators Arteriolar vasodilators	Hydralazine, minoxidil	Lupus-like syndrome may occur with hydralazine; minoxidil may cause severe volume retention	Sometimes for hypertension refractory to β-blocker/thiazide diuretic combination; in combination with a diuretic and often a β-blocker
Arteriolar and venule vasodilator	Sodium nitroprusside	Excessive decrease in blood pressure may occur	

−are similar in action to propranolol and block both β_1- and β_2-adrenoceptors.

−**nadolol** has extended duration of action.

−**pindolol, carteolol, and penbutolol** have partial agonist activity (sympathomimetic).

c. **Metoprolol [Lopressor], atenolol [Tenormin], and acebutolol [Sectral]**

−are relatively selective for β_1-adrenoceptors.

−**acebutolol** has partial agonist activity.

2. α-Adrenoceptor antagonists

−**lower total peripheral resistance** by preventing stimulation (and consequent vasoconstriction) of α-receptors, which are located predominantly in resistance vessels of the skin, mucosa, intestine, and kidney. They **reduce pressure** by dilating resistance and conductance vessels.

a. **Prazosin [Minipress], terazosin [Hytrin], and doxazosin [Cardura]**

−are α_1-**selective antagonists.**

−are used in treating **hypertension,** especially in the presence of **CHF**.

−are often administered with a diuretic and a β-adrenoceptor antagonist.

−may produce initial orthostatic hypotension. Other adverse effects are minimal.

b. **Phentolamine [Regitine] and phenoxybenzamine [Dibenzyline]**

−antagonize α_1- and α_2-adrenoceptors.

−are used primarily in treating **hypertension** in the presence of **pheochromocytoma**.

3. Labetalol [Normodyne, Trandate]

−is an α- and β-adrenoceptor antagonist.

−reduces heart rate and contractility, slows AV conduction, and decreases peripheral resistance.

−is available for both oral and IV administration.

−is useful for treating hypertensive emergencies and in the treatment of **hypertension of pheochromocytoma**.

−does not cause reflex tachycardia.

E. ACE inhibitors

−reduce vascular resistance and blood volume; lower blood pressure by decreasing total peripheral resistance.

−include **captopril** [Capoten], **enalapril** [Vasotec], **lisinopril** [Prinivil, Zestril], and **ramipril** [Altace].

−are useful in treating **mild to severe hypertension**.

F. Calcium-channel blocking agents

−inhibit entry of calcium into cardiac and smooth muscle cells; lower blood pressure by reducing peripheral resistance.

−include **verapamil, nifedipine, nicardipine, isradipine** [DynaCirc], and **diltiazem**.

−are effective in the treatment of **mild to moderate hypertension**.

−when combined with a β-adrenoceptor antagonist, may lower blood pressure to a greater extent than when either class of drug is administered separately.

G. Other drugs

1. Centrally acting sympathomimetic agents

−reduce peripheral resistance, inhibit cardiac function, and increase pooling in capacitance venules.

a. Methyldopa [Aldomet]

−has active metabolite, α-**methylnorepinephrine,** a potent false neurotransmitter.

−activates presynaptic inhibitory α-adrenoceptors and postsynaptic α_2-receptors in the CNS and reduces sympathetic outflow. It decreases total peripheral resistance.

−reduces pressure in standing and supine positions.

−is used to treat **mild to moderate hypertension;** is often added to the regimen when a diuretic alone is not successful.

−produces adverse effects that include drowsiness, dry mouth, and gastrointestinal upset. Sexual dysfunction may occur and reduce compliance.

b. Clonidine [Catapres]

−stimulates postsynaptic α_2-adrenoceptors in the CNS and causes reduction in total peripheral resistance.

−is useful in treating **all degrees of hypertension;** is often added to the diuretic regimen.

−commonly produces drowsiness, dry mouth, and constipation.

−is available as a transdermal patch [Catapres-TTS] that allows weekly dosing.

c. Guanabenz acetate [Wytensin]

−activates central α-adrenoceptors and inhibits sympathetic outflow from the brain, which results in **reduced blood pressure**.

−is used in **mild to moderate hypertension,** most commonly in combination with a diuretic.

−most commonly produces **sedation** and **dry mouth** as adverse effects.

2. Adrenergic neuronal blocking drugs

a. Guanethidine monosulfate [Ismelin] and guanadrel sulfate [Hylorel]

−**deplete norepinephrine concentrations** to reduce norepinephrine release.

−reduce cardiac output and total peripheral vascular resistance.

−do not cross the blood–brain barrier. **Guanadrel** has a more rapid onset and a shorter duration of action than **guanethidine**.

−are used for patients with **severe refractory hypertension**.

−commonly produce **orthostatic and postexercise hypotension**. They may cause severe hypertension in patients with pheochromocytoma.

−may be reversed or blocked by drugs that prevent catecholamine reuptake (e.g., cocaine, tricyclic antidepressants).

b. Reserpine

–eliminates norepinephrine release in response to nerve impulse by preventing vesicular uptake. It depletes norepinephrine from sympathetic nerve terminals in the periphery and in the adrenal medulla.

–is used in **mild to moderate hypertension.**

–most commonly produces **gastrointestinal disturbances. Mental depression,** sometimes severe, may result, especially with high doses; is contraindicated in patients with a history of depression.

3. Agents that block catecholamine synthesis

a. Metyrosine (α-methyltyrosine) [Demser]

–**inhibits tyrosine hydroxylase** and thus prevents formation of dopa.

–is useful in the treatment of **pheochromocytoma-induced hypertension;** it is not useful in essential hypertension.

–most commonly produces **sedation.**

b. Pargyline

–is a **monoamine oxidase inhibitor** no longer in prevalent use because of **severe adverse effects.**

4. Trimethaphan [Arfonad]

–is a **ganglionic-blocking agent.**

–blocks postsynaptic action of acetylcholine at nicotinic receptors.

–is short-acting and is administered intravenously in **hypertensive crises,** especially for initial control in **acute dissecting aortic aneurysm.**

–may be used during surgery to decrease blood pressure to minimize blood loss.

5. Vasodilators

–**relax smooth muscle** and **lower total peripheral resistance,** thereby lowering blood pressure.

–**use is declining** as a result of newer modalities, such as ACE inhibitors and calcium-channel blocking agents, which are more effective with fewer adverse effects.

a. Hydralazine [Apresoline]

–reduces blood pressure directly by **relaxing arteriolar muscle.**

–**must be administered with a diuretic** to counteract sodium and water retention. Risk of tachycardia is reduced by administration with a β-adrenoceptor antagonist.

–is used to treat **chronic hypertension** and in **hypertensive crises** accompanying acute glomerular nephritis or eclampsia.

–may cause lupus-like syndrome.

b. Minoxidil [Loniten]

–reduces **total peripheral resistance.** Accompanying increase in heart rate and output and fluid retention is controlled by administration with a β-adrenoceptor antagonist and a diuretic.

–is useful for long-term therapy of **refractory hypertension.**

–produces **hirsutism,** an advantage in formulations that are now used to reverse male-pattern baldness.

c. Sodium nitroprusside [Nipride, Nitropress]

–dilates both resistance and capacitance vessels; increases heart rate but not output.

–is the preferred agent for use in **hypertensive emergencies** because of its rapid action. Continuous infusion is necessary to maintain effects.

–is usually administered with **furosemide**.

–on initial infusion, may cause excessive vasodilation and hypotension.

–can be converted to cyanide and thiocyanate. Accumulation of cyanide and risk of toxicity is minimized by concomitant administration of **sodium thiosulfate**.

d. Diazoxide [Hyperstat]

–is used intravenously to reduce blood pressure rapidly, usually in an emergency situation.

–is administered with **furosemide** to prevent fluid overload.

–is **declining in use** because of unpredictable action and adverse effects.

e. Tolazoline [Priscoline]

–is a direct-acting vasodilator that produces transient α-adrenoceptor blockade.

–is used to treat **persistent pulmonary hypertension of the newborn** if oxygen and mechanical ventilation do not relieve hypoxemia.

–most frequently produces hypotension as adverse effect and may require **dopamine** to counteract this action.

Review Test

Directions: Each of the numbered items or incomplete statements in this section is followed by answers or by completions of the statement. Select the **one** lettered answer or completion that is **best** in each case.

1. Potential adverse effects of furosemide treatment include which one of the following?

(A) Ototoxicity
(B) Hypokalemia
(C) Metabolic alkalosis
(D) Hypovolemia
(E) All of the above

2. Which one of the following drugs can be used to reduce ventricular preload?

(A) Norepinephrine
(B) Nitroglycerin
(C) Hydralazine
(D) Verapamil

3. Which one of the following agents binds to the aldosterone receptor?

(A) Propranolol
(B) Amiloride
(C) Furosemide
(D) Spironolactone
(E) Acetazolamide

4. Which of the following conditions can be treated successfully with osmotic diuretics?

(A) Hypercalcemia
(B) Congestive heart failure (CHF)
(C) Pulmonary edema
(D) Acute renal failure

5. Which one of the following drugs reduces renin secretion?

(A) Spironolactone
(B) Clonidine
(C) Captopril
(D) Allopurinol

6. Furosemide acts by which one of the following mechanisms?

(A) Inhibits reabsorption of NaCl in distal convoluted tubule
(B) Inhibits action of aldosterone
(C) Inhibits Na^+ absorption in the cortical collecting tubule
(D) Inhibits NaCl reabsorption in ascending loop of Henle

7. In the kidney, which one of the following is inhibited by thiazide diuretics?

(A) Sodium chloride reabsorption in the early part of the distal convoluted tubule
(B) Water removal from intracellular space by osmosis
(C) Reabsorption of Ca^{2+}
(D) Aldosterone action on the nephron
(E) Excretion of Cl^-

8. Which one of the following conditions is associated with digitalis toxicity?

(A) Tinnitus
(B) Pleural effusions
(C) Bradycardia
(D) Constipation

9. Digitalis increases myocardial contractility. Which of the following actions is associated with this effect?

(A) Activates adenylate cyclase
(B) Inactivates the Na^+ channel
(C) Activates the slow Ca^{2+} channel
(D) Inhibits Na^+,K^+-ATPase

10. Nitroglycerin is useful for the treatment of angina pectoris because of its ability to

(A) decrease intracellular Ca^{2+}
(B) block catecholamine release
(C) decrease ventricular preload and arterial afterload
(D) inhibit guanylate cyclase and resultant cyclic guanine nucleotides

11. Which of the following drugs is most likely to produce arrhythmias as an adverse effect?

(A) Quinidine
(B) Lidocaine
(C) Dobutamine
(D) Methyldopa

12. Which of the following drugs can induce a syndrome similar to systemic lupus erythematosus?

(A) Tocainide
(B) Hydralazine
(C) Quinidine
(D) Nifedipine
(E) Amrinone

13. Which of the following drugs can be used to suppress ventricular tachycardia?

(A) Digoxin
(B) Nitroprusside
(C) Atropine
(D) Lidocaine

14. Which of the following statements concerning calcium-channel blockers is correct?

(A) Can relax skeletal muscle
(B) Can increase cardiac automaticity
(C) Can decrease myocardial contractility
(D) Can be administered safely in the presence of hepatic disease

15. Which one of the following drugs may be useful in the management of pulmonary edema associated with acute left ventricular failure?

(A) Osmotic diuretic (mannitol)
(B) Vasopressin
(C) Ca^{2+}-channel blocker (verapamil)
(D) Loop diuretic (furosemide)

16. Which one of the following is the mechanism of action of lovastatin?

(A) Increase 7-α-hydroxylase activity
(B) Inhibit HMG-CoA reductase
(C) Increase lipoprotein lipase
(D) Inhibit hormone-sensitive lipase
(E) Increase lecithin–cholesterol acyltransferase

17. Which of the following agents will increase myocardial contractility with the least effect on total peripheral resistance?

(A) Epinephrine
(B) Phenylephrine
(C) Terbutaline
(D) Dobutamine
(E) Carbachol

18. Acetazolamide may be useful in treating which one of the following conditions?

(A) Congestive heart failure
(B) Cirrhosis of the liver
(C) Edema of pregnancy
(D) Glaucoma
(E) Hypertension

19. Probenecid inhibits which one of the following processes?

(A) Secretion of weak organic bases
(B) Secretion of weak organic acids
(C) Na^+ excretion
(D) Na^+ reabsorption
(E) Ca^{2+} reabsorption

20. Vasopressin can be useful in treating which one of the following conditions?

(A) Congestive heart failure
(B) Hypertension
(C) Some forms of diabetes insipidus
(D) Glaucoma

21. In some patients, metoprolol is preferred rather than propranolol because

(A) metoprolol's action on α-adrenoceptors adds to its hypotensive effects
(B) only metoprolol is active if given orally
(C) metoprolol is less likely to cause bronchoconstriction
(D) metoprolol is less likely to cause myocardial depression
(E) only metoprolol interferes with renin release

22. Severe psychological depression is most likely to occur as an adverse effect of which of the following drugs?

(A) Terbutaline
(B) Propranolol
(C) α-Methyldopa [Aldomet]
(D) Reserpine
(E) Guanethidine

23. Which of the following is a reasonable estimate of the $t_{1/2}$ of digoxin in a normal individual?

(A) 30 seconds
(B) 8 minutes
(C) 4 hours
(D) 1.5 days
(E) 3 weeks

24. Ventricular tachycardia associated with an acute myocardial infarction (MI) is best managed by intravenous administration of which of the following drugs?

(A) Dobutamine
(B) Digitalis
(C) Quinidine
(D) Lidocaine
(E) Atropine

25. Arrhythmias secondary to hyperthyroidism are best controlled with which of the following agents?

(A) Verapamil
(B) Propranolol
(C) Digitalis
(D) Bretylium
(E) Tocainide

26. Digitalis is a useful adjunct to quinidine in the treatment of atrial flutter. Digitalis can

(A) offset the negative inotropic effects of quinidine
(B) reduce preload
(C) induce peripheral vasodilation
(D) decrease conduction through the atrioventricular (AV) node
(E) increase the plasma concentration of quinidine

27. Nitroprusside toxicity is caused by which of the following actions?

(A) Conversion to thiocyanate
(B) Negative inotropic activity
(C) Precipitation in the skin
(D) Long half-life
(E) Lack of vasodilator activity

28. Which of the following conditions may be caused by a nonselective β-adrenoceptor antagonist?

(A) Sinus tachycardia
(B) Hyperglycemia
(C) Bronchospasm
(D) Hypertension
(E) Hyperthyroidism

29. Atropine is used to treat bradycardias because of its ability to

(A) block Ca^{2+} channels
(B) block muscarinic cholinergic receptors
(C) activate β-adrenergic receptors
(D) increase myocardial contractility
(E) dilate blood vessels

30. Nitroglycerin is given sublingually to

(A) decrease vasodilator side effects such as flushing and headache
(B) decrease renal excretion
(C) bypass the coronary circulation
(D) improve compliance
(E) avoid hepatic first-pass metabolism

31. Verapamil produces which one of the following effects?

(A) Decreased intracellular cAMP
(B) Decreased myocardial contractility
(C) Accelerated reactivation of the Na^+ channel
(D) Decreased intracellular K^+
(E) Increased conduction velocity

32. Digitalis increases myocardial contractility by which one of the following properties?

(A) Decreased vagal tone
(B) Increased the heart rate
(C) Decreased the conduction velocity
(D) Increased intracellular Ca^{2+}

33. Quinidine can increase conduction through the AV node by

(A) stimulating catecholamine release
(B) inhibiting phase 3 repolarization
(C) activating the Na^+ channel
(D) decreasing vagal tone
(E) increasing myocardial contractility

34. Which one of the following conditions is the most common manifestation of lidocaine toxicity?

(A) Arrhythmias
(B) CNS disturbances
(C) Drug fever
(D) Hypertension
(E) Hypokalemia

35. Digitalis is useful in the management of which one of the following conditions?

(A) Ventricular fibrillation
(B) Cardiac standstill
(C) Second-degree heart block
(D) Sick sinus syndrome
(E) Congestive heart failure

36. All of the following agents may be associated with hypokalemia EXCEPT

(A) hydrochlorothiazide
(B) furosemide
(C) amiloride
(D) indapamide

37. Renin secretion is increased by all of the following EXCEPT

(A) angiotensin II
(B) decreased Na^+ in kidney cortex
(C) decreased blood pressure
(D) increased sodium at the distal tubule
(E) stimulation of sympathetic activity

38. Chlorothiazide can be useful in the treatment of all of the following disorders EXCEPT

(A) hypertension
(B) congestive heart failure
(C) prevention of renal calcium stones
(D) hypokalemia
(E) edema

39. Guanethidine is associated with all of the following EXCEPT

(A) depletion of neuronal stores of norepinephrine
(B) treatment of moderate to severe hypertension
(C) significant postural hypotension
(D) crossing of the blood–brain barrier
(E) reduction in cardiac output

40. All of the following are signs and symptoms of digitalis toxicity EXCEPT

(A) anorexia and nausea
(B) generalized malaise
(C) cardiac arrhythmias
(D) drug fever
(E) disorientation and visual disturbances

41. All of the following drugs can be useful in controlling the ventricular response rate in atrial flutter or fibrillation EXCEPT

(A) procainamide
(B) verapamil
(C) propranolol
(D) lidocaine
(E) quinidine

42. Niacin administration is associated with all of the following EXCEPT

(A) inhibition of lipolysis
(B) treatment of pellagra
(C) decreased very-low density lipoprotein (VLDL) synthesis
(D) lowered blood pressure
(E) reduced plasma triglyceride and cholesterol

43. Administration of clofibrate leads to all of the following EXCEPT

(A) decreased circulating triglyceride levels
(B) decreased lipolysis
(C) displacement of warfarin bound to albumin
(D) increased lipoprotein lipase activity
(E) significantly reduced plasma cholesterol levels

44. Administration of cholestyramine leads to all of the following EXCEPT

(A) enhanced chylomicron production
(B) enhanced excretion of bile
(C) decreased circulating cholesterol
(D) enhanced receptor-mediated endocytosis of low-density lipoprotein (LDL)

Directions: Each group of items in this section consists of lettered options followed by a set of numbered items. For each item, select the **one** lettered option that is most closely associated with it. Each lettered option may be selected once, more than once, or not at all.

Questions 45–47

Match each of the drugs below with the most appropriate description of its mechanism of action

(A) An aminoglycoside antibiotic that inhibits absorption of bile acids
(B) Sequesters bile acids
(C) Increases activity of lipoprotein lipase
(D) Inhibitor of 3-hydroxy-3-methylglutaryl-coenzyme A reductase (HMG-CoA reductase)
(E) Inhibitor of xanthine oxidase

45. Lovastatin

46. Gemfibrozil

47. Cholestyramine

Questions 48–52

Match each of the drugs below with the most appropriate description of its mechanism of action.

(A) Blocks slow calcium channel indirectly by interacting with P_1 receptors
(B) β_1-Adrenoceptor antagonist
(C) Activates guanylate cyclase
(D) Inhibitor of Na^+,K^+-ATPase
(E) α-Adrenoceptor agonist

48. Clonidine

49. Adenosine

50. Digoxin

51. Esmolol

52. Isosorbide dinitrate

Answers and Explanations

1–E. Furosemide can produce hypovolemia, as well as hypokalemia due to enhanced K^+ secretion and alkalosis due to enhanced H^+ secretion. Ototoxicity is dose-related and occurs more commonly in individuals with renal impairment.

2–B. Vasodilators such as nitroglycerin decrease venous resistance. Net effect is reduced ventricular preload. Norepinephrine increases peripheral resistance and diastolic blood pressure. Hydralazine reduces blood pressure by relaxing arteriolar muscle. Calcium channel blockers such as verapamil decrease contractile force and decrease cardiac afterload.

3–D. Only spironolactone is a structural analog of aldosterone and binds to the mineralocorticoid receptor. Propranolol is a β-adrenoceptor antagonist. Amiloride, although also a potassium-sparing diuretic that acts at the collecting tubule, is not structurally related to aldosterone. Furosemide is a high-ceiling diuretic; acetazolamide is a carbonic anhydrase inhibitor.

4–D. Osmotic diuretics are used chiefly in preventing acute renal failure. They may increase extracellular volume and are contraindicated in CHF and pulmonary edema.

5–B. Sympathetic stimulation elevates renin release. Thus, drugs such as clonidine that inhibit sympathetic activity will reduce renin release.

6–D. High-ceiling diuretics such as furosemide and ethacrynic acid reduce NaCl reabsorption in the loop of Henle. Thiazide diuretics reduce NaCl reabsorption in the early distal part of the nephron. Aldosterone analogs interfere with aldosterone action. Amiloride and triamterene act, independent of mineralocorticoids, to reduce Na^+ absorption in the collecting tubule.

7–A. Thiazide diuretics inhibit NaCl reabsorption in the distal convoluted tubule. Although thiazide diuretics reduce intracellular water, the reduction is linked to the increased excretion of Na^+ (and Cl^-) rather than osmosis. Thiazide diuretics increase the absorption of Ca^{2+}. They do not affect aldosterone action.

8–C. Digitalis has a narrow therapeutic index and can induce nearly every type of arrhythmia. It is associated with gastrointestinal disturbances that include diarrhea.

9–D. Digitalis and other cardiac glycosides inhibit Na^+,K^+-ATPase. Effects on Ca^{2+} are either indirect or by activation of Ca^{2+} entry.

10–C. Vasodilation by nitroglycerin affects both venous and arterial vascular beds. Nitroglycerin does not inhibit catecholamine release. Activation of guanylate cyclase imitates the cascade of events that leads to relaxation of vascular smooth muscle.

11–A. Quinidine can cause ventricular arrhythmias, quinidine syncope (as a result of ventricular tachycardia), and prolonged Q–T interval. Lidocaine and dobutamine (at moderate doses) have a very low level of cardiotoxicity. Methyldopa reduces sympathetic outflow and peripheral resistance.

12–B. Because of their tendency to produce adverse effects such as the production of antihydralazine antibodies (which manifest as a lupus-like syndrome) on chronic use, use of many classic vasodilators is diminishing.

13–D. Lidocaine is useful as a treatment for ventricular tachycardia. Digoxin, an inotropic agent, and nitroprusside, a vasodilator, are useful in treating CHF. Atropine, which blocks the effects of acetylcholine to elevate sinus rate and conduction velocity, can be useful in treating bradyarrhythmias.

14–C. Calcium-channel blockade is effective on the slow calcium channel of the heart. These agents (e.g., verapamil) produce negative inotropic effects and are peripheral vasodilators. Hepatic disease decreases drug metabolism and may result in toxic levels.

15–D. Loop diuretics treat CHF by reducing acute pulmonary edema. Osmotic diuretics are contraindicated in CHF. Vasopressin acts to conserve body water. Negative inotropic effects of calcium channel–blocking agents render them unsuitable for treating this disease.

16–B. Lovastatin inhibits cholesterol biosynthesis by inhibiting 3-hydroxy-3-methylglutaryl-coenzyme A reductase (HMG-CoA reductase).

17–D. Dobutamine increases myocardial contractility, but has little effect on total peripheral resistance. Epinephrine and terbutaline decrease peripheral resistance by activating β_2-adrenoceptors in the vascular bed of skeletal muscle. Phenylephrine activates α-adrenoceptors, which results in increased peripheral resistance. Carbachol activates muscarinic cholinoceptors in vascular smooth muscle resulting in vasodilation.

18–D. Acetazolamide is a carbonic anhydrase inhibitor. This enzyme is present in most tissues in huge excess. In the eye, this enzyme produces high concentrations of bicarbonate in the aqueous humor. Inhibition of carbonic anhydrase reduces the rate of aqueous humor formation, with a resultant decrease in intraocular pressure.

19–B. Probenecid was developed to inhibit the secretion of the weak organic acid penicillin, which, when first discovered, was in extremely short supply.

20–C. Vasopressin is "antidiuretic" and therefore would not be useful in treating CHF, hypertension, or glaucoma. It has use in treating ADH-sensitive diabetes insipidus.

21–C. Metoprolol is a selective β_1-receptor antagonist that is less likely to produce bronchospasm than the nonselective agent propranolol.

22–D. Although minor depression may occur as a result of administration of some of the other drugs, such as propranolol, mental depression can be quite severe with reserpine; the drug is contraindicated in individuals with a history of depression.

23–D. The long half-life of digoxin contributes to a delay in reaching steady state, which, in the absence of a loading dose, may take up to 1 week to attain. Use of a relatively large loading dose promotes earlier attainment of therapeutic levels.

24–D. Lidocaine is the best agent for management of ventricular tachycardia associated with acute MI. Dobutamine, digitalis, quinidine, and atropine can all induce tachyarrhythmias. Lidocaine does not slow conduction and has little effect on atrial function.

25–B. Hyperthyroidism apparently increases β-adrenoceptors. β-adrenoceptor antagonists such as propranolol can actually decrease symptoms of hyperthyroidism.

26–D. Quinidine acts to prolong refractoriness and slow conduction rather than as a negative inotropic agent. The ability of digitalis to decrease conduction through the AV node makes its effects compatible with quinidine to reduce atrial flutter. Digitalis does not produce vasodilation or affect the plasma concentration of quinidine.

27–A. Cyanide accumulation can be minimized by administration of sodium thiosulfate, which is a limiting factor in the metabolism of cyanide.

28–C. Due to the presence of β_2-adrenoceptors in bronchial smooth muscle, nonselective β-adrenoceptor antagonists (e.g., propranolol) can lead to life-threatening bronchoconstriction in patients with asthma or obstructive pulmonary disease.

29–B. Atropine produces cholinergic blockade at the sinoatrial node, thus increasing heart rate.

30–E. Nitrates undergo large first-pass metabolism due to high-capacity organic nitrate reductase in the liver. The sublingual route is preferred for rapid delivery of nitroglycerin.

31–B. Calcium channel–blocking agents such as verapamil decrease contractile force and slow conduction through the AV node. They do not interact with Na^+ channels or alter intracellular K^+.

32–D. Inhibition of Na^+,K^+-ATPase by digitalis reduces normal exchange of intracellular Ca^{2+} for extracellular Na^+, resulting in an increased Ca^{2+} concentration within the cell.

33–D. Quinidine depresses all muscles, leading to a decrease in vagal tone and sometimes skeletal weakness, especially in individuals with myasthenia gravis. Quinidine has no effect on catecholamine release, on the Na^+ channel, or on contractility. It reduces the rate of phase 0 and phase 4 depolarization, rather than phase 3 repolarization.

34–B. Although lidocaine has few cardiotoxic effects, it often results in CNS disturbances, such as drowsiness or hallucinations, in the therapeutic range.

35–E. Due to its ability to increase cardiac contractility, digitalis is a principal drug in the treatment of CHF. It is also useful for certain arrhythmias, including atrial fibrillation and flutter, but would not be useful for ventricular fibrillation because it reduces preload.

36–C. Amiloride is a potassium-sparing diuretic and interferes with K^+ secretion in the collecting tubule. It is associated with hyperkalemia.

37–A. Renin releases angiotensin I, which is converted enzymatically to angiotensin II and angiotensin III. Angiotensin II controls release of aldosterone.

38–D. One of the major side effects of thiazide diuretics is loss of K^+; they are inappropriate treatment for hypokalemia.

39–D. Guanethidine acts only on the periphery and does not cross the blood–brain barrier.

40–D. Digitalis can cause anorexia, nausea, generalized malaise, cardiac arrhythmias, disorientation, and visual disturbances. It does not cause drug fever.

41–D. Lidocaine does not slow conduction and has little effect on atrial function.

42–D. Niacin does not reduce blood pressure.

43–B. Clofibrate activates lipoprotein lipase, thus increasing lipolysis. It has little effect on plasma cholesterol.

44–A. Cholestyramine is a bile acid sequestrant; it does not enhance chylomicron production.

45–D. Lovastatin is a cholesterol biosynthesis inhibitor that acts by inhibiting HMG-CoA reductase.

46–C. Gemfibrozil is a clofibrate analog that acts to decrease plasma concentration of VLDL cholesterol by increasing the activity of lipoprotein lipase.

47–B. Cholestyramine is a bile acid sequestrant that acts in the intestine, exchanging chloride for bile salts and preventing enterohepatic reutilization of bile acids.

48–E. Clonidine activates α_2-receptors, reduces sympathetic tone, and lowers blood pressure by decreasing peripheral resistance.

49–A. Adenosine indirectly inhibits calcium channel flux by acting at specific adenosine, or purinergic (P_1), receptors.

50–D. Cardiac glycosides such as digoxin inhibit Na^+,K^+-ATPase, resulting in increased intracellular Na^+ and decreased intracellular K^+.

51–B. Esmolol is a β_1-specific adrenoceptor antagonist.

52–C. Isosorbide is a nitrate that activates guanylate cyclase and produces vasodilation.

4

Drugs Acting on the Central Nervous System

I. Sedative–Hypnotic Drugs

A. Definitions

1. Sedation is characterized by decreased anxiety, motor activity, and mental acuity.

2. Hypnosis is characterized by an increased tendency to sleep.

B. Benzodiazepines

—are the drugs of choice to treat **anxiety** (**sedative action**) and **insomnia** (**hypnotic action**) because of their great margin of safety. Other available nonbenzodiazepine sedative–hypnotic agents produce a dose-dependent continuum of central nervous system (CNS) depression, leading ultimately to coma and death.

—have similar therapeutic actions. However, some benzodiazepines are marketed for specific therapeutic purposes.

—are classified according to their elimination half-life. Therapeutic use is dictated on the basis of relative lipid solubility, biotransformation, and elimination half-life.

1. Structure and mechanism of action

—are heterocyclic 1,4-benzodiazepines with an electronegative group at position 7 of the benzene ring (halogen, nitro) and a phenyl ring substitution at position 5 (Figure 4.1).

—facilitate γ-aminobutyric acid (GABA)-mediated inhibition of neuronal activity, particularly in the limbic and cortical areas of the CNS. They bind to a benzodiazepine receptor (α subunit) that is part of, but distinct from, the GABA$_A$ receptor–chloride channel complex ($\alpha_2\,\beta_2$ heterotetramic channel).

—allosterically increase GABA affinity and the frequency of GABA-stimulated chloride channel opening, chloride conductance, and neuronal hyperpolarization; also prevent depolarization by excitatory neurotransmission. **Buspirone** [Buspar], a nonbenzodiazepine, second-generation anxiolytic, is a serotonin ($5HT_{1A}$)-receptor antagonist.

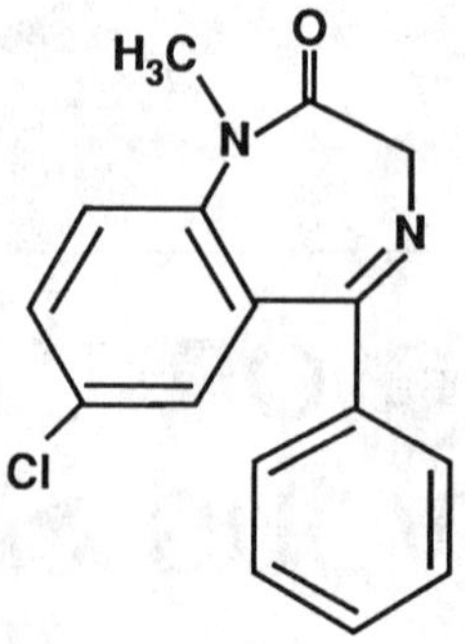

Figure 4.1. Structure of diazepam.

—can be antagonized by certain β-carbolines, some of which may be endogenous. When administered without benzodiazepines, these "inverse agonists" cause anxiety and can induce seizures.

2. **Pharmacologic properties** (Table 4.1)

    a. Generally, benzodiazepines are administered orally to treat anxiety and sleep disorders. **Chlordiazepoxide, diazepam,** and **lorazepam** can be given intramuscularly (deltoid). After oral administration, plasma concentrations peak in 1–4 hours.

    b. Benzodiazepines are extensively bound to plasma proteins (no reported clinical interactions).

Table 4.1. Benzodiazepine Indications

Drug and Half-life	Primary Indications
Short-acting ($t_{1/2} < 5$ hr)	
Midazolam [Versed]	Preanesthetic
Triazolam [Halcion]	Hypnotic, preanesthetic
Intermediate-acting ($t_{1/2}$ 5–24 hr)	
Alprazolam [Xanax]	Anxiolytic, antidepressant*
Clonazepam [Klonopin]	Anticonvulsant
Estazolam [ProSom]	Hypnotic
Lorazepam [Ativan]	Anxiolytic, hypnotic, preanesthetic
Oxazepam [Serax]	Anxiolytic
Temazepam [Restoril]	Hypnotic
Long-lasting ($t_{1/2} > 24$ hr)	
Chlordiazepoxide [Librium][†]	Anxiolytic, preanesthetic
Clorazepate [Tranxene][†‡]	Anxiolytic
Diazepam [Valium][†]	Anxiolytic, preanesthetic, anticonvulsant
Flurazepam [Dalmane]	Hypnotic
Halazepam [Paxipam][†]	Anxiolytic
Prazepam [Centrax][†‡]	Anxiolytic
Quazepam [Doral]	Hypnotic

*For panic disorders.
[†]Converted to the long-acting, active metabolite.
[‡]Pro-drug.

c. Onset of action after a single dose is related to the degree of lipid solubility (e.g., **diazepam** and **clorazepate** actions occur in 30–60 minutes).

d. Duration of action after a single dose is also related to the relative degree of lipid solubility and, for some, biotransformation to active metabolites. Active metabolites, particularly **desmethyldiazepam,** result from acid hydrolysis in the stomach (as with **clorazepate**) or hepatic microsomal oxidation (*N*-dealkylation, aliphatic hydroxylation) and extend the half-life ($t_{1/2}$) of some benzodiazepines to as long as 140 hours. Benzodiazepines with long half-lives are more likely to cause cumulative and residual effects.

e. Redistribution from the brain to peripheral tissues is an important factor in terminating the actions of the most highly soluble benzodiazepines (**midazolam** > **flurazepam** > **diazepam** and **desmethyldiazepam** > other benzodiazepines).

f. Biotransformation (ring hydroxylation and glucuronidation) to inactive metabolites is the most important factor for terminating the actions of less lipid-soluble benzodiazepines. These are excreted by the kidney.

g. Clearance of benzodiazepines is decreased in the elderly and in patients with liver disease. In these patients, doses should be reduced. Also, **lorazepam** and **oxazepam** may be used in these patients because these agents are inactivated only by glucuronidation.

h. With **chronic therapy,** the rate and extent of accumulation of benzodiazepines and metabolites or their disappearance after discontinuing administration is directly related to elimination half-life and clearance.

3. Therapeutic uses (see Table 4.1)

a. Generalized anxiety disorders are characterized by severe apprehension, tension, and uneasiness that disrupt normal function.
  (1) Buspirone relieves anxiety without the sedation, hypnosis, or general CNS depression or drug abuse liability of the benzodiazepines.
  (2) It may be the drug of choice for treating **chronic anxiety,** particularly in the elderly, who are more susceptible to the CNS depressant action of benzodiazepines.

b. Situational anxiety (e.g., frightening medical or dental procedures)

c. Panic disorders and agoraphobia; alprazolam is the benzodiazepine of choice.

d. Insomnia is characterized by difficulty in falling or staying asleep or inadequate duration of sleep.
  (1) Triazolam is used to initiate sleep because of its rapid onset and ability to decrease sleep latency.
  (2) Flurazepam and **temazepam,** which have longer durations of action, are used to sustain sleep.

e. Seizures
  (1) Diazepam, given by intravenous (IV) infusion, is preferred for status epilepticus and drug- or toxin-induced seizures. **Lorazepam,**

which is longer acting, is an alternative to diazepam and is the drug of choice in the pediatric population because it does not undergo biotransformation.

(2) **Clonazepam** and **clorazepate** are used as adjuncts for absence, myoclonic, and atonic seizures.

f. Preanesthetic medication

(1) Shorter-acting benzodiazepines are preferred for their anxiolytic, sedative, and amnestic actions prior to surgery, endoscopy, or bronchoscopy. They do not produce full surgical anesthesia.

(2) **Midazolam,** a water-soluble, rapidly acting benzodiazepine, is less irritating than other benzodiazepines given by IV route for anesthetic induction.

g. Muscle relaxation; diazepam is used to treat spontaneous muscle spasms, spasms associated with endoscopy, and spasticity of cerebral palsy.

h. Withdrawal from CNS depressants; long-acting benzodiazepines such as diazepam are used to treat or prevent the withdrawal syndrome of physical dependence associated with shorter-acting benzodiazepines and other sedative–hypnotic drugs, including alcohol and barbiturates.

4. Adverse effects and contraindications

−commonly produce **daytime drowsiness** and **ataxia** that may impair judgment and interfere with motor skills. These effects are more likely with long-acting benzodiazepines.

−may cause **rebound insomnia** on discontinuation.

−**accumulate in fetus** during the first trimester of pregnancy.

−infrequently cause confusion in the elderly, blurred vision, hypotension, tremor, constipation, and anterograde amnesia.

−cause rare paradoxical excitement.

−enhance **CNS depression** when taken in **combination** with other **drugs** that depress the CNS, most notably **alcohol**.

5. Tolerance and dependence

a. Tolerance develops to sedative–hypnotic action of benzodiazepines but not to anxiolytic action. Exhibit cross-tolerance with other sedative–hypnotic agents, including **alcohol**.

b. Abuse potential is low compared to other classes of sedative–hypnotic drugs; abuse is more frequent in patients with a history of substance abuse.

c. Signs of withdrawal after chronic benzodiazepine use may include **anxiety, insomnia, gastrointestinal disturbances, headache,** and **tremor**. Perceptual distortions, delusions, and seizures also have been reported. Withdrawal occurs sooner and is more severe after abruptly discontinuing shorter-acting benzodiazepines; doses should be tapered.

d. Cross-dependence with other sedative–hypnotic agents, including **barbiturates** and **alcohol,** has been noted.

e. Buspirone has negligible abuse, dependence, or CNS depression potential and has no cross-tolerance or cross-dependence with other CNS depressants.

C. Other sedative–hypnotics

—with few exceptions, have been supplanted by benzodiazepines for treatment of anxiety and sleep disorders.

1. Barbiturates

—include **amobarbital** [Amytal], **pentobarbital** [Nembutal], and **secobarbital** [Seconal] (see also section X).

—interact with the binding site on the **GABA-receptor–chloride channel complex** that is separate from the benzodiazepine receptor.

—at low doses, allosterically prolong GABA-induced opening of chloride channels and enhance GABA-inhibitory neurotransmission; at higher doses, have GABA-mimetic activity (open chloride channel independently of GABA).

—are limited for use by strong sedation, rapid tolerance, drug interactions, abuse potential, and lethality in overdose.

2. Meprobamate [Equanil, Miltown, Meprospan]

—is marketed as an **anxiolytic** but has strong **sedative** properties.

—has effects similar to those of barbiturates, including withdrawal syndrome.

3. Chloral hydrate

—acts by a mechanism thought to be similar to that of **ethanol**.

—has a **rapid onset** and short duration of action. Is rapidly metabolized (reduced) in the liver to its active form, **trichloroethanol,** which is extensively bound to plasma proteins and may displace other drugs, including **phenytoin** and anticoagulants, and potentiate their action.

—is used to treat **insomnia,** particularly in children, the elderly, and institutionalized patients.

—is less likely to cause paradoxical excitement than benzodiazepines. May cause gastrointestinal disturbances; **chloral hydrate** has an unpleasant taste and odor that can be masked.

—tolerance develops to hypnotic action.

—is contraindicated in patients with renal or hepatic impairment, cardiac disease, or gastritis.

II. Antipsychotic Drugs

—demonstrate no therapeutic differences between classes. They are selected for use primarily on the basis of associated adverse effects.

—for the most part, show little correlation between plasma levels and therapeutic action. Plasma levels are monitored primarily for compliance.

—in most cases, are highly lipophilic and highly bound to plasma proteins with **long half-lives** (10–20 hours). They are metabolized by liver microsomal oxidation and conjugation.

A. Chemical structure and classification (Table 4.2)

—are often classified according to their oral milligram potency. High-potency drugs (piperazine phenothiazines or thioxanthenes and **haloperidol**) are more likely to produce acute extrapyramidal reactions. Low-potency drugs (aliphatic phenothiazines or thioxanthenes and piperidine phenothiazines) are more likely to produce sedation and hypotension.

Table 4.2. Classification, Potency, and Adverse Effects of Antipsychotic Drugs

Drug and Classification	Oral Dosage Range (mg/day)	Extrapyramidal Effects*	Autonomic Effects	Sedation
Aliphatic phenothiazines				
Chlorpromazine [Thorazine, generic]	100–1000	+ +	+ + +	+ + +
Triflupromazine [Vesprin]	50–150	+ +	+ + +	+ + +
Piperidine phenothiazines				
Thioridazine [Mellaril, generic][†]	100–800	+	+ + +	+ + +
Mesoridazine [Serentil][†]	50–400	+	+ + +	+ + +
Piperazine phenothiazines				
Trifluoperazine [Stelazine, generic]	10–60	+ + +	+ +	+ +
Fluphenazine [Prolixin, Permitil][‡]	5–20	+ + + +	+ +	+ +
Perphenazine [Trilafon]	16–64	+ + +	+ +	+ +
Acetophenazine [Tindal]	80–120	+ + +	+	+ +
Aliphatic thioxanthene				
Chlorprothixene [Taractan]	100–600	+ +	+ + +	+ + +
Piperazine thioxanthene				
Thiothixene [Navane, generic]	2–120	+ + +	+ +	+ +
Butyrophenone				
Haloperidol [Haldol, generic]	2–20	+ + + +	+	+
Other heterocyclic drugs				
Molindone [Moban][†]	20–200	+ + +	+ +	+ +
Loxapine [Loxitane]	20–250	+ + +	+ +	+ +
Clozapine [Clozaril][†**]	25–400	+	+ + +	+ + +

*Excluding tardive dyskinesia.
[†]No antiemetic action.
[‡]Esterification (enanthate or decanoate) results in depot form.
**Agranulocytosis in up to 3% of patients.

1. Phenothiazines and thioxanthenes

—are classified chemically according to the structure of their carbon side-chains (R_1 = aliphatic, piperidine, piperazine), which consist of a tertiary amine nitrogen separated from the phenothiazine or thioxanthene nucleus by three carbon atoms (Figure 4.2).

2. Butyrophenones

—include **haloperidol,** the only butyrophenone approved for use as an antipsychotic drug.

3. Other heterocyclic drugs

—include **clozapine,** which may be useful for treatment-resistant patients.

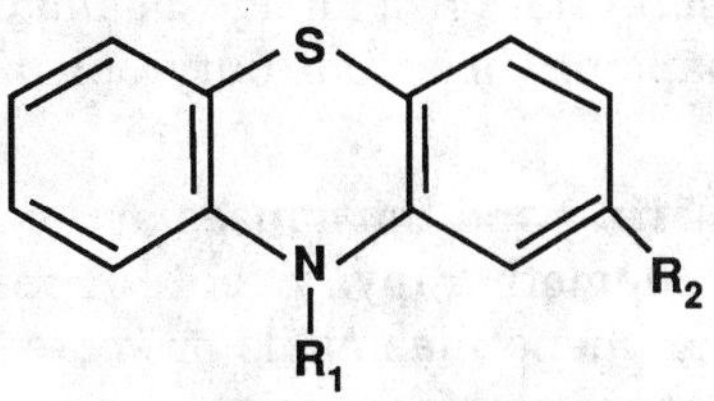

Phenothiazine nucleus

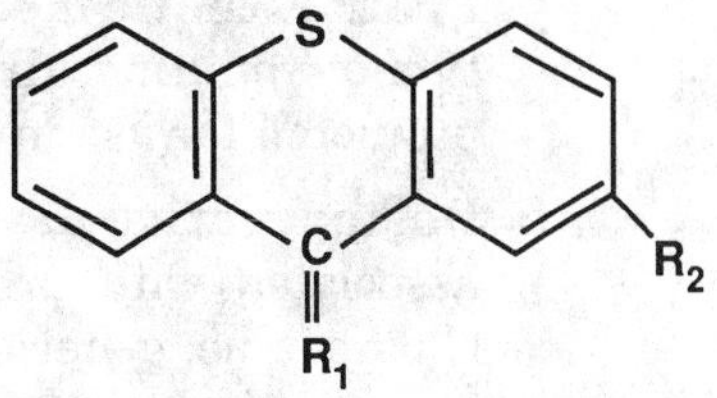

Thioxanthene nucleus

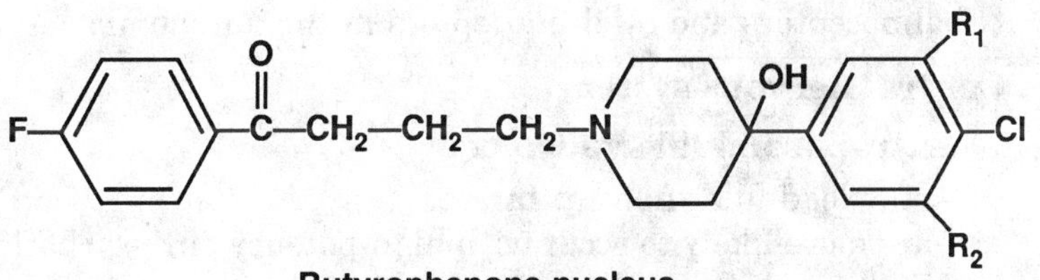

Butyrophenone nucleus

Figure 4.2. Structures of phenothiazine, thioxanthene, and butyrophenone nuclei in antipsychotic drugs.

B. Mechanism of action

- –is correlated best with antagonist activity at postjunctional dopamine (D_2)-receptors where activation results in inhibition of adenylate cyclase activity. Antipsychotic drugs are also antagonists at prejunctional dopamine (D_2)-receptors, where activation inhibits dopamine release. Antagonist actions at other recently discovered dopamine receptor subtypes (D_3–D_5) may also be relevant to therapeutic action.
- –inhibit dopamine neurotransmission in the mesolimbic and mesocortical areas of the CNS.

C. Therapeutic uses

1. Schizophrenia

- –produce immediate quieting action with decreased symptoms of thought disorders, paranoid features, delusions, hostility, and hallucinations (positive symptoms).
- –have less effect on negative symptoms (withdrawal, apathy, and blunted affect).
- –curb acute psychotic attacks and delay subsequent relapses. Antipsychotic effects typically take several weeks or longer to occur.

2. Other therapeutic uses

a. Acute **mania**

b. **Atypical psychotic disorders** (e.g., following surgery or myocardial infarction)

c. **Tourette's syndrome,** which is treated by **haloperidol or pimozide** [Orap]

d. **Ballismus,** which is treated by **haloperidol**

e. **Huntington's disease**

f. Intractable **hiccups** or **vomiting**

g. **Preanesthetic medication** for potentiation of analgesia and prevention of vomiting; **droperidol** [Inapsine], a potent butyrophenone, is promoted for use in anesthesia.

h. **Postoperative nausea** and **vomiting** and the nausea and vomiting associated with pregnancy and chemotherapy; **prochlorperazine** [Compazine, generic], a piperazine phenothiazine, is promoted solely as an antiemetic agent. **Droperidol** is also used as an antiemetic.

D. **Adverse effects and contraindications** (see Table 4.2)

—are associated with antagonist activity at dopamine receptors, histamine receptors, and serotonin receptors in the CNS, and with antagonist action at cholinoceptors and α-adrenoceptors in the autonomic nervous system.

1. **Central nervous system**

a. **Extrapyramidal syndromes**

—may lead to **noncompliance**.

—are more likely to occur with high-potency antipsychotic drugs; least likely with **thioridazine** and **clozapine**.

—can sometimes spontaneously remit.

—can be controlled by **anticholinergic drugs** (e.g., **benztropine, biperiden**) or by reducing the antipsychotic drug dose.

(1) **Acute dystonia,** facial grimacing and torticollis, often elicited immediately or soon after beginning drug therapy.

(2) **Akathisia** (feeling of stress, compulsion to be in motion); generally develops during first 2 weeks of treatment and is often confused with an increase in psychotic tension.

(3) **Parkinsonian-like syndrome** (tremor, rigidity, bradykinesia); may develop within weeks to months after drug treatment due to dopamine–receptor antagonist activity in the nigrostriatal pathway.

b. **Tardive dyskinesia**

—is primarily **orofacial choreiform movements (tics)** but occasionally includes the trunk.

—may be the result of a developing **supersensitivity of postjunctional dopamine receptors** in the striatum.

—generally occurs after **months to years of drug exposure;** may be precipitated or exacerbated by discontinuation of therapy.

—is induced by all antipsychotic drugs except clozapine and is **often irreversible**.

—has an estimated incidence of 10%–20%. More likely to occur in elderly or institutionalized patients who receive chronic, high-dose therapy.

—is predisposed by prophylactic use of anticholinergic drugs.

c. **Toxic-confusional state**

—is more likely with low-potency drugs.

d. **Sedation**

—may be mild to severe. Tolerance to the effect is likely to develop.

e. **Seizures**

—lower seizure threshold; may precipitate or unmask epilepsy.

f. Neuroleptic malignant syndrome

–is characterized by autonomic instability, muscle rigidity, diaphoresis, and profound hyperthermia.

–occurs in 1% of patients, but is associated with a 5%–20% mortality rate.

–is more common with high-potency antipsychotic drugs.

–is **treated** by **discontinuing drug therapy** and initiating **supportive measures: Bromocriptine** to overcome dopamine-receptor blockade and **dantrolene** to reduce muscle rigidity.

2. Autonomic nervous system

a. α-Adrenoceptor blockade

–causes **orthostatic hypotension,** as a result of peripheral vasodilation; central depression of the vasomotor center may also contribute. May be severe and may result in reflex tachycardia. Elderly patients and those with heart disease are more at risk. Tolerance to this effect may develop.

–causes **impotence** and inhibition of ejaculation (10% of patients).

b. Muscarinic–cholinoceptor blockade

–produces an atropine-like effect resulting in **dry mouth** and **blurred vision**.

–may also produce constipation, tachycardia, and difficulty in urination leading to urine retention.

–more rarely causes paralytic ileus and severe bladder infections.

–**elderly patients** are more at **risk,** and tolerance to these effects may develop.

3. Endocrine and metabolic disturbances

–are generally **transient**.

–include the following, which are due to dopamine (D_2)-receptor antagonist activity in the pituitary, which results in hyperprolactinemia, and other neuroendocrine reactions: in **women—spontaneous or induced galactorrhea, loss of libido, delayed ovulation and menstruation,** or **amenorrhea; in men—gynecomastia, impotence,** and **persistent priapism. Clozapine** causes little elevation in prolactin levels.

–also produce **edema and weight gain,** which are thought to be due to histamine– or serotonin–receptor antagonist activity.

4. Rare idiosyncratic effects

a. Withdrawal-like syndrome

–is characterized by **nausea, vomiting, insomnia,** and **headache** in 30% of patients, especially those receiving low-potency antipsychotics.

–is possibly due to prolonged cholinoceptor blockade.

–may persist for up to 2 weeks.

–symptoms can be reduced with **tapering of drug dosage**.

b. Cardiac arrhythmias

–result from a quinidine-like effect; local anesthetic activity with an increased likelihood of heart block.

–are more common with low-potency antipsychotics.

–are often due to **overdose**. Also may lead to conduction block and sudden death.

c. Blood dyscrasias

–are **rare**. **Clozapine** may induce **agranulocytosis** in up to 3% of patients and is used only when other drug classes have been shown to be ineffective.

d. Cholestatic jaundice

–is caused primarily by **chlorpromazine**.

e. Photosensitivity

–is specific to **chlorpromazine;** includes dermatitis (5%) and rash, sunburn, and pigmentation and may be irreversible. **Chlorpromazine** and high-dose **thioridazine** also produce **retinitis pigmentosa**.

E. Overdose

–is rarely fatal except when caused by **thioridazine** or **mesoridazine,** which may result in drowsiness, agitation, coma, ventricular arrhythmias, heart block, or sudden death.

F. Drug interactions

–CNS depressants (e.g., sedative–hypnotics, opioids, antihistamines) potentiate sedative effects.

–inhibit **levodopa** effectiveness (reduce dopamine interaction with dopamine receptors in the CNS) in Parkinson's disease.

–produce additive anticholinergic effects with tricyclic antidepressants, antiparkinsonian drugs, and other drugs with anticholinergic activity.

–block uptake of **guanethidine** into sympathetic nerve endings and decrease antihypertensive activity.

–block α-receptors and reduce antihypertensive action of **clonidine** and **α-methyldopa**.

III. Antidepressant Agents

–have no therapeutic differences between classes (i.e., tricyclic antidepressants, the newer second-generation antidepressants, or monoamine oxidase [MAO] inhibitors).

–are selected for use primarily on the basis of associated adverse effects.

–may take several weeks to demonstrate therapeutic responses.

A. Chemical structure and classification (Table 4.3)

1. **Tricyclic antidepressants** are three-ring structures resembling the phenothiazine antipsychotics, with either a secondary or tertiary amine side-chain (Figure 4.3).

2. Newer **second-generation antidepressants** often have unconventional ring structures.

3. **MAO inhibitors** are classified as hydrazides or nonhydrazides.

a. **Phenelzine** [Nardil] and **isocarboxazid** [Marplan] are hydrazides that irreversibly inhibit MAO. These drugs are used infrequently because of their hepatotoxicity.

Table 4.3. Relative Biochemical Activity of Antidepressant Drugs

Drug and Classification	Inhibition of Norepinephrine Reuptake	Inhibition of Serotonin Reuptake	Antimuscarinic Activity	Antiadrenergic Activity	Antihistamine Activity
Tricyclic Antidepressants					
Tertiary amines					
Amitriptyline [Elavil, others]	+	+++	++++	+++	++++
Imipramine [Tofranil, others]	+	+	++	++	+
Trimipramine [Surmontil]	+		++	++	+++
Doxepin [Sinequan, others]	++	+	++	++	+++
Clomipramine [Anafranil]	+	+++	++	+	+
Secondary amines					
Desipramine [Norpramin, Pertofrane, generic]	++		+	+	
Nortriptyline [Aventyl, Pamelor]	+++	+/-	++	++	+
Protriptyline [Vivactil]	+++	+/-	++	+	
Newer Cyclic Antidepressants					
Dibenzoxazepine					
Amoxapine [Asendin]*	++			+	+/-
Tetracyclic					
Maprotiline [Ludiomil]	++		+	+	++
Bicyclic					
Fluoxetine [Prozac]		+++			
Triazolopyridine					
Trazodone [Desyrel, generic]	+	+		+	+/-

*Some dopamine-receptor antagonist activity.

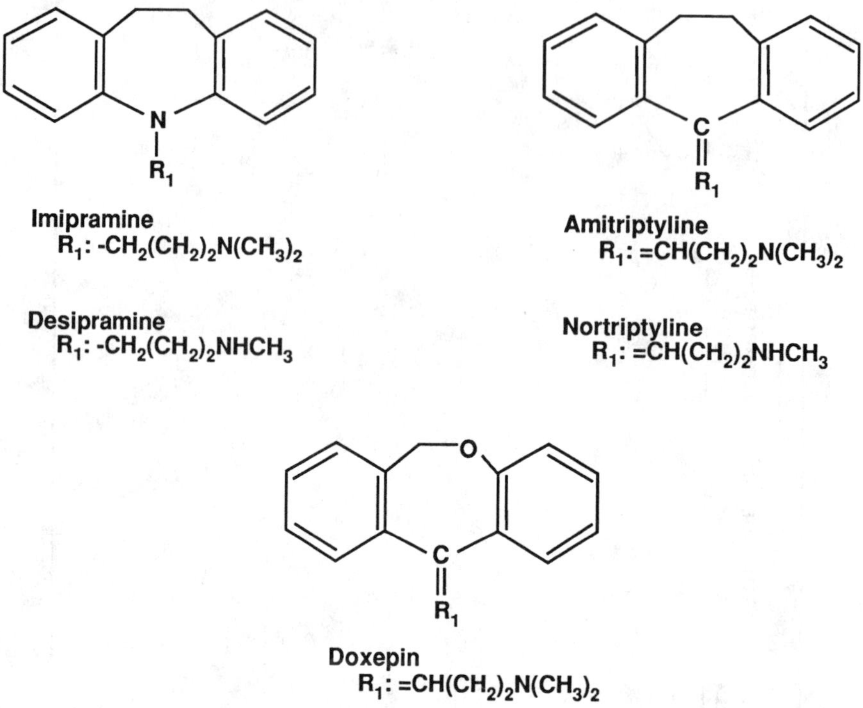

Imipramine
R_1: -CH$_2$(CH$_2$)$_2$N(CH$_3$)$_2$

Amitriptyline
R_1: =CH(CH$_2$)$_2$N(CH$_3$)$_2$

Desipramine
R_1: -CH$_2$(CH$_2$)$_2$NHCH$_3$

Nortriptyline
R_1: =CH(CH$_2$)$_2$NHCH$_3$

Doxepin
R_1: =CH(CH$_2$)$_2$N(CH$_3$)$_2$

Figure 4.3. Structures of selected tricyclic antidepressants.

   b. Tranylcypromine [Parnate] is a nonhydrazide structurally similar to dextroamphetamine and is a reversible but long-lasting MAO inhibitor.

B. Mechanism of action (see Table 4.3)

   1. According to the **biogenic amine hypothesis** of depression, endogenous unipolar depression is correlated with **decreased levels** and **activity** of **norepinephrine** or **serotonin** (5-hydroxytryptamine, or 5HT) in the CNS.

     a. Most **tricyclic antidepressants and second-generation antidepressants** restore the effective endogenous activity of norepinephrine or serotonin by acutely reducing their active reuptake into prejunctional nerve endings.

     b. MAO inhibitors inhibit the activity of the **enzymes MAO-A** and **MAO-B,** which degrade biogenic amines, and thereby increase CNS levels of norepinephrine and serotonin.

   2. Chronic antidepressant therapy is associated with the down-regulation of postjunctional β-adrenoreceptors, 5HT-receptors, cyclic AMP (cAMP) levels, and a concomitant decreased activity of biogenic amines correlated with the delayed therapeutic response.

   3. Antagonist activity of antidepressants at adrenoceptors, muscarinic cholinoceptors, and others accounts for many of their **adverse effects**.

C. Pharmacologic properties
  —are highly **lipid-soluble**.

—are **incompletely** and **slowly absorbed** due to extensive first-pass metabolism and enterohepatic recirculation; MAO inhibitors are readily absorbed and so are not given parenterally.

—are metabolized by ring **hydroxylation** and glucuronide **conjugation,** or by **demethylation;** monodemethylation of some tricyclic antidepressant tertiary amines results in active secondary amine metabolites. Hydrazide MAO inhibitors are inactivated by acetylation; genetically slow acetylators may show exaggerated effects.

—have **variable half-lives** (0.5–3 days).

—are extensively bound to plasma proteins.

—demonstrate tenuous relationship of plasma levels to therapeutic response. **Plasma levels** are used primarily to monitor compliance and toxicity.

D. Therapeutic uses

1. Unipolar endogenous depression

—elevate mood, increase physical activity and mental alertness, increase appetite, increase sexual drive, improve sleep patterns, and reduce preoccupation with morbid thoughts.

—are effective in 70% of patients.

—MAO inhibitors are used rarely, usually when tricyclic antidepressants are ineffective; also used in **narcolepsy,** but this use is controversial.

2. Bipolar endogenous depression

—is treated with antidepressants given in combination with **lithium.**

3. Obsessive–compulsive disorder

—is treated with **clomipramine**.

4. Schizoaffective disorders

5. Paranoid schizophrenia

—is treated with antidepressants given in **combination** with **antipsychotic agents**.

6. Chronic pain

—are often used for pain of unknown origin.

—may work directly on pain pathways, but mechanism is unknown.

7. Nocturnal enuresis

—are used only as a last resort, and only for patients over age 6.

E. Adverse effects and contraindications (see Table 4.3)

1. CNS

a. Sedation

—is produced particularly by tertiary amines, probably due to CNS antihistaminic (H_1) action; **trazodone** is highly sedating for unknown reasons, and **fluoxetine** produces little sedation.

b. Mania

—results from "switch" reaction in patients with bipolar disorder.

c. Stimulation

—is marked by agitation, increased motor activity, insomnia, tremor, and excitement.

−may be experienced as dysphoria; most likely with **fluoxetine** and **bupropion,** sometimes with secondary amines.

d. Confusion and delirium

−is a central anticholinergic effect; is more common in the elderly.

e. Agitation and psychosis

−may worsen in psychotic patients.

f. Seizures

−occur occasionally due to lowered seizure threshold.

−are more common with tertiary amines and **bupropion;** risk with **maprotiline** may be 4% at high therapeutic doses.

g. Movement disorders

−are occasionally produced by **amoxapine,** due to dopamine−receptor antagonist activity.

h. Headache

−is caused by **fluoxetine, bupropion,** and drugs with low anticholinergic activity.

2. Cardiovascular system

a. Orthostatic hypotension

−is probably due to peripheral α_1-adrenoceptor blockade; may be severe. Tolerance often occurs.

b. Tachycardia, conduction defects, and arrhythmias

−are particularly **common with overdose;** patients with preexisting heart block or compensated cardiac output are at risk; risk is highest with imipramine and lowest with fluoxetine, trazodone, bupropion, and MAO inhibitors.

3. Gastrointestinal tract

a. Constipation

−is due to muscarinic-cholinoceptor antagonist activity, which more rarely may precipitate paralytic ileus.

b. Gastric irritation

−includes nausea and heartburn; is caused by **trazodone** or **fluoxetine**.

4. Autonomic nervous system

−reflects muscarinic−cholinoceptor activity. **Trazodone, fluoxetine,** and **bupropion** have less adverse anticholinergic activity. Tolerance to these effects may develop.

−commonly produces **dry mouth, blurred vision,** and **difficulty in urination**.

−more rarely may precipitate narrow-angle glaucoma or cause urine retention.

−are more common in the **elderly**.

5. Other adverse effects and contraindications
   —tricyclic antidepressants often produce **weight gain; fluoxetine** often produces **weight loss**.
   —cause **sexual dysfunction; trazodone** occasionally causes **priapism**.
   —produce **hematologic changes,** including hemolytic anemia and agranulocytosis.
   —cause **allergic reactions** and **obstructive jaundice**.
   —**amoxapine** has additional adverse effects similar to those of antipsychotics.

F. Overdose and toxicity
   1. Overdose of **tricyclic antidepressants** produces severe anticholinergic signs, respiratory depression, arrhythmias, shock, seizures, coma, and death. Treatment is supportive and includes gastric lavage with activated charcoal; propranolol, lidocaine, or phenytoin for arrhythmias; benzodiazepines for seizures; and bicarbonate to correct acidosis and to increase drug binding to plasma proteins.
   2. Uncommon results of overdose of **MAO inhibitors** include agitation, hyperthermia, seizures, hypotension or hypertension, and rare hepatotoxicity (hydrazides) with 20% to 25% mortality rate.

G. Drug interactions
   1. Tricyclic antidepressants
   —result in **additive depression** with CNS depressants such as **alcohol** and **barbiturates**.
   —**block uptake of guanethidine** into sympathetic nerve endings and decrease antihypertensive action.
   —block α-adrenoceptors and reduce the antihypertensive action of **clonidine** and α-**methyldopa**.
   —**decrease absorption** of **levodopa** (L-dopa) through their anticholinergic activity.
   —have a rare interaction with MAO inhibitors, causing seizures, hyperpyrexia, and hypertensive crisis.
   —have additive **anticholinergic effects** with antiparkinsonian drugs, antipsychotic drugs, and other drugs with anticholinergic activity.

   2. MAO inhibitors
   —may result in **hypertension** and rarely, in subarachnoid bleeding when **combined** with indirectly acting sympathomimetics (e.g., **amphetamine** and **tyramine** from foods). These reactions are due to the release of increased stores of catecholamines.
   —can potentiate the effect of high doses of directly acting sympathetic amines.
   —may cause **severe agitation** and **hyperthermia** in the presence of **opioids**.
   —may cause hyperthermia, hypertension, seizures, and death in the presence of tricyclic antidepressants. Tricyclic antidepressants should be administered before MAO inhibitors or with them, but not after.
   —result in additive **sedation** and **CNS depression** in the **presence** of **barbiturates, alcohol,** and **opioids**.

IV. Lithium

A. Structure and mechanism of action

—is an endogenous monovalent cation with no known physiologic role. Mechanism of action is unknown. Has reported effects on nerve conduction, release and synthesis of biogenic amines, and calcium and phospholipid metabolism.

B. Pharmacologic properties

—is eliminated almost entirely by the kidney; 80% is reabsorbed in the proximal tubule.

—has a narrow therapeutic index; plasma levels must be monitored continuously.

C. Therapeutic uses

1. Acute mania or bipolar (manic-depressive) disorder

—normalizes mood in 60%–80% of patients. Onset of therapeutic effect takes 2–3 weeks; antipsychotics are often used in initial stages of disease to control acute agitation.

—**carbamazepine,** an anticonvulsant, has been used successfully as an adjunct when lithium therapy is inadequate or not tolerated; dose is similar to that used for epilepsy; mechanism of action is unknown.

2. Prophylaxis of bipolar disorder

—is often administered with a tricyclic antidepressant.

3. Alternative to tricyclic antidepressants in recurrent depression with or without mania

D. Adverse effects

—are common at therapeutic doses of 0.5–1.4 mmol/L or slightly higher.

—include **diarrhea, tremor, polydipsia,** and **weight gain**.

—produces **polyuria.** Occurs as the kidney becomes unresponsive to antidiuretic hormone (reversible). More rarely, decreased renal function occurs with long-term treatment, similar to nephrogenic diabetes insipidus.

—produces **benign, reversible thyroid enlargement** by reducing tyrosine iodination and synthesis of thyroxine. More rarely causes hypothyroidism.

—is contraindicated during the first trimester of pregnancy because of risk of fetal congenital abnormalities. Breast feeding is not recommended because lithium is secreted in breast milk.

E. Toxicity

1. **> 2mmol/L:** Confusion (important first sign of toxicity), drowsiness, vomiting, ataxia, dizziness, and severe tremors

2. **> 2.5 mmol/L:** Clonic movements of the limbs, seizures, circulatory collapse, and coma

3. **Treatment** includes discontinuing lithium administration, hemodialysis, and use of anticonvulsants.

4. Sodium depletion is increased by low-salt diet, **thiazide diuretics, furosemide, ethacrynic acid,** or severe vomiting or diarrhea. This increases renal reabsorption of lithium.

5. Renal clearance is decreased by some nonsteroidal anti-inflammatory drugs (e.g., **indomethacin** and **phenylbutazone**).

V. Opioid Analgesics and Antagonists

A. Definitions

1. **Opioids** are drugs with morphine-like activity that reduce pain and induce tolerance and physical dependence. They are also referred to as narcotic analgesics.

2. **Opiates** are drugs derived from opium (e.g., morphine, heroin), a powdered, dried exudate of the fruit capsule (poppy) of the plant *Papaver somniferum*. Opium alkaloids (e.g., **thebaine**) are used to make semisynthetic opioids. Others are prepared **synthetically** (e.g., **meperidine, methadone**).

3. **Opiopeptins** are endogenous peptides that have opioid activity; they include endorphins, enkephalins, and dynorphins.

   —are localized in discrete areas of the CNS, pituitary, autonomic nervous system, pancreas, adrenal gland, and gastrointestinal tract.

   —are derived from distinct polypeptide precursors:

   a. **Pro-opiomelanocortin:** Contains β-endorphin, adrenocorticotropic hormone (ACTH), and β-melanocyte-stimulating hormone

   b. **Proenkephalin:** Contains *met*-enkephalin and *leu*-enkephalin

   c. **Prodynorphin:** Contains dynorphin A and B and neoendorphin α and β

B. Mechanism of action

1. **Opioids** are believed to mimic the effects of endogenous opiopeptins by interaction with several **distinct receptors** (μ, κ, δ). Each opioid receptor may have distinct subtypes (e.g., μ1, μ2). Opioids with mixed agonist–antagonist properties may act as agonists at one opioid receptor and as antagonists at another.

   a. **μ Receptors** = supraspinal analgesia, respiratory depression, euphoria, physical dependence

   b. **κ Receptors** = spinal analgesia, sedation, miosis

   c. **δ Receptors** = significance unclear; perhaps contributes to analgesia

2. Opioids **inhibit prejunctional release of numerous neurotransmitters** (e.g., the release of substance P in the spinal cord); they also inhibit neurotransmitter-stimulated calcium influx and adenylate cyclase activity.

C. Tolerance and physical dependence

1. **Tolerance**

   —occurs gradually with repeated administration; a larger opioid dose is necessary to produce the same initial effect.

   —is due to a direct effect of opioids on neurons in the CNS (cellular tolerance).

   —varies in degree. **Substantial** tolerance to analgesia, euphoria, and respiratory depression. **Minimal** tolerance to constipation, seizures, miosis, and antagonist activity.

   —can be conferred from one opioid agonist to others (**cross-tolerance**).

2. Physical dependence

—occurs with the development of tolerance to opioids.

a. Abstinent withdrawal

—is a syndrome revealed with discontinuation of opioid administration.

—is characterized by lacrimation, rhinorrhea, yawning, sweating, restlessness, dilated pupils, goose bumps (**"cold turkey"**); anorexia, irritability, tremor, diarrhea, flushing, cramps, muscle spasms (**"kicking the habit"**).

—peaks at 48–72 hours.

—is generally not life-threatening, except in dependent neonates.

—can be reversed by re-administration of opioid.

b. Precipitated withdrawal

—is induced by administration of an opioid antagonist such as **naloxone**.

—peaks sooner than abstinent withdrawal and is more severe.

—is more difficult to reverse with opioid agonists than abstinent withdrawal.

D. Prototype: morphine

1. Chemical structure (Figure 4.4)

—is a **phenanthrene alkaloid** with a phenylmethyl-piperidine ring structure. Substitutions at the C-3-phenolic position, the C-6-hydroxyl position, or the N-17-nitrogen in the piperidine ring markedly change its potency or convert it to a compound that is an antagonist or has both agonist and antagonist activity (mixed agonist–antagonist).

2. Pharmacologic properties

—is usually given **parenterally,** but can be given orally or rectally.

—is **erratically absorbed**.

—undergoes extensive first-pass metabolism with glucuronide conjugation. (Morphine-6-glucuronide may possess analgesic activity.) Dosage adjustment necessary in hepatic insufficiency.

—has $t_{1/2}$ of 2–3 hours; duration of action is 3–6 hours.

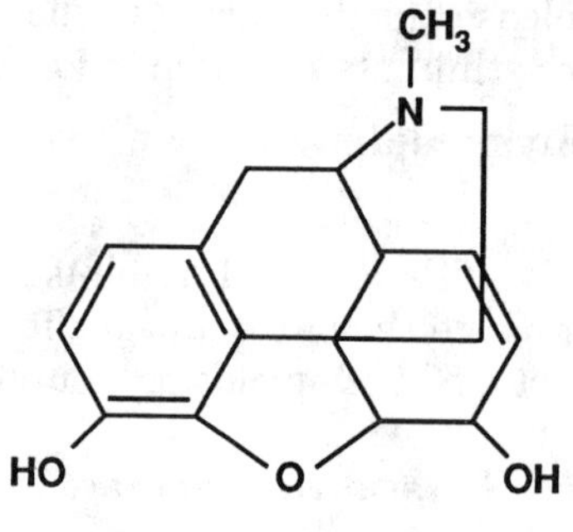

Figure 4.4. Structure of morphine.

3. Therapeutic uses (Table 4.4)

   a. Analgesia
   - **morphine** (also **meperidine** and **hydromorphone**) is used for analgesia in severe preoperative and postoperative pain as well as pain of terminal illness; is used to treat pain of trauma, burns, cancer, acute myocardial infarction (MI), and renal or biliary colic.
   - produces analgesia by increasing threshold for sensation of pain. Perception of pain is dissociated from the sensation, but there is significant interpatient variability in this effect.
   - decreases the continuous, moderate-to-severe dull aching pain that is associated with visceral damage. Higher doses are necessary for intermittent sharp pain.
   - occurs without loss of consciousness.

   b. Euphoria, decreased anxiety and a floating sensation; occasionally a paradoxical dysphoric effect

   c. Sedation, marked by drowsiness, inability or decreased ability to concentrate, and loss of recent memory
   - places ambulatory patients at risk for accidents.
   - is useful for the relief of **anxiety** in frightening disorders, such as MI and terminal illness.

   d. Depression of cough reflex; codeine used when not controlled by nonopioids
   - produce direct depression of the cough center in the medulla.
   - is depressed by both L-isomers and D-isomers of opioids (D-isomers are without analgesic action).
   - requires doses lower than for analgesia; reduced coughing may lead to pneumonia when opioids are used for analgesia, particularly when respiration is compromised.

   e. Anesthesia applications
   (1) Preanesthetic medication or supplement to anesthetic agents during surgery
   (a) Opioids are used for analgesic and sedative or anxiolytic effects.

Table 4.4. Indications for Morphine and Other Opioids

Indication	Opioid Used
Analgesia	Morphine, meperidine, hydromorphone
Dyspnea	Morphine
Diarrhea	Morphine, diphenoxylate, codeine, and loperamide
Cough	Codeine when not controlled by nonnarcotic cough suppressants
Preanesthesia	Fentanyl often used for its short duration of action (1–2 hr)
Regional anesthesia	Morphine
Cardiovascular surgery	High-dose fentanyl as primary anesthetic because it produces minimal cardiac depression
Withdrawal or maintenance therapy	Methadone, substitution for treatment of opioid dependence; clonidine, an α-adrenoceptor agonist, is also used for withdrawal because it suppresses autonomic components

(b) Fentanyl is used often for its short duration of action (1–2 hours).

(2) Regional anesthesia

(a) Long-lasting analgesia of **morphine** mediated through action on spinal cord (epidural or intrathecal administration)

(b) Reduced incidence of adverse effects but often delayed respiratory depression, nausea, and vomiting

(3) High-dose **fentanyl** is used as primary anesthetic in **cardiovascular surgery** because of minimal cardiac depression.

f. Withdrawal or maintenance therapy

(1) Methadone substitution is used as treatment of opioid dependence.

(2) Clonidine (α-adrenoceptor agonist) is also used for withdrawal as it suppresses autonomic components.

g. Opioids are used to treat **diarrhea** because of their constipating effect.

–are often used after ileostomy or colostomy (**diphenoxylate, codeine, loperamide**) at a dose lower than for analgesia.

4. Adverse effects and contraindications

a. Respiratory depression

–is due to direct inhibition of the respiratory center in the brain stem and to decreased sensitivity of the respiratory center to CO_2 with decreased hypoxic drive; leads to decreased respiratory rate, minute volume, and tidal exchange.

(1) Opioids are contraindicated if there is preexisting decrease in respiratory reserve (e.g., emphysema) or excessive respiratory secretions (e.g., obstructive lung disease).

(2) Depression of respiration may be responsible for the beneficial effect of **morphine** when used to treat dyspnea (from pulmonary edema secondary to acute left ventricular failure). **Morphine** relieves feeling of shortness of breath by an unclear mechanism; may be due to depression of the respiratory center (and CNS response to hypoxic drive), decreased peripheral resistance or preload, or decreased anxiety of patient regarding impaired respiration.

(3) Cerebral vasodilation results from the increased Pco_2 caused by respiratory depression and may result in increased cerebral vascular pressure. **Morphine** is contraindicated in patients with head injury due to cerebral vasodilation induced by respiratory depression, which may lead to altered brain function and death.

(4) Because they cause fetal respiratory depression and dependence, opioids should be used cautiously during pregnancy.

(5) Clinical or accidental overdose with respiratory depression may be treated with ventilation; may be sufficient for treatment of respiratory depression or coma. Opioid antagonists will reverse respiratory depression.

b. Nausea and vomiting

–is caused by the direct stimulation of the chemoreceptor trigger zone; also a direct vestibular component.

−is blocked by dopamine-receptor antagonists.

−is self-limiting due to subsequent direct inhibition by morphine of the vomiting center.

c. Physical or psychological dependence should not be an excuse for inadequate therapy.

d. Miosis

(1) Stimulation of the Edinger-Westphal nucleus of the oculomotor nerve results in "pinpoint" pupils in complete darkness. This is mediated by acetylcholine and blocked by atropine.

(2) During severe respiratory depression and asphyxia, miosis may revert to mydriasis.

e. Pneumonia is a potential result of reduced cough reflex.

f. Mental clouding and drowsiness put ambulatory patients at risk.

g. Hypotension

−inhibits the vasomotor center in the brain stem, causing peripheral vasodilation; also inhibits compensatory baroreceptor reflexes and increases histamine release.

−opioids should be used cautiously in patients in shock or with reduced blood volume. The elderly are particularly susceptible.

−vasodilation and subsequent decreased cardiac preload is of therapeutic benefit when morphine is used for pain of MI. **Pentazocine** and **butorphanol** increase preload and are contraindicated for pain of MI.

h. Constipation

−results from decreased coordinated gastrointestinal motility and increased anal sphincter tone.

−is due to both the CNS and peripheral action of **morphine**.

i. Pain from biliary or urinary spasm

−results from increased intrabiliary duct pressure due to increased tone of smooth muscle (spasm) and the sphincter of Oddi of the biliary tract.

−may result in paradoxical increase in pain when used to alleviate the pain associated with the passing of urinary or biliary stones if the opioid dose is insufficient to induce centrally mediated analgesia.

j. Urine retention

−is due to decreased renal plasma flow, increased tone, decreased coordinated contractility of the ureters and bladder, increased urethral sphincter tone, and inattention to the urinary reflex.

−**catheterization** is necessary in some instances.

−opioids should be used cautiously in patients with prostatic hypertrophy or urethral stricture.

k. Increased release of antidiuretic hormone

l. Prolonged labor is due to block of the contractile effect of oxytocin on the uterus and reduction of uterine muscle tone.

5. Drug interactions

a. CNS depressants add to or potentiate respiratory depression.

b. Antipsychotics and antidepressants potentiate sedation.

    c. MAO inhibitors produce severe respiratory depression, restlessness, excitement, fever, and seizures, particularly with **meperidine**.

E. Other strong opioid agonists

  1. Hydromorphone [Dilaudid], oxymorphone [Numorphan], and heroin

    —are **phenanthrenes** with actions similar to **morphine**.

    a. Oxymorphone has little antitussive activity.

    b. Heroin (not approved for clinical use) is more lipid-soluble and faster-acting than **morphine;** it is rapidly metabolized in the brain to its active metabolites, morphine and monoacetylmorphine.

  2. Meperidine [Demerol]

    —is a phenylpiperidine with indications similar to morphine.

    —has a shorter duration of action than morphine.

    —may cause less constipation and vomiting and less fetal respiratory depression than morphine. **Overdose** may cause **seizures**.

    —causes severe restlessness, excitement, and fever when administered with MAO inhibitors.

    —may result in **mydriasis** and **tachycardia** due to weak anticholinergic activity.

    —has no effect on the cough reflex.

  3. Fentanyl [Sublimaze]

    —is a phenylpiperidine with a shorter duration of action (20 minutes) than morphine.

    —is administered IV as a preanesthetic medication for preoperative and postoperative pain.

    —is used in **high doses** as a **primary anesthetic** for cardiovascular surgery because it produces minimal cardiac depression.

    —is used to supplement the analgesia and sedative–hypnotic effects of nitrous oxide and halothane—"balanced anesthesia." Morphine also is used for this indication.

    —is infrequently used in combination product **fentanyl/droperidol** [Innovar] to induce neuroleptanalgesia; permits a wakeful state when patient cooperation is needed (intubations, minor surgical procedures, changing burn dressings); droperidol is a butyrophenone.

    —may cause severe muscle rigidity when administered rapidly by IV.

  4. Methadone [Dolophine]

    —is a phenylheptylamine.

    —is administered orally and has a longer duration of action than **morphine**.

    —is associated with less severe withdrawal syndrome than **morphine** and often is substituted for other opioids for treatment of physical dependence.

F. Weak agonists

  1. Codeine

    —is a phenanthrene used for moderate pain. **Dihydrocodeine, oxycodone,** and **hydrocodone** (phenanthrenes) also are used to treat moderate pain. **Codeine** is used at lower doses for diarrhea and cough.

–is orally effective and undergoes less first-pass metabolism than morphine.

–is associated with less respiratory depression than morphine and has less dependence liability. **Overdose** produces **seizures**.

2. Propoxyphene [Darvon]

–is a phenylheptylamine. The dextro isomer is used as an **analgesic;** however, it has less efficacy than codeine.

–is associated with possible **tolerance** and **dependence**.

–may cause **seizures** at high doses.

3. Diphenoxylate/atropine [Lomotil] and loperamide [Imodium]

–are phenylpiperidines; **diphenoxylate** is a derivative of **meperidine**. **Atropine** is combined with **diphenoxylate** to discourage self-administration.

–are used only for **symptomatic treatment of diarrhea**. Insolubility limits parenteral use and penetration into CNS. Have little dependence liability.

–**difenoxin** [Motofen] is also available; it is an active metabolite of **diphenoxylate**.

G. Mixed agonist–antagonists

1. Pentazocine [Talwin]

–is a benzomorphan derivative, the prototype of opioids with both agonist (κ-receptor) and antagonist (μ-receptor) activity or partial agonist activity at the μ-receptor.

–is used for **moderate pain**.

–has less dependence liability than morphine.

–can precipitate withdrawal.

–occasionally causes dysphoria, hallucinations, and depersonalization.

2. Nalbuphine [Nubain], buprenorphine [Buprenex], butorphanol [Stadol], and dezocine [Dalgan]

–are classified as phenanthrenes (**nalbuphine, buprenorphine**), a morphinan derivative (**butorphanol**), and an aminotetralin (**dezocine**).

–have the same actions as **pentazocine**.

H. Opioid antagonists

–are competitive antagonists of opioids; include **naloxone** [Narcan] and **naltrexone** [Trexan], which are formed, respectively, by allyl and methylcyclopropyl substitutions at the *N*-17-methyl group of morphine.

–will precipitate opioid withdrawal and reverse opioid-induced toxicity.

–differ in duration of action. **Naloxone** action ranges from 1–4 hours; **naltrexone** duration is 10 hours.

I. Antitussives

–include **dextromethorphan** [Benylin DM] and **levopropoxyphene**.

–are isomers of opioids that, like codeine, are used for their antitussive activity as over-the-counter **cough medications,** but have no analgesic or addictive properties. Some **constipation** and **sedation** have been noted.

VI. Antiparkinsonian Drugs

A. Idiopathic parkinsonian disease

–is characterized by resting tremor, rigidity, bradykinesia, loss of postural reflexes and, occasionally, behavioral manifestations.

–is caused by the progressive degeneration of dopamine neurons in the substantia nigra, which leads to a decreased inhibition by **dopamine** of excitatory cholinergic neurons in the basal ganglia.

–may be idiopathic or drug-induced.

B. Therapeutic goal

–because it is not possible to reverse the degenerative process, drugs are used to correct the **imbalance** of **dopamine** and **acetylcholine activity** in the basal ganglia.

C. Levodopa (L-dopa) [Dopar, Larodopa] and levodopa/carbidopa [Sinemet]

1. Mechanism of action

–is levorotatory isomer of dopa that is decarboxylated in the CNS to **dopamine** (which does not cross the blood–brain barrier), where it activates postjunctional dopamine (D_2)-receptors in the basal ganglia.

2. Pharmacologic properties

–is **rapidly absorbed**. Absorption is delayed by food and influenced by the rate of gastric emptying and pH.

–requires **high doses** (unless administered with a peripheral decarboxylase inhibitor such as **carbidopa**), because 95% is metabolized to dopamine in the periphery.

3. Therapeutic effects

a. Clinical improvement, including major improvement in functional capacity and quality of life, occurs after several weeks of treatment in 75% of patients.

b. Tremor is more resistant to therapy, and there is little improvement of **dementia**.

c. Therapeutic effects of therapy last for about 2–5 years. It is believed that neuronal regeneration progresses to the extent that the remaining functional neurons are unable to process enough exogenous L-dopa to compensate for decreased endogenous dopamine levels.

4. Adverse effects and contraindications

a. Dyskinesias

–are the major limiting factor in therapy.

–occur in 80% of patients and are characterized by repetitive involuntary gross movements.

–may be relieved by **decreasing** the dose of **levodopa,** but parkinsonian symptoms may increase.

b. Akinesias

–are characterized by decreased voluntary movement, which lasts for a few minutes or several hours.

(1) End-of-dose akinesia: Decreasing the dose and increasing the frequency of administration may relieve symptoms.

(2) "On-off" akinesia: Unexpected loss of mobility may be a signal that the efficacy of **levodopa** is waning.

(3) Akinesia paradoxica: Freezing of movement often following an episode of dyskinesia and often precipitated by stress.

c. Behavioral effects

−include occasional anxiety, insomnia, and early-onset psychosis due to exacerbation of preexisting psychotic problem. Also, occasional late-onset (2 years) dream alterations (vivid dreams, nightmares), visual hallucinations, and drug-induced psychoses characterized by paranoia and confusional states.

d. Nausea and vomiting

−occurs in 80% of patients; attenuated if levodopa is taken with carbidopa, with food or in divided doses, or with nonphenothiazine antiemetics such as cyclizine.

−is due to direct **effects** of dopamine on the **gastrointestinal tract** and on the **chemoreceptor trigger zone in the CNS**. Tolerance to nausea and vomiting may develop.

e. Cardiovascular effects

−include orthostatic hypotension, occasional hypertension and, rarely, tachycardia, arrhythmias, and atrial fibrillation due to increased circulating catecholamines; some tolerance may develop.

f. Contraindications

−is contraindicated in patients with **psychosis, narrow-angle glaucoma,** and **peptic ulcer disease**.

5. Drug interactions

a. Therapeutic action is reduced by **antipsychotic** or **antiemetic drugs** that block dopamine receptors.

b. Gastrointestinal absorption is decreased by **tricyclic antidepressants** and other drugs with anticholinergic activity.

c. Should not be used with nonselective **MAO inhibitors,** such as **tranylcypromine,** which inhibit both MAO-A and MAO-B. This **combination** can cause a **severe hypertensive crisis** and **hyperthermia**.

d. Peripheral levels decreased by pyridoxine (**vitamin B$_6$**), which increases the activity of dopa decarboxylase and increases conversion of levodopa to dopamine in the periphery.

e. Natural aromatic **amino acids** (tryptophan, histidine, phenylalanine, tyrosine) decrease absorption of levodopa.

6. Carbidopa (α-methyldopahydrazine)

a. Carbidopa is an L-amino acid decarboxylase inhibitor that does not cross the blood–brain barrier and has little effect of its own.

b. In the presence of carbidopa, less **levodopa** is metabolized in the periphery; therefore, therapeutic dose of levodopa can be reduced by up to 80%, and nausea and vomiting and adverse cardiovascular effects are decreased.

D. Bromocriptine [Parlodel] and pergolide [Permax]

—are dopamine-receptor agonists.

—are an alternative to levodopa when it is not tolerated. Often given in combination with levodopa for optimal treatment; more effective than amantadine or anticholinergic drugs. Bromocriptine also is used to treat **lactation, infertility, amenorrhea,** or **galactorrhea** caused by hyperprolactinemia, and it is an **adjunct** in treatment of **pituitary tumors** associated with hyperprolactinemia or acromegaly.

—are as effective as levodopa when given in high doses but are not as long lasting due to suspected desensitization of dopamine receptors.

—have the same adverse effects, cautions, and contraindications as levodopa.

E. Amantadine [Symmetrel]

—is an **antiviral drug** that increases the release of dopamine in the CNS by an unknown mechanism.

—is useful in the early stages of **parkinsonism** or as an **adjunct to levodopa** therapy. Therapeutic effect may diminish in a few weeks.

—is **excreted unchanged;** renal function should be monitored to prevent toxicity, particularly in the elderly.

—is associated with occasional headache, confusion, hallucinations, and peripheral edema. Long-term use may lead to discoloration of skin (**livedo reticularis**) or, more rarely, urine retention and congestive heart failure. **Overdose** may cause a **toxic psychosis and seizures**.

F. Selegiline [Eldepryl, Deprenyl]

—is an MAO inhibitor selective for MAO-B that decreases dopamine metabolism in the CNS and prolongs its action.

—is used as an adjunct to **levodopa** therapy.

—delays progression of neuronal degeneration; however, this action is controversial.

G. Benztropine [Cogentin], trihexyphenidyl [Artane], and other anticholinergic drugs and antihistamine with anticholinergic activity

—suppress overactivity of cholinergic neurons in the basal ganglia; have somewhat greater ratio of CNS to peripheral activity.

—are often used in initial stages of **mild parkinsonism,** particularly in younger patients, or in combination with **levodopa.** They have significant effect on tremor and rigidity but little effect on akinesia and postural reflexes. These drugs are effective in 25% of patients, many of whom become refractory.

—are associated with occasional restlessness, sedation, confusion, mood changes, dry mouth, mydriasis, constipation, tachycardia, and arrhythmias.

—are contraindicated in patients with prostatic hypertrophy, paralytic ileus, or narrow-angle glaucoma.

VII. Antiepileptic Drugs

A. Drug treatment of seizures

—are effective for about 80% of epileptic patients. (Epilepsy occurs in approximately 1% of the American population.) Lifelong treatment is not always necessary.

—are mostly **well absorbed** and have **long plasma half-lives** (6–36 hours). May take weeks to establish adequate drug plasma levels and to determine adequacy of therapeutic improvement. Lack of compliance is responsible for many treatment failures.

—are most **effective** and have the least adverse effects when used as **monotherapy**. Addition of a second drug to the therapeutic regimen should be gradual, as should discontinuance of the initial drug before substitution of an alternative drug, because **status epilepticus** may occur on withdrawal.

—can extensively bind to plasma proteins and can induce hepatic metabolism. These activities are associated with many adverse effects.

—usually have teratogenic potential during the first trimester of pregnancy. This may call for the reduction or termination of therapy during pregnancy or before planned pregnancy. However, maternal seizures also present risk to the fetus.

—also may be used to treat seizures that result acutely from various neurologic disorders, as well as from metabolic disturbances, trauma, and exposure to certain toxins.

B. Classification of epilepsies

—are **chronic seizure disorders** characterized by either focal or generalized abnormal neuronal discharges. Drug selection, based on seizure classification, is listed below in the order of general choice.

1. Partial (focal) seizures

    a. Simple: Localized discharge; consciousness unaltered

    b. Complex: Localized discharge that becomes widespread; may lose consciousness

        (1) Carbamazepine, phenytoin

        (2) Phenobarbital, primidone

        (3) Valproic acid

2. Generalized seizures

    a. Major motor or tonic–clonic (grand mal): Dramatic bilateral movements with either clonic jerking of the extremities or tonic rigidity of the entire body; accompanied by loss of consciousness.

        (1) Carbamazepine, valproic acid

        (2) Phenytoin, phenobarbital

    b. Minor motor seizures

        (1) Absence (petit mal): Sudden onset of altered consciousness that lasts 10–45 seconds; up to hundreds of seizures per day; begins in childhood or adolescence.

            (a) Ethosuximide

            (b) Valproic acid

            (c) Clonazepam/clorazepate

        (2) Myoclonic: Lightning-like jerks of one or more extremities occurring singly or in bursts of up to a hundred; accompanied by alteration of consciousness.

        (3) Atonic: Sudden onset of altered consciousness and loss of postural tone that lasts less than 30 seconds.

            (a) Valproic acid (only with concurrent absence seizure)

(b) Clonazepam/clorazepate

(c) Corticotropin, prednisone

3. **Status epilepticus:** Prolonged seizure (> 20 minutes) of any of the types previously described. The most common is life-threatening generalized tonic–clonic status epilepticus.

   –**diazepam** or **lorazepam** followed by **phenytoin** or IV **phenobarbital**.

C. Mechanism of action

1. **Carbamazepine, valproic acid,** and **phenytoin** block sodium channels and inhibit generation of action potentials.

2. **Phenobarbital, clonazepam, clorazepate, diazepam,** and **lorazepam** facilitate GABA-mediated inhibition of neuronal activity; **phenobarbital** also blocks glutamate-mediated excitation.

3. **Ethosuximide** reduces low-threshold T-type Ca^{2+} current that provides pacemaker activity in the thalamus.

4. **Acetazolamide** inhibits carbonic anhydrase and increases accumulation of CO_2.

D. Phenytoin [Dilantin]

1. **Pharmacologic properties**

   –is a diphenyl-substituted **hydantoin**.

   –has variable interpatient oral absorption (30%–95%) but relatively constant absorption for the individual patient. Rate and extent depend on formulation.

   –is extensively (90%) bound to plasma proteins.

   –is metabolized primarily by microsomal enzymes by parahydroxylation and glucuronide conjugation; $t_{1/2}$ is approximately 24 hours at therapeutic doses. In some patients, metabolic enzymes become saturated at low doses and $t_{1/2}$ increases as plasma concentration increases.

2. **Adverse effects and toxicity**

   a. **Common:** Gingival hyperplasia and hirsutism, often precluding use in children; at high blood levels, nystagmus, ataxia, and diplopia.

   b. **Occasional:** Coarsening of facial features and osteomalacia after chronic use

   c. **Rare:** Idiosyncratic reactions requiring drug discontinuance (e.g., exfoliative dermatitis; blood dyscrasias, including aplastic anemia)

3. **Drug interactions**

   a. **Stimulates hepatic metabolism** by enzyme induction and reduces plasma concentrations of numerous drugs, including carbamazepine, valproic acid, ethosuximide, primidone, tetracyclines, chloramphenicol, rifampin, oral anticoagulants, oral contraceptives, and quinidine.

   b. **Plasma concentrations increased** by drugs that inhibit hepatic metabolism (e.g., cimetidine, isoniazid).

   c. **Plasma concentration decreased** by drugs that stimulate hepatic metabolism (e.g., carbamazepine, phenobarbital).

      d. Displaced from plasma proteins by phenylbutazone, benzodiazepines, sulfonamides, oral anticoagulants, aspirin, and valproic acid, and in renal and hepatic failure.

      e. Valproic acid may increase or decrease blood levels of **phenytoin**.

E. Carbamazepine [Tegretol]

  1. Pharmacologic properties

    –is a **tricyclic compound** related to **imipramine** with some three-dimensional similarities to phenytoin.

    –has good oral absorption with interpatient variability in rate; plasma protein binding (70%) not clinically significant; its dihydro-derivative of metabolism has anticonvulsant activity.

    –induces microsomal enzymes and increases its own hepatic clearance. Autometabolism requires gradual dosage adjustment early in therapy.

    –is the drug of choice to treat **trigeminal neuralgia** and other **pain syndromes;** also is used to treat **bipolar** (manic-depressive) **disorders**.

  2. Adverse effects and toxicity

    a. Common: Diplopia, ataxia, gastrointestinal disturbances; sedation at high doses

    b. Occasional: Hypernatremia

    c. Rare idiosyncratic reactions: Blood dyscrasias and exfoliative dermatitis

    d. May exacerbate minor motor seizures

  3. Drug interactions

    a. Increases hepatic clearance of phenytoin, valproic acid, clonazepam, and primidone.

    b. Plasma concentration increased by drugs that inhibit hepatic metabolism (e.g., cimetidine, chloramphenicol, dicumarol, isoniazid, sulfonamides, phenylbutazone, trimethoprim, and erythromycin).

F. Phenobarbital [Luminal] and primidone [Mysoline]

  –for further discussion, see sedative–hypnotic drugs, section I, and drugs of abuse, section X.

  1. Phenobarbital is used most often for infants. Paradoxic hyperactivity and shortened attention span are not uncommon in children and the elderly.

  2. Primidone, although not a barbiturate, is structurally related to **phenobarbital**. It is well absorbed, active itself, and also partially and slowly metabolized to **phenobarbital**. Adverse effects include sedation and gastrointestinal disturbances.

G. Ethosuximide [Zarontin]

  –is a **succinimide** that is structurally similar to the hydantoins

  –although effective in fewer patients with **absence seizures** than **valproic acid,** is the drug of choice because of its greater safety.

  –produces gastrointestinal disturbances, fatigue, headache, and dizziness.

  –**phensuximide** [Milontin] and **methsuximide** [Celontin] are congeners with limited utility.

H. Valproic acid (dipropylacetic acid) [Depakene] and divalproex sodium [Depakote]

1. Pharmacologic properties

–has good oral absorption. Depakote is a 1:1 enteric formulation of **valproic acid** and **valproate sodium** that is absorbed more slowly.

–is 90% plasma protein-bound; displaces and is displaced by **phenytoin** and **aspirin**.

–inhibits its own hepatic metabolism and the metabolism of other drugs (e.g., **phenytoin, carbamazepine,** and **phenobarbital**).

2. Adverse effects and toxicity

a. Common: Gastrointestinal disturbances

b. Uncommon: Weight gain or loss, hair loss, tremor at high doses

c. Rare: Idiosyncratic pancreatitis and idiosyncratic hepatotoxicity; may be fatal and are more common in infants and in patients using multiple anticonvulsants

I. Other anticonvulsant agents

1. Benzodiazepines include **clonazepam** [Klonopin] and **clorazepate** [Tranxene], IV **diazepam** [Valium], and **lorazepam** [Ativan]. Sedation and tolerance limit chronic use.

2. Acetazolamide [Diamox] is a diuretic used for all types of seizures. Rapid development of tolerance limits use.

3. Corticotropin and prednisone are drugs of choice for **infantile spasms**. Use is severely limited by adverse effects.

VIII. General Anesthetics

A. Overview of general anesthetics

1. General anesthesia

–is characterized by a loss of consciousness, analgesia, amnesia, skeletal muscle relaxation, and inhibition of autonomic and sensory reflexes.

–the ideal anesthetic should induce anesthesia smoothly and rapidly, be rapidly reversible, and be without adverse effects. No available agent has all of these properties.

2. Balanced anesthesia

–refers to a combination of drugs used to take advantage of their individual properties while attempting to minimize their adverse actions.

–in addition to inhalation anesthetics and neuromuscular junction (NMJ)-blocking drugs, other drugs such as barbiturates, opioids, and benzodiazepines are administered preoperatively, intraoperatively, and postoperatively to ensure smooth induction, analgesia, sedation, and smooth recovery.

3. Stages and planes of anesthesia

–is the progression of physical signs that indicate the depth of anesthesia. Newer, more potent agents progress through these stages rapidly and therefore the stages are often obscured. Further, mechanical ventilation and the use of adjunct drugs also obscure the signs indicating the depth of anesthesia.

  a. Stage I: Analgesia, amnesia

  b. Stage II: Loss of consciousness (may be excitement)

  c. Stage III: Surgical anesthesia (The loss of the eyelash reflex and a pattern of respiration that is regular in rate and depth are the most reliable signs of stage III, surgical anesthesia.)

  (1) Plane I: Unresponsive to surgical stimulation, moist and mobile eyes and constricted pupils, intercostal ventilation

  (2) Plane II: Dry and immobile eyes and mid-dilated pupils, onset of lower intercostal paralysis with increased diaphragmatic ventilation

  (3) Plane III: Absence of corneal reflex and further pupil dilation, skeletal muscle relaxation, intercostal paralysis, and total diaphragmatic breathing

  (4) Plane IV: Maximal pupil dilation, apnea, and circulatory depression

  d. Stage IV: Medullary paralysis and failure of circulation

B. Inhalation anesthetics

1. Halothane, enflurane, and isoflurane

  −are the most commonly used inhalation anesthetics (all are halogenated volatile liquids).

  −produce dose-related decreases in alveolar ventilation and response to carbon dioxide; consequently, assisted or controlled ventilation is usually necessary during surgical anesthesia.

  −produce a dose-related decrease in sympathetic activity and in cardiovascular function.

  −concentrations of halogenated inhalation anesthetics that produce good skeletal muscle relaxation generally produce unacceptable cardiovascular depression; consequently, neuromuscular junction-blocking drugs are commonly used for surgical muscle relaxation. Also, they are generally administered with **nitrous oxide,** which decreases the extent of cardiovascular and respiratory depression at equivalent anesthetic depths.

2. Mechanism of action

  −are thought to alter membrane ion channel conductance or neurotransmitter storage or release and increase the threshold for neuronal firing.

  −may interact directly with hydrophobic sites on protein channels.

  −may interact indirectly by increasing membrane fluidity.

  −according to Meyer-Overton principle, anesthetic potency correlates with lipid solubility.

3. Potency

  a. Minimum alveolar concentration, or **MAC,** is a relative term defined as the minimum alveolar concentration at steady state (measured in volume/volume percent) results in immobility in 50% of patients when exposed to a noxious stimulus, such as a surgical incision.

  b. The **lower the MAC value the more potent the agent;** for example, **nitrous oxide** has a MAC of more than 100, indicating that immobility can only be achieved under hyperbaric conditions.

  c. MAC is an **additive function**.

d. MAC decreases with increasing age, pregnancy, hypothermia, and hypotension, and decreases in the presence of adjuvant drugs, such as other general anesthetics, opioids, sedative–hypnotics, or other CNS depressants.

4. Solubility

a. The **rate** at which the partial pressure of an inhalation anesthetic reaches equilibrium between various tissues (particularly the CNS) and inspired air depends primarily on the **solubility of the drug in blood**. At equilibrium, the partial pressure of the anesthetic is the same in all biophases. However, the concentration of drug in tissues varies depending on the solubility of the anesthetic in the tissue.

b. The **relative solubility** of an inhalation anesthetic in blood relative to air is defined by its **blood–gas partition coefficient (lambda)**. Relatively few molecules of an anesthetic with a low solubility in blood are necessary to increase its partial pressure in blood. This results in its rapid equilibrium in the CNS and a rapid induction of and recovery from anesthesia.

(1) Increasing the **anesthetic concentration** in inspired air will increase the rate of induction.

(2) Increased **rate and depth of ventilation,** such as produced by mechanical hyperventilation or CO_2 stimulation, will increase the partial pressure more rapidly for anesthetics with intermediate or high blood solubility.

(3) Changes in the **rate of pulmonary blood flow** to and from the lungs will change the rate of rise of arterial tension, particularly for anesthetic agents with intermediate-to-low solubility. Increased pulmonary flow from, for example, increased cardiac output, decreases the rate of rise in partial pressure by presenting a larger volume of blood into which the anesthetic can dissolve. Conversely, decreased pulmonary flow, such as occurs during shock, increases the rate of induction of anesthesia.

(4) The less soluble an anesthetic, the more rapid its elimination and the recovery from anesthesia. For **soluble anesthetics,** the longer the exposure the longer the time to recovery because of accumulation of anesthetic in various tissues.

5. Pharmacology of commonly used inhalation anesthetics

a. Nitrous oxide (N_2O) (MAC = 100 +; lambda = 0.5)

—is an anesthetic gas that lacks sufficient potency to produce surgical anesthesia. It has good analgesic and sedative properties but no skeletal muscle relaxant properties.

—is used as the sole agent in **brief procedures,** in the **second stage of labor,** and as a sedative with local anesthetics for **regional anesthesia**.

—is often used in **combination** with other inhalation anesthetics to increase their rate of uptake and to add to their analgesic activity while reducing their adverse effects. When given in large volumes, it increases the volume of uptake of a second blood-soluble gas such as halothane (second-gas effect) which then speeds the induction of anesthesia.

–is often supplemented in balanced anesthesia with sedative-hypnotics, analgesics, and skeletal muscle relaxants.

–is commonly associated with postoperative nausea and vomiting.

–depresses levels of methionine synthase with chronic exposure (e.g., recreational use). This may cause vitamin B_{12} deficiency and result in neuropathy or leukopenia.

b. Halothane [Fluothane] (MAC = 0.8; lambda = 2.4)

–produces relatively **rapid induction** with little excitation.

–has fair **analgesic** and **skeletal muscle relaxant properties;** has excellent **hypnotic properties**.

–is associated with **cardiovascular system depression,** primarily resulting in decreased cardiac output and increased ventricular filling pressure with a minor effect on vascular resistance.

–sensitizes the heart to catecholamines, producing ventricular arrhythmias; catecholamines should be administered cautiously.

–may result in **hepatotoxicity,** possibly due to reactive free radical metabolite. However, incidence is extremely rare (1 in 10,000–30,000).

c. Enflurane [Ethrane] (MAC = 1.7; lambda = 1.9)

–produces relatively **rapid induction** and **recovery** with little excitation.

–is **pungent,** which may result in breath holding or coughing; less acceptance by children than halothane.

–produces good **analgesia** and **hypnosis**.

–at high concentrations, produces **CNS stimulation** with mild twitching or tonic–clonic movements; hypocapnia exaggerates these effects.

–does not produce sensitization of the heart to catecholamines.

–is associated with **cardiovascular system depression,** primarily resulting in decreased cardiac output and increased ventricular filling pressure, with a little more decrease in vascular resistance than halothane.

d. Isoflurane [Forane] (MAC = 1.2; lambda = 1.2)

–produces **rapid induction** and **emergence**.

–is more **pungent** and **irritating** than enflurane with less acceptance by children.

–has good **analgesic** and **sedative** effects.

–is associated with dose-dependent depression of the cardiovascular system, primarily resulting in decreased vascular resistance, with less decrease in cardiac output than halothane.

e. Methoxyflurane [Penthrane] (MAC = 0.2; lambda = 13.0)

–is rarely used in humans but is a popular **veterinary anesthetic**.

–is highly metabolized with resultant dose-related fluoride-induced nephrogenic diabetes insipidus.

6. Additional adverse effects of inhalation anesthetics

a. May be associated with an increased **risk of spontaneous abortion** and **teratogenicity**.

      b. Increase cerebral blood flow, which may increase intracranial pressure. Patients with brain tumor or head injury are at risk.

      c. Halothane, enflurane, and **isoflurane** are **uterine relaxants,** which is a useful property for fetal manipulations during delivery. However, use may **increase postpartum bleeding** or bleeding during therapeutic abortion.

C. Intravenous anesthetics and preanesthetic drugs

  1. Ultra-short-acting barbiturates: thiopental and methohexital

      –see also sedative–hypnotic drugs, section I, and drugs of abuse, section X.

      –are administered IV to **induce or supplement sedation and hypnosis** during anesthesia; result in a smooth, pleasant, and rapid induction.

      –have no analgesic or muscle relaxant properties.

      –have a short duration of action (15 minutes) due to redistribution from highly vascular tissue, particularly brain tissue, to less vascular tissues such as muscle and adipose tissue.

  2. Benzodiazepines and intermediate-acting barbiturates

      –include **diazepam** and **midazolam,** benzodiazepines that may be administered orally or IV (see also sedative–hypnotic drugs, section I, and the barbiturates pentobarbital and secobarbital, section X C 3).

      –are used for **sedation** and to reduce **anxiety.** The **benzodiazepines** are supplanting the use of **barbiturates** because they are safer and produce anterograde amnesia.

    a. Diazepam

      –has a slow onset of action, unpredictable dose-response relationship, and long duration of hypnosis.

      –produces minimal cardiovascular depression and is used with opioids in cardiac patients.

      –causes **phlebitis;** reduces lower esophageal pressure and may increase gastric reflux.

    b. Midazolam

      –has a rapid onset of action and a more predictable dose-response relationship than diazepam and produces more cardiovascular depression.

      –produces excellent amnesia.

    c. Lorazepam

      –has minimal effects on respiration and the cardiovascular system.

  3. Opioids: fentanyl, morphine, meperidine, and pentazocine

      –see Opioid Analgesics and Antagonists, section V.

      –are administered preoperatively to **reduce pain** or to **produce sedation.** Use for sedation is being supplanted by the **benzodiazepines.**

      –are used at high doses to achieve **general anesthesia,** particularly for cardiac surgery. **Fentanyl** has replaced **morphine** for use in cardiac surgery.

      –increase the risk of preoperative and postoperative nausea and vomiting.

    a. Fentanyl produces minimal cardiovascular depression at high doses. Rapid IV infusion may cause spasm of respiratory muscles (**wooden rigidity**).

    b. Fentanyl/droperidol [Innovar] is an illogical combination of a short-duration opioid and long-acting butyrophenone. It is used rarely for diagnostic and therapeutic procedures such as **burn dressings** and **cardiac catheterization**.

4. Etomidate [Amidate]

    –is a **nonbarbiturate anesthetic** used for rapid-onset, short-duration hypnosis.

    –has **no analgesic effects** and results in minimal cardiorespiratory depression.

    –produces the following **adverse effects:** pain at injection site, unpredictable and often severe myoclonus, suppression of adrenocortical function (with continued use), and postoperative nausea and vomiting.

5. Propofol [Diprivan]

    –is administered IV for rapid-onset, short-duration hypnosis. Emergence from anesthesia is due to redistribution from brain to peripheral tissue.

    –produces **no analgesia**.

    –produces the following **adverse effects:** pain at injection site and systemic hypotension from decreased systemic vascular resistance.

6. Ketamine [Ketalar]

    –produces an effect similar to neuroleptanalgesia in which patients feel dissociated from their surroundings (**dissociative anesthesia**).

    –has an analgesic effect on superficial pain but not visceral pain. Also has amnestic action.

    –is a potent bronchodilator; useful in **asthmatics**.

    –is used primarily for **infants and children**. In adults, frequently results in distortions of reality, terrifying dreams, and delirium.

    –**increases blood pressure, heart rate,** and **cardiac output** (vagal inhibition and sympathetic stimulation).

    –**increases intracranial pressure;** contraindicated for patients with tumors and head injuries.

7. Anticholinergic drugs: atropine, scopolamine, and the quaternary ammonium compound glycopyrrolate [Robinul]

    –are rarely used except in infants and small children.

    –are used to **decrease salivation and bronchial secretions,** and to protect against bradycardia and hypotension caused by neuromuscular junction-blocking drugs such as **succinylcholine**.

    –decrease tone of the lower esophageal sphincter, which may increase the risk of reflux.

    –may prolong postoperative drowsiness or confusion.

IX. Local Anesthetics

A. Overview of local anesthetics

    –produce a transient and reversible loss of sensation (**analgesia**) in a circumscribed region of the body without loss of consciousness. Smaller nonmyelinated dorsal root type C nerve fibers and lightly myelinated delta type A nerve fibers, which carry pain and temperature sensations (and also sympathetic type C unmyelinated postganglionic nerve fibers), are blocked before larger, heavily myelinated type A fibers, which transmit sensory propioception and motor functions.

—are generally either esters or amides, usually linked to a lipophilic aromatic group and to a hydrophilic, ionizable tertiary amine. Most are weak bases with pK_a values between 8 and 9, and at physiologic pH are primarily in the charged, cationic form.

—are selected therapeutically based on the duration of drug action (short = 20 minutes; intermediate = 1–1.5 hour; long = 2–4 hours), effectiveness at the administration site and potential for toxicity.

B. Mechanism of action

1. The cationic charged form of local anesthetics interacts with open Na^+ channels on the inner aspect of the axonal membrane during nerve excitation to **block sodium current** and **increase the threshold for excitation**.

2. This results in a dose-dependent decrease in impulse conduction and in the rate of rise and amplitude of the action potential. This is more pronounced in rapidly firing axons where Na^+ channels are more often in an open configuration.

3. **Blockade** is voltage-dependent and time-dependent.

C. Pharmacologic properties

1. Administration and absorption

a. Local anesthetics are administered generally by **infiltration into tissues to bathe local nerves,** by injection directly around nerves and their branches, and by injection into epidural or subarachnoid spaces.

b. The **rate and extent of absorption** into and out of nerves is important in determining the rate of onset of action and termination of action and the potential for systemic adverse effects. This rate is correlated with the relative lipid solubility of the uncharged form and is influenced by the dose and the drug's physicochemical properties, as well as by tissue blood flow and drug binding.

c. **Coadministration** of the vasoconstrictor **epinephrine** (1:200,000 or less) with a local anesthetic of short or intermediate duration of action reduces systemic absorption of the local anesthetic and prolongs its action. Epinephrine should not be coadministered for nerve block in areas supplied with end-arteries, because it may cause ischemia or necrosis, and should be used cautiously in patients in labor or in those with thyrotoxicosis or cardiovascular disease. All **local anesthetics** (except cocaine) are **vasodilators** at therapeutic doses.

2. Metabolism

a. Some ester-type local anesthetics are rapidly hydrolyzed by plasma cholinesterase and thus have very short plasma half-lives. Metabolic rate is decreased in patients with decreased or genetically atypical cholinesterase.

b. Amide-type local anesthetics are metabolized by hepatic microsomal enzymes. Metabolic rate is decreased in patients with liver disease or decreased hepatic blood flow.

D. Specific drugs and their therapeutic uses

1. Amides

a. Lidocaine [Xylocaine]
   –the prototype, has an intermediate duration of action.
   –is generally preferred for **infiltration block** and **epidural anesthesia**.

b. Mepivacaine [Carbocaine]
   –has an **intermediate duration of action** longer than lidocaine, but has actions similar to lidocaine.
   –is not used topically.
   –causes less drowsiness and sedation than lidocaine.

c. Prilocaine [Citanest]
   –has actions similar to lidocaine but is less toxic. Not used topically or for subarachnoid anesthesia.
   –should not be used in patients with cardiac or respiratory disease or with idiopathic or congenital methemoglobinemia because toluidine metabolites may produce methemoglobin. Methemoglobinemia can be reversed by administration of **methylene blue**.

d. Bupivacaine [Marcaine, Sensorcaine]
   –has a **long duration of action**.
   –is generally preferred for **infiltration block** and **epidural anesthesia**.

e. Etidocaine [Duranest]
   –is long-acting and is rarely used for infiltration and peripheral nerve block, and epidural anesthesia.
   –may cause motor block before or without sensory block.

2. Esters

a. Procaine [Novocain]
   –is **short-acting** and is not effective topically.

b. Chloroprocaine [Nesacaine]
   –is very rapidly metabolized by plasma cholinesterase and has less reported toxicity than **procaine**.

c. Cocaine
   –is a **short-acting,** naturally occurring alkaloid used only for **topical anesthesia of mucous membranes**.
   –systemically, will **block uptake of catecholamines** into nerve terminals and may induce intense vasoconstriction. **Adverse effects** include euphoria, CNS stimulation, tachycardia, restlessness, tremors, seizures, and arrhythmias.
   –should be used cautiously for patients with hypertension, cardiovascular disease, thyrotoxicosis, or with other drugs that potentiate catecholamine activity.
   –is a **controlled substance** that is subject to abuse.

d. Tetracaine [Pontocaine]
   –is **long-acting** but has a **slow onset** of action (> 10 minutes).

−is often preferred for **spinal anesthesia**.

−is not generally used for peripheral nerve block, infiltration block, or lumbar epidural nerve block.

e. Dibucaine [Nupercainal]

−is **long-acting** but has a **slow onset** of action (15 minutes).

−is used only for **topical and spinal anesthesia**.

f. Benzocaine [Americaine] and butamben picrate [Butesin]

−are used topically only to treat sunburn, minor burns, and pruritus.

3. Other local anesthetics

a. Dyclonine [Dyclone]

b. Pramoxine [Tronothane]

E. Adverse effects and toxicity

−are usually the result of overdose or inadvertent injection into the vascular system. Systemic effects are most likely to occur with administration of the amide class.

1. CNS

−include light-headedness, dizziness, restlessness, tinnitus, visual disturbances, and tremor. **Lidocaine** and **procaine** may cause sedation and sleep.

−at **high blood concentrations,** produce nystagmus, shivering, tonic–clonic seizures, respiratory depression, coma, and death.

−are treated by maintenance of airway and assisted ventilation, IV **diazepam** for seizures (or prophylactically), and **succinylcholine** to suppress muscular reactions.

2. Cardiovascular system

a. **Bradycardia** from block of cardiac sodium channels and depression of pacemaker activity

b. **Hypotension** from arteriolar dilation and decreased cardiac contractility

3. Allergic reactions

−include rare rash, edema, and anaphylaxis. Usually associated with ester-type drugs that are derivatives of *para*-aminobenzoic acid.

X. Drugs of Abuse

A. Overview

1. Most drugs of abuse act on the CNS to modify the user's mental state.

2. **Chronic use** leads to psychological or physical dependence, or both. May result in the development of tolerance.

3. **Complications** related to parenteral drug administration under unsterile conditions or to the coadministration of adulterants are extremely **common**. These include transmission of viral hepatitis, HIV infection, and various bacteria and fungi, as well as the development of cellulitis, thrombophlebitis, endocarditis, and local and systemic abscesses.

B. Definitions

1. **Drug abuse:** Nonmedical use of a drug that is deemed unacceptable by society.

2. **Drug addiction:** Overwhelming preoccupation with the procurement and use of a drug.

3. **Tolerance:** Decreased intensity of a response to a drug following its continued administration. A larger dose often can produce the same initial effect.

   a. **Metabolic tolerance (pharmacokinetic or dispositional tolerance):** The rate of drug elimination increases with chronic use due to stimulation of its own metabolism.

   b. **Cellular tolerance (pharmacodynamic or functional tolerance):** Biochemical adaptation or homeostatic adjustment of cells to the continued presence of a drug. May be due to a change in the levels, storage, or release of specific neurotransmitters in the CNS, or to changes in the number or activity of their receptors.

   c. **Cross-tolerance:** Tolerance to one drug confers tolerance to other drugs in the same drug class.

4. **Dependence:** Psychological, physiologic, or biochemical need to continue to take a drug.

   a. **Psychological dependence:** Overwhelming compulsion to take a drug to maintain a sense of well-being; generally precedes physical dependence but does not necessarily lead to it

   b. **Physical dependence:** Necessity to continue drug use to avoid withdrawal (abstinent) syndrome.

   c. **Cross-dependence:** Ability of one drug to substitute for another drug in the same drug class to maintain a dependent state or prevent withdrawal.

C. CNS depressants (see also section I)

1. **Ethanol**

   a. **Mechanism of action**

   —is unknown. May be related to changes in membrane fluidity with changes in membrane functions. Also has a direct action on the neuronal GABA-receptor system.

   b. **Acute pharmacologic effects**

   (1) **General CNS depression**

      (a) At a **low-to-moderate dose,** general CNS depression occurs with disinhibition of inhibitory CNS pathways, resulting in decreased anxiety with slurred speech, ataxia, and impaired judgment.

      (b) At a **moderate-to-toxic dose,** further CNS depression results in sedative effects, with a further decrease in mental acuity and motor function.

      (c) At a **toxic dose,** CNS depression results in anesthetic action with profound respiratory depression.

(d) **Acute toxicity with respiratory depression** is a serious medical emergency. Patient may require respiratory support, gastric lavage and possibly hemodialysis, restoration of fluid balance, and treatment of metabolic acidosis and hypothermia.

(2) **Cutaneous vasodilation**
   −is due to probable effects on the vasomotor and thermoregulatory centers, and possibly also by a direct action on vascular smooth muscle.

(3) **Diuresis**
   −is due to an increase in plasma fluid volume and the inhibition of antidiuretic hormone release from the posterior pituitary.

(4) **Uterine smooth muscle relaxation**

(5) **Depressed myocardial contractility**

c. **Chronic pharmacologic effects**
   −increase risk of morbidity and mortality.

   (1) **Cirrhosis**
      (a) Hepatic oxidative metabolism of **ethanol** increases NADH:NAD ratio in the liver, which may account, in part, for altered hepatic metabolism and for accumulation of fat in the liver and eventual cirrhosis.
      (b) Other contributing factors to liver disease may include reduced glutathion as a free radical scavenger and direct acetaldehyde toxicity.

   (2) **Pancreatitis and gastritis**
      −produce increased pancreatic and gastric secretions and decreased gastrointestinal mucosal defense barriers, which may increase the incidence of gastritis.

   (3) **Wernicke's encephalopathy and Korsakoff's psychosis**
      −may result, in part, from **thiamine deficiency** secondary to malnutrition.

   (4) **Fetal alcohol syndrome**
      −results from **maternal abuse;** a fetal syndrome characterized by retarded growth, microencephaly, poorly developed coordination, and also possible mental retardation and congenital heart abnormalities.

   (5) **Other chronic effects**
      −include nutritional deficiency, cancer of the gastrointestinal tract, cardiomyopathy, arrhythmias, and peripheral neuropathy with paresthesias of the hands and feet.

d. **Pharmacologic properties**
   −is **rapidly absorbed** from the stomach and small intestine and is rapidly distributed in total body water. Absorption is delayed by food.
   −is oxidized to acetaldehyde by the liver cytosolic enzyme **alcohol dehydrogenase,** with the generation of NADH. Acetaldehyde is further oxidized by mitochondrial **aldehyde dehydrogenase** to acetate, which can be further metabolized to CO_2 and H_2O.

   (1) Women demonstrate less activity of a stomach alcohol dehydrogenase than men, with resulting higher blood alcohol levels after oral administration.

(2) Ninety percent of absorbed **ethanol** is **oxidized** by the **liver;** remainder is excreted in urine or through the lungs.

(3) Hepatic metabolism shows **zero-order kinetics** (in the adult, approximately 6–8 g (7.5–10 mL) of alcohol is metabolized/hr).

(4) At elevated blood concentrations, **ethanol** may also be oxidized by liver microsomal enzymes, which may be induced with chronic use.

e. Therapeutic uses

–is used as an antiseptic or as a solvent for other drugs.

f. Drug interactions

(1) Additive CNS depressant activity is produced with other **CNS depressants**.

(2) **Acute ethanol use** decreases the metabolism of many drugs by its inhibitory effects on liver metabolism or blood flow.

(3) **Chronic ethanol use** increases the metabolism of numerous drugs by induction of liver microsomal enzymes.

g. Tolerance and dependence

(1) Tolerance to intoxicating and euphoric effects develops with chronic use; this is related to neuronal adaptation and also to some increased metabolism. Little tolerance develops to the potentially lethal action of **ethanol**.

(2) **Physical dependence and withdrawal syndrome**

(a) **Symptoms** occurring over 1–2 days include anxiety, hyperexcitability, weakness, intestinal cramps, hyperreflexia, confusion, delusions, visual hallucinations, delirium, and tremulousness (**delirium tremens**), and seizures. Can be life-threatening in debilitated individuals.

(b) In addition to maintenance and nutritional therapy and long-term psychological support, treatment may include prevention or reversal of seizures with a **benzodiazepine** or **phenytoin,** and administration of a long-acting benzodiazepine as a substitute for **alcohol,** followed by gradual dose reduction over several weeks.

(c) **Disulfiram** [Antabuse] is used as an adjunct in the treatment of **alcoholism**.

–inhibits **aldehyde dehydrogenase,** resulting in the accumulation of toxic levels of acetaldehyde with nausea, vomiting, flushing, headache, sweating, hypotension, and confusion lasting up to 3 hours.

–can be toxic in the presence of small amounts of alcohol (e.g., the amount in some OTC preparations).

–is absorbed rapidly; peak effect takes 12 hours; elimination is slow so that its action may persist for several days.

2. Methanol (wood alcohol)

–is metabolized by alcohol dehydrogenase to formaldehyde, which is then oxidized to formic acid, which is **toxic**.

–produces blurred vision and other visual disturbances when poisoning has occurred. In severe poisoning, bradycardia, acidosis, coma, and seizures are common. In addition to other supportive measures, dialysis and bicarbonate are used for acidosis. Treatment of **methanol toxicity** includes **administration of ethanol** to slow the conversion of methanol to formaldehyde (**ethanol** has a higher affinity for alcohol dehydrogenase).

3. **Barbiturates** (see also section I C 1)

a. **Chemical structure and classification** (Table 4.5)
  −are **weak organic acids** (substituted barbituric acid).
  −are classified according to rate of onset and duration of therapeutic action.

b. **Pharmacologic properties**
  (1) **Redistribution** is responsible for short duration of highly lipid-soluble barbiturates (e.g., **thiopental**).
  (2) **Metabolism** (oxidation and conjugation in the liver) and **excretion** are more important determinants for less lipid-soluble barbiturates.
  (3) **Extensively bound to serum albumin.** At least 25% of phenobarbital dose is excreted unchanged. Alkalinization of the urine enhances excretion and shortens its duration of action.

c. **Therapeutic uses** (see Table 4.5)
  (1) Use as sedative–hypnotics is almost obsolete (pentobarbital is still used to a limited extent); have been replaced by the benzodiazepines.
  (2) **Phenobarbital** is still widely used as an **anticonvulsant**.
  (3) **Thiopental** (and other ultra-short-acting barbiturates) is used as an IV anesthetic.
  (4) **Phenobarbital** and **pentobarbital** are used for detoxification from sedative–hypnotic drugs.

d. **Adverse effects, drug interactions, and contraindications**
  −produce **drowsiness** at hypnotic doses; can interfere with motor and mental performance.
  −potentiate the **depressant effects** of other CNS depressants or drugs with CNS depressant activity, such as antidepressants.

Table 4.5. Classification and Indications of Barbiturates

Drug and Classification	Indications
Ultra-short-acting Thiopental [Pentothal] Methohexital [Brevital] Thiamylal [Surital]	Intravenous general anesthesia
Intermediate-acting Amobarbital [Amytal] Pentobarbital [Nembutal] Secobarbital [Seconal]	Preanesthetic medication and regional anesthesia; sedation and hypnosis (largely supplanted by benzodiazepines)
Long-acting Phenobarbital [Luminal] Mephobarbital [Mebaral]	Seizure disorders; withdrawal syndrome from sedative–hypnotics; congenital hyperbilirubinemia and neonatal jaundice (enhance bilirubin metabolism by induction of microsomal enzymes)

–induce **hepatic enzymes** (cytochrome P-450) and increase their own metabolism or the metabolism of numerous other drugs such as **digitoxin, phenytoin, warfarin,** and **phenylbutazone**.

–increase porphyrin synthesis by induction of hepatic δ-aminolevulinic acid synthase and can precipitate acute intermittent porphyria (1:10,000).

–produce **dose-related respiratory depression with cerebral hypoxia,** possibly leading to coma or death; results from abuse or suicide attempt. **Treatment** includes ventilation, gastric lavage, hemodialysis, osmotic diuretics, and alkalinization of urine for phenobarbital.

–are contraindicated in patients with pulmonary insufficiency.

–depress the medullary vasomotor center with circulatory collapse.

–hepatic and renal disease may prolong barbiturate action.

–use with **MAO inhibitors** potentiates CNS depression.

e. Tolerance and dependence

–abuse and psychological dependence are more likely with the short-acting drugs (e.g., **pentobarbital, secobarbital**). Abuse potential is greater than with the benzodiazepines.

(1) Tolerance

(a) Neuronal adaptation (pharmacodynamic) and enzyme induction (pharmacokinetic) contribute to the development of tolerance.

(b) Cross-tolerance occurs with other CNS depressants, including benzodiazepines and **ethanol**.

(c) Tolerance develops less readily to the potentially lethal respiratory depression.

(2) Physical dependence

(a) Withdrawal symptoms include restlessness, anxiety, insomnia, nausea, aches, pains, paresthesias, sensory hypersensitivity, delusions, hallucinations, muscle weakness, fasciculation, and potentially life-threatening status epilepticus, tonic–clonic seizures, delirium, and coma.

(b) Cross-dependence with other CNS depressants is seen.

(c) For smoother **withdrawal, phenobarbital** is sometimes substituted for shorter-acting agents.

D. CNS stimulants

1. Cocaine and amphetamines

–also include **methamphetamine** [Desoxyn], **dextroamphetamine** [Dexedrine], **phenmetrazine,** [Preludin], **methylphenidate** [Ritalin], **DOM** ("STP"), and **MDMA** ("Ecstasy").

a. Mechanism of action

(1) IV administration or smoking results in intense euphoria ("rush") and increased intensity of other pharmacologic responses.

(2) Cocaine blocks reuptake of catecholamines, particularly dopamine, into nerve terminals in the mesolimbic pathway.

(3) Amphetamine increases release and decreases prejunctional neuronal reuptake of catecholamines, including norepinephrine and dopamine.

–exhibits some direct sympathomimetic action and weakly inhibits MAO.

–at low doses, stimulates the reticular activating system and induces cortical arousal. Increases wakefulness, alertness, self-confidence, and ability to concentrate. Increases motor activity and sexual urge and decreases appetite.

b. Pharmacologic properties

–**cocaine** is snorted or smoked ("crack"); **amphetamine** is taken orally, IV, or smoked (**methamphetamine** crystals, "ice").

(1) Cocaine is more rapidly absorbed and has a much shorter duration of action (1–2 hours) than **amphetamine**.

(2) Smoking "ice" results in a longer-lasting pharmacologic action than smoking "crack."

(3) Cocaine is metabolized by plasma and liver cholinesterase; genetically slow metabolizers are more likely to show severe adverse effects.

c. Therapeutic uses

(1) Amphetamine (controversial): Narcolepsy, obesity, attention-deficit hyperactivity disorder in children

(2) Cocaine: Topical anesthesia

d. Adverse effects and contraindications

–usually occur after repeated IV administration or smoking ("spree," "run"), or after overdose; are due to **excessive sympathomimetic activity**. Include the following:

(1) Anxiety, inability to sleep, hyperactivity, and stereotypic behavior (and sometimes dangerous behavior), often followed by exhaustion ("crash") with increased appetite, and increased sleep with disturbed sleep patterns—**withdrawal pattern**.

(2) Toxic psychosis

–is marked by paranoia and tactile and auditory hallucinations.

–is usually reversible, but may be permanent.

(3) Necrotizing arteritis

–is produced by **amphetamine**.

–sometimes results in brain hemorrhage and renal failure.

(4) Overdose

–results in tachycardia, hypertension, hyperthermia, and tremor.

–possibly causes hypertensive crisis with cerebrovascular hemorrhage.

–occasionally produces seizures, coronary vasospasm, cardiac arrhythmias, MI, shock, and death.

–is more likely with "crack" and "ice."

e. Tolerance and dependence

(1) Extremely strong psychological dependence

(2) Tolerance that may reach extraordinary levels

(3) Withdrawal-like syndrome; includes long periods of sleep, increased appetite, and mental depression

2. Nicotine

–is a constituent of tobacco, along with various gases (carbon monoxide, nitrosamines, hydrogen cyanide, sulfur-containing compounds, and ketones), and particulate matter.

a. Mechanism of action

–causes biphasic CNS stimulation and sedation; biphasic release of adrenal catecholamines; stimulation or inhibition of heart rate and blood pressure; skeletal muscle relaxation; and increased tone, motor activity, and secretions of the gastrointestinal tract.

–mimics the action of ACh at cholinergic nicotinic receptors of ganglia, skeletal muscle, and the CNS.

b. Pharmacologic properties

–is a volatile liquid alkaloid that is well absorbed from the lung after smoking and is rapidly distributed.

–is rapidly metabolized in the liver and eliminated by the kidney; $t_{1/2}$ is approximately 1 hour; is excreted into breast milk.

c. Adverse effects

–contributes to cancer of the lungs, oral cavity, bladder, and pancreas; obstructive lung disease; coronary artery disease; peripheral vascular disease; acceleration of atherosclerosis; and increased incidence of abortion.

d. Tolerance and dependence

(1) Tolerance

–develops rapidly and is long-lasting.

–is primarily cellular tolerance with some metabolic tolerance.

–may be due to changes in the activity of peripheral and CNS nicotinic receptors.

(2) Dependence

–produces strong psychological dependence.

–**withdrawal-like syndrome** occurs within 24 hours and persists for weeks or months. Dizziness, tremor, increased blood pressure, craving, irritability, anxiety, restlessness, difficulty in concentration, drowsiness, headache, sleep disturbances, increased appetite, gastrointestinal complaints, nausea, and vomiting may occur.

e. Nicotine polacrilex

–is a nicotine resin contained in a **chewing gum** [Nicorette] that has some therapeutic value for avoiding withdrawal symptoms while patient undergoes behavioral modification to overcome psychological dependence.

–because of potential nicotine overdose, the **gum** or **nicotine patch** should be used with **caution** in patients who continue to use cigarettes. **Clonidine** also has been used with some reported success.

E. Hallucinogens (psychodysleptics, psychotomimetics)

1. LSD (*d*-lysergic acid diethylamide), mescaline, psilocybin, and belladona alkaloids

a. **LSD** is an extremely **potent synthetic drug** that when taken orally causes altered consciousness, euphoria, increased sensory awareness ("mind expansion"), perceptual distortions, and increased introspection.

b. The **mechanism of psychotomimetic effects** is **unknown,** but it may be related to the action of LSD at prejunctional serotonin receptors to inhibit the release of serotonin in the CNS.

    c. Sympathomimetic activity includes pupillary dilation, increased blood pressure, and tachycardia.

    d. Adverse effects include "flashback," panic reactions, misjudgment, suicide, and psychosis; anticholinergic drugs or benzodiazepines are used to treat confusion and flashbacks.

    e. Rapid and high degree of tolerance to behavioral effects; **cross-tolerance** with **mescaline** and **psilocybin,** hallucinogens that are less potent than LSD; no physical dependence.

2. Phencyclidine (PCP)

    –is a **veterinary anesthetic** used initially in humans as a dissociative anesthetic (replaced by **ketamine**).

    –is taken orally and IV and is also "snorted" and smoked.

    –produces euphoria, hallucinations, changed body image, and increased sense of isolation and loneliness; impairs judgment and increases aggressiveness. Behavioral actions are thought to be related to either increased activity of dopamine (due to inhibition of dopamine reuptake) or to allosteric antagonist activity at receptors for the excitatory amino acid glutamate.

    –also has sympathomimetic and cholinergic activity.

    –**overdose** may result in seizures, respiratory depression, cardiac arrest, and coma; treatment includes emesis, maintenance of respiration, control of seizures (with **diazepam**), and therapy directed at behavioral manifestations, possibly including antipsychotic drug therapy.

F. Marijuana

1. Active ingredient is **Δ-9 tetrahydrocannabinol;** mechanism of action is unknown.

2. Initial phase consists of euphoria, uncontrolled laughter, loss of sense of time, depersonalization, and increased introspection. **Second phase** includes relaxation, dreamlike state, sleepiness, and difficulty in concentration.

3. Physiological effects include increased pulse rate, tachycardia, and characteristic reddening of the conjunctiva.

4. Therapeutically used to decrease intraocular pressure for treatment of **glaucoma**. Analog **dronabinol** [Marinol] is used as an antiemetic in **cancer chemotherapy**.

5. Tolerance and psychological or physical **dependence** are difficult to demonstrate.

6. Adverse effects related to chronic use are controversial. Include:

    a. Chronic effects similar to cigarette smoking

    b. Exacerbation of preexisting paranoia or psychosis

    c. "Amotivational syndrome"

    d. Impairment of short-term memory

    e. Disturbances of the immune, reproductive, and thermoregulatory systems

Review Test

Directions: Each of the numbered items or incomplete statements in this section is followed by answers or by completions of the statement. Select the **one** lettered answer or completion that is **best** in each case.

1. Epinephrine is often used in combination with local anesthetics to

(A) increase the duration of action of local anesthetics
(B) increase the rate of redistribution of local anesthetics from the injection site
(C) enhance the metabolism of local anesthetics by plasma cholinesterase
(D) decrease the effects of local anesthetics on Type A nerve fibers
(E) all of the above

2. Which of the following statements concerning the pharmacology of local anesthetics is true?

(A) Type C nerve fibers are generally affected first
(B) The ester class of local anesthetics is more likely than the amide class to cause hypersensitivity reactions
(C) The amide class of local anesthetics is more likely than the ester class to cause systemic effects
(D) The therapeutic action of local anesthetics is due to sodium channel blockade
(E) All of the above

3. Morphine is used therapeutically

(A) to suppress the withdrawal syndrome associated with the chronic use of alcohol
(B) to induce miosis
(C) to treat severe constipation
(D) to relieve pain associated with a heart attack
(E) all of the above

4. Which of the following adverse effects is caused by thioridazine?

(A) Constipation
(B) Orthostatic hypotension
(C) Sedation
(D) Tardive dyskinesia
(E) All of the above

5. The rigidity of parkinsonian syndrome may be reduced by which of the following drugs?

(A) Benztropine
(B) Bromocriptine
(C) Selegiline
(D) Pergolide
(E) All of the above

6. Which of the following statements concerning lithium is true?

(A) Lithium is used to control agitation associated with schizophrenia
(B) Retention of lithium is enhanced by a high-sodium diet
(C) Early signs of lithium toxicity may include tremors
(D) The onset of lithium action occurs within 24 hours
(E) All of the above

7. Which of the following effects is produced by tricyclic antidepressant drugs?

(A) Increase in antihypertensive effect of guanethidine
(B) Hypertensive crisis
(C) Increased absorption of an oral dose of levodopa
(D) Precipitation of narrow-angle glaucoma
(E) All of the above

8. Which of the following conditions might lengthen the induction time of general anesthetics?

(A) Circulatory shock
(B) Pulmonary emphysema
(C) Preanesthetic medication with diazepam
(D) Raising the anesthetic concentration in the inspired air
(E) All of the above

9. Benzodiazepines differ from barbiturates in that benzodiazepines

(A) Facilitate the action of GABA on neuronal chloride channels
(B) Have anticonvulsant activity
(C) May induce physical dependence
(D) Have a higher margin of safety than barbiturates

10. Which of the following agents is the primary drug for treatment of major motor seizures and partial seizures?

(A) Clonazepam
(B) Ethosuximide
(C) Carbamazepine
(D) Trimethadione
(E) All of the above

11. Benzodiazepines are used therapeutically for all of the following indications EXCEPT

(A) panic disorder
(B) schizophrenia
(C) status epilepticus
(D) insomnia
(E) ethanol withdrawal

12. Which of the following effects is produced by morphine?

(A) Relief of dyspnea accompanying pulmonary edema
(B) Decreased sensitivity of the respiratory center to CO_2
(C) Miosis that can be blocked by atropine
(D) Vasodilation of cerebral blood vessels
(E) All of the above

13. Which one of the following conditions may be produced by frequent administration of high-dose chlorpromazine?

(A) Lens opacities
(B) Skin pigmentation
(C) Obstructive jaundice
(D) Tardive dyskinesia
(E) All of the above

14. Which of the following drugs may produce orthostatic hypotension?

(A) Imipramine
(B) Morphine
(C) Chlorpromazine
(D) Tranylcypromine
(E) All of the above

15. How does haloperidol differ from trifluoperazine?

(A) Is more therapeutically efficacious as an antipsychotic
(B) Is less likely to produce sedation
(C) Is a phenothiazine
(D) Is less likely to produce parkinsonian syndrome
(E) All of the above

16. Which of the following phrases best describes the mechanism of action of carbidopa?

(A) Increases dopa decarboxylase activity
(B) Reduces levodopa-induced nausea and vomiting
(C) Reduces levodopa-induced dyskinesias
(D) Increases dopamine synthesis in the liver
(E) All of the above

17. Which of the following statements concerning barbiturates is true?

(A) Barbiturates can increase bleeding time when administered to patients taking anticoagulants
(B) Barbiturates are contraindicated in patients with acute intermittent porphyria
(C) Patients tolerant to the therapeutic actions of barbiturates are also tolerant to the analgesic effect of morphine
(D) Barbiturates are used to prevent withdrawal symptoms associated with heroin dependence
(E) All of the above

18. Which of the following effects is associated with benzodiazepines?

(A) Paradoxical excitement
(B) Ataxia
(C) Sedation
(D) Amnesia
(E) All of the above

19. Which of the following statements concerning ethyl alcohol is true?

(A) Exerts an antidiuretic effect
(B) Is metabolized to acetaldehyde by alcohol dehydrogenase
(C) Reduces the rate of methanol metabolism to its toxic products
(D) Can suppress the heroin withdrawal syndrome
(E) All of the above

20. Which of the following conditions is treated with benztropine?

(A) Parkinsonian disorders
(B) Manic-depressive disorders
(C) Huntington's disease
(D) Tardive dyskinesia
(E) All of the above

21. A hypertensive crisis is most likely to result from the action of drugs from which one of the following drug classes?

(A) Tricyclic antidepressants
(B) Barbiturates
(C) Opioids
(D) MAO inhibitors
(E) All of the above

22. Which of the following statements concerning local anesthetics is true?

(A) Local anesthetics accelerate nerve impulse conduction
(B) Local anesthetics are often used in combination with diuretic drugs that restrict their diffusion from nerves and prolong their action
(C) Cocaine is the only local anesthetic that causes vasoconstriction
(D) Local anesthetics bind to the closed sodium channels on the outside of neurons
(E) All of the above

23. Which of the following agents may be considered the drug of choice for the treatment of absence seizures?

(A) Phenytoin
(B) Phenobarbital
(C) Carbamazepine
(D) Ethosuximide

Directions: Each group of items in this section consists of lettered options followed by a set of numbered items. For each item, select the **one** lettered option that is most closely associated with it. Each lettered option may be selected once, more than once, or not at all.

Questions 24–27

Match each of the descriptions below with the appropriate drug.

(A) Loperamide
(B) Codeine
(C) Naloxone
(D) Methadone
(E) Dextromethorphan

24. Weak-to-moderate opioid agonist with a higher ratio of oral to parenteral activity than morphine

25. Antitussive with no dependence liability

26. Opioid-receptor antagonist

27. Strong opioid agonist that has a longer duration of action and produces a less intense withdrawal syndrome than morphine

Questions 28–31

Match the agent below with the phrase that most closely describes its mechanism of action.

(A) Inhibits reuptake of biogenic amines into nerve endings
(B) Blocks dopamine receptors
(C) Blocks muscarinic cholinoceptors
(D) Inhibits dopa decarboxylase

28. Haloperidol

29. Benztropine

30. Imipramine

31. Thioridazine

Questions 32–35

Match each of the pharmacologic effects with the drug most closely related to it.

(A) Cocaine
(B) LSD
(C) PCP
(D) Marijuana

32. Aggressive behavior
33. Action at serotonin receptors
34. Vasoconstriction
35. Reddening of the conjunctiva

Answers and Explanations

1–A. Epinephrine causes local vasoconstriction, thus prolonging the action of local anesthetics by limiting their diffusion away from their site of action.

2–E. All of the statements are true.

3–D. Morphine is used to relieve the pain associated with myocardial infarction. It can suppress the opioid withdrawal syndrome but not the withdrawal syndrome associated with other classes of CNS depressants. Morphine and other opioids induce constipation and can be used to treat diarrhea. Miosis is an adverse effect of morphine.

4–E. Thioridazine, one of the low-potency antipsychotic drugs known as phenothiazines, is more likely to cause constipation, orthostatic hypotension, and sedation than the high-potency antipsychotic drugs such as trifluoperazine or haloperidol. Almost all antipsychotic drugs may cause tardive dyskinesia, but extrapyramidal effects are least likely to occur with the use of thioridazine and clozapine.

5–E. Each drug listed either increases dopamine or decreases acetylcholine neurotransmission in the nigrostriatal tract to restore the balanced activity of these endogenous substances in the parkinsonian patient.

6–C. Severe tremors, along with confusion, drowsiness, vomiting, ataxia, and dizziness, are an early sign of lithium toxicity. Retention of lithium may be enhanced by a low-sodium diet because sodium competes with lithium for reuptake in the kidney. Onset of lithium action may take a week or more; the drug is used to normalize mood in patients with mania or bipolar disorder.

7–D. Tricyclic antidepressants can precipitate narrow-angle glaucoma through their muscarinic–cholinoceptor antagonist activity. They may cause hypotension and may block neuronal uptake of guanethidine and thus decrease its antihypertensive action. They also may decrease gastrointestinal absorption of levodopa.

8–B. Emphysema decreases anesthetic exchange. Circulatory shock decreases pulmonary blood flow, thereby increasing the rate of reduction. Raising the anesthetic concentration in the inspired air will increase the rate of transfer to the blood and the rate of induction. Diazepam increases the depth of respiration; opioids, such as morphine, decrease it.

9–D. Benzodiazepines are much safer than barbiturates because they cause minimal CNS depression. Both drug classes facilitate the action of GABA, although by different mechanisms of action. They are both used to prevent seizures, and both can result in physical dependence with long-term use.

10–C. Carbamazepine (or valproic acid) is the drug of choice for major motor (tonic–clonic) seizures and for partial (focal) seizures. Clonazepam is used to treat minor motor seizures, and ethosuximide is indicated for absence seizures.

11–B. Benzodiazepines are not used to treat schizophrenia. Alprazolam is the benzodiazepine of choice in the treatment of panic disorder, and IV diazepam is preferred for status epilepticus and to prevent withdrawal syndrome associated with CNS depressants such as ethanol. Triazolam, flurazepam, and temazepam are indicated for insomnia.

12–E. Morphine produces all of the above effects. It decreases the sensitivity of the respiratory center to CO_2 and directly inhibits the respiratory center, leading to respiratory depression. This effect on respiration may be responsible for morphine's beneficial effect when used to treat dyspnea and for cerebral vasodilation. Morphine produces miosis by stimulation or the Edinger-Westphal nucleus of the oculomotor nerve; this is mediated by acetylcholine and can be blocked by atropine.

13–E. Chlorpromazine is associated with all of these adverse effects. Because of its numerous adverse effects, some authorities consider it to be an obsolete antipsychotic agent.

14–E. Antipsychotic drugs, such as chlorpromazine, and antidepressants, such as imipramine and tranylcypromine, produce orthostatic hypotension as a result of α-adrenoceptor blockade. Morphine produces hypotension by inhibition of the vasomotor center in the brain stem, which causes peripheral vasodilation.

15–B. Haloperidol, a butyrophenone, has the same therapeutic efficacy as other antipsychotic drugs. It is a high-potency drug that is more likely than a low-potency antipsychotic drug, such as triflupromazine, to result in a parkinsonian-like syndrome and is less likely to result in sedation.

16–B. Carbidopa inhibits peripheral dopa decarboxylase activity, resulting in reduced conversion of levodopa to dopamine. Administration of less levodopa to treat parkinsonian disorder reduces the incidence of peripheral adverse effects such as nausea and vomiting, but not centrally mediated effects such as dyskinesia.

17–B. Barbiturates induce liver microsomal enzymes that increase porphyrin synthesis and increase the metabolism and inactivation of certain anticoagulants. Barbiturates show cross-dependence with other sedative–hypnotic drugs but not with opioids.

18–E. Short-acting benzodiazepines are used as preanesthetic medications because of their anxiolytic, sedative, and amnestic effects. Daytime drowsiness and ataxia are commonly produced by benzodiazepines and may impair judgment and interfere with motor skills. Paradoxical excitement is a rare adverse effect of these drugs.

19–C. Ethyl alcohol is used to treat methanol toxicity because it slows the conversion of methanol to formaldehyde through its greater affinity for alcohol dehydrogenase. Ethyl alcohol has diuretic activity. Disulfiram inhibits acetaldehyde dehydrogenase, not alcohol dehydrogenase. There is no cross-dependence between ethyl alcohol and opioids.

20–A. Benztropine, a cholinoceptor antagonist, is used to treat parkinsonian disorders. It has no effect on or may exacerbate manic-depressive disorders, Huntington's disease, or tardive dyskinesia.

21–D. MAO inhibitors such as tranylcypromine may precipitate a hypertensive crisis when used in the presence of certain foods that contain tyramine, or in the presence of certain sympathomimetic agents. Note also that opioids, particularly meperidine, may also (although rarely) precipitate a hypertensive crisis when used with MAO inhibitors.

22–C. All local anesthetics except cocaine are vasodilators. Epinephrine, a vasoconstrictor, is administered with local anesthetics to reduce systemic absorption and prolong their action. Local anesthetics bind to the open sodium channel on the inner aspect of the axonal membrane. This results in a dose-dependent decrease in nerve impulse conduction.

23–D. Ethosuximide is the drug of choice for absence seizures. Carbamazepine, phenytoin, and phenobarbital are used to treat partial seizures and tonic-clonic seizures; phenytoin is also used to treat status epilepticus.

24–B. Unlike morphine, codeine is well absorbed by the oral route.

25–E. Unlike the antitussive codeine, dextromethorphan has no analgesic or addictive properties.

26–C. Naloxone is a competitive antagonist at all opioid receptors.

27–D. Methadone is often substituted for other opioids for treatment of physical dependence.

28–B. Haloperidol is a competitive antagonist at dopamine receptors.

29–C. Benztropine is a competitive antagonist at muscarinic cholinoceptors.

30–A. In addition to inhibiting reuptake of biogenic amines, imipramine has some anticholinergic activity that accounts for some of its adverse effects.

31–B. In addition to being a competitive antagonist at dopamine receptors, thioridazine has some anticholinergic activity that accounts for some of its adverse effects.

32–C. PCP typically impairs judgment and increases aggressiveness, perhaps by increasing the activity of dopamine or by allosteric antagonist activity at receptors for the excitatory amino acid glutamate.

33–B. It is believed that the psychomimetic effects of LSD are related to its action at prejunctional serotonin receptors to inhibit the release of serotonin.

34–A. Cocaine, a controlled substance subject to abuse, is the only local anesthetic that produces vasoconstriction.

35–D. Effects of marijuana use include increased pulse rate, tachycardia, and characteristic reddening of the conjunctiva.

5

Autacoids, Ergots, Anti-inflammatory Agents, and Immunosuppressive Agents

I. Histamine and Antihistamines

A. Histamine (Figure 5.1)

—is a small molecule produced by decarboxylation of the amino acid histidine, catalyzed by the enzyme L-histidine decarboxylase in a reaction that requires pyridoxal phosphate.

1. Synthesis

—is found in many tissues, including the brain. Stored and found in the highest amounts in mast cells and basophils. **Mast cells,** which are especially abundant in the respiratory tract, skin (especially hands and feet), gastrointestinal tract, and blood vessels, store histamine in a granule bound in a complex with heparin, adenosine triphosphate (ATP), and an acidic protein.

—**release** can occur by two processes:

a. Energy- and Ca^{2+}-independent release (displacement)

—induced by drugs such as **morphine, tubocurarine, guanethidine,** and amine antibiotics. In addition, mast cell damage is caused by noxious agents such as venom or by mechanical trauma that can release histamine.

b. Energy- and Ca^{2+}-dependent degranulation reaction

—release from mast cells is induced by immunoglobulin E (IgE) fixation to mast cells (**sensitization**) and subsequent exposure to specific antigen; complement activation (IgG- or IgM-mediated) may also induce degranulation.

2. Mechanism of action

a. Histamine (H_1) receptors

—are found in the brain, heart, bronchi, gastrointestinal tract, and vascular smooth muscles.

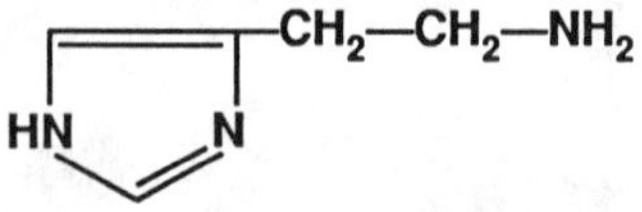

$$\text{HN}\underset{\text{N}}{\overset{\text{CH}_2-\text{CH}_2-\text{NH}_2}{\boxed{}}}$$

Figure 5.1. Structure of histamine.

−the mechanism coupling stimulation of the H_1-receptor to biological response is not clear. Most evidence supports a role for altered Ca^{2+} flux and the phosphatidylinositol system; some evidence suggests that H_1 effects are mediated by changes in cyclic GMP (cGMP).

b. Histamine (H_2)-receptors

−are found in brain, heart, and parietal cells.
−response is coupled to cyclic AMP (cAMP).

c. Histamine (H_3)-receptors

−are found in the central nervous system (CNS) and peripheral nervous system (PNS) at presynaptic nerve terminals.
−stimulation of H_3-receptors on nerve cells causes a decrease in histamine release; presence on vagal nerve may cause decreased acetylcholine (ACh) release.

B. Histamine agonists

1. Prototypes

−include **histamine, betazole** [Histalog], and **impromidine**.

a. Betazole has approximately tenfold greater activity at H_2-receptors than at H_1-receptors.

b. Impromidine is an investigational agent; ratio of H_2:H_1 activity is about 10,000.

2. Uses

−are primarily diagnostic. Are used in **allergy testing** to assess histamine sensitivity, and in **test of gastric secretory function** (have been largely supplanted for this use by **pentagastrin** [Peptavlon], a synthetic peptide analog of gastrin with fewer adverse effects).

3. Adverse effects

−can be quite severe; include flushing, burning sensation, hypotension, tachycardia, and bronchoconstriction.

C. Histamine (H_1)-receptor antagonists

−are competitive inhibitors at the H_1-receptor.

1. Classification

a. First-generation agents

(1) Alkylamines

−include **chlorpheniramine** and **brompheniramine**.
−produce slight sedation.
−are the antihistamines used most frequently in the United States.

(2) Ethanolamines

−include **dimenhydrinate, diphenhydramine, doxylamine, and clemastine** [Tavist].

　　　　　　　　　　–produce marked **sedation; doxylamine** marketed only as a
　　　　　　　　　　sleeping aid.
　　　　　　　　　　–also act as **antiemetics**.
　　　　　　　　(3) Ethylenediamines
　　　　　　　　　　–include **pyrilamine, antazoline,** and **tripelennamine**.
　　　　　　　　　　–produce moderate **sedation** and **gastrointestinal upset**.
　　　　　　　　(4) Piperazines
　　　　　　　　　　–include **meclizine** and **cyclizine**.
　　　　　　　　　　–produce marked **adverse gastrointestinal effects** and **moder-
　　　　　　　　　　ate sedation**.
　　　　　　　　　　–are **antiemetics**.
　　　　　　　　(5) Phenothiazines
　　　　　　　　　　–include **promethazine** and **cyproheptadine**.
　　　　　　　　　　–produce marked **sedation**.
　　　　　　　　　　–are **antiemetics**.
　　　　　　　　　　–are also weak α-adrenoceptor antagonists.
　　　　b. Second-generation (nonsedating) agents
　　　　　　　(1) Piperidine: terfenadine [Seldane]
　　　　　　　　　–produces little sedation; poor penetration into the CNS.
　　　　　　　(2) Benzimidazole: astemizole [Hismanal]
　　　　　　　　　–is less sedating.

　　2. Pharmacologic properties (Table 5.1)
　　　　–are well absorbed after oral administration; effects are usually seen in 30
　　　　minutes (maximal effects at 1–2 hours); duration of action 3–6 hours.
　　　　–are lipid-soluble; most first-generation agents cross the blood–brain bar-
　　　　rier, a property reduced with second-generation agents.
　　　　–are metabolized in the liver; many induce microsomal enzymes and alter
　　　　their own metabolism and that of other drugs.

　　3. Pharmacologic actions
　　　　–many, especially the **ethanolamines, phenothiazines,** and **ethylene-
　　　　diamines,** have muscarinic-cholinergic antagonist activity.
　　　　–most are effective local anesthetics, probably due to a blockade of sodium
　　　　channels in excitable tissues. **Dimenhydrinate** and **promethazine** are
　　　　potent local anesthetics.
　　　　–relax histamine-induced contraction of bronchial smooth muscle and
　　　　have limited use in allergic bronchospasm.
　　　　–block the vasodilator action of histamine.

Table 5.1. Major Pharmacologic Properties of H_1-Receptor Antagonists

Drug Class	Duration of Action	Antihistamine Potency	Anticholinergic Potency	Antiemetic Potency	Sedative Effect
Alkylamines	4–25 hr	+ + +	+ +	Marginal	+ +
Ethanolamines	4–6 hr	+ +	+ + +	+ + +	+ +
Ethylenediamines	4–6 hr	+	+ +	Marginal	+
Piperazines	4–24 hr	+ +	+ +	+ + +	+
Phenothiazines	4–24 hr	+/+ + +	+ + +	+ + + +	+ + +
Second-generation agents	12–24 hr	+ + +	Marginal	None	Marginal

   —inhibit histamine-induced increases in capillary permeability.
   —block mucus secretion and sensory nerve stimulation.
   —frequently cause CNS depression (marked by sedation, decreased alertness, and decreased appetite). In children and some adults, stimulate the CNS.

   4. Therapeutic uses

   a. Treatment of **allergic rhinitis and conjunctivitis;** are also used to treat the common cold based on their anticholinergic properties, but they are only marginally effective for this use. **Diphenhydramine** also has an antitussive effect not mediated by H_1-receptor antagonism.

   b. Treatment of **urticaria and atopic dermatitis**

   c. Sedatives; several (**doxylamine, diphenhydramine**) are marketed as over-the-counter (OTC) sleep aids.

   d. Prevention of **motion sickness**

   e. Appetite suppressants

   5. Adverse effects

   —produce sedation (synergistic with alcohol and other depressants), dizziness, and loss of appetite.
   —can cause gastrointestinal upset, nausea, and constipation or diarrhea.
   —produce anticholinergic effects (dry mouth, blurred vision, and urine retention).

D. Histamine (H_2)-receptor antagonists

   —include **cimetidine, ranitidine, famotidine,** and **nizatidine**.
   —are competitive antagonists at the H_2-receptor, which predominates in the gastric parietal cell.
   —are used in the treatment of gastrointestinal disorders.
   —promote healing of **gastric and duodenal ulcers** and are used to treat hypersecretory states such as **Zollinger-Ellison syndrome**.

E. Inhibitor of histamine release: cromolyn [Intal]

   —is a poorly absorbed salt; must be administered by **inhalation**.
   —inhibits the release of histamine and other autacoids from the mast cell.
   —is used prophylactically in the treatment of **asthma**.
   —produces adverse effects that are usually confined to the site of application; include sore throat and dry mouth.

II. Serotonin and Serotonin Antagonists

A. Serotonin (5-hydroxytryptamine, 5HT)

   1. Biosynthesis and distribution

   —is synthesized from the amino acid L-tryptophan by hydroxylation and decarboxylation.
   —approximately 90% is found in the enterochromaffin cells of the gastrointestinal tract. Much of the remaining 10% is found in the platelets; small amounts are found in other tissues, including the brain. Platelets acquire serotonin from the circulation during passage through the intestine by a specific and highly active uptake mechanism.
   —is stored in granules as a complex with adenosine triphosphate (ATP).
   —major breakdown product is **5-hydroxyindoleacetic acid (5-HIAA)**.

2. Mechanism of action

—acts on several classes of 5HT-receptors, which are located on cell membranes of many tissues:

a. 5HT$_1$ (subtypes 5HT$_{1A}$ through 5HT$_{1E}$); stimulation contracts arterial smooth muscle, especially in carotid circulation; at presynaptic sites, neuronal serotonin release is inhibited.

b. 5HT$_2$; stimulation causes contraction of vascular and intestinal smooth muscle and increases microcirculation and vascular permeability; stimulation on platelet membranes causes platelet aggregation; in the CNS, this receptor mediates hallucinogenic effects.

c. 5HT$_3$; stimulation in the *area postrema* causes nausea and vomiting; stimulation on peripheral sensory neurons causes pain.

B. Serotonin antagonists and agonists

1. Cyproheptadine [Periactin]

—is a potent H$_1$-receptor antagonist of the phenothiazine class; blocks both 5HT$_1$ and 5HT$_2$ receptors.

—is used most frequently to limit diarrhea and intestinal spasms produced by **serotonin-secreting carcinoid tumors** and postgastrectomy **dumping syndrome**.

—produces sedation and anticholinergic actions.

2. Sumatriptan

—is a 5HT$_{1D}$-receptor agonist.

—promotes contraction of vessels in carotid circulation, with minimal effects on other organs.

—is used for treatment of **acute migraine**.

3. Ondansetron [Zofran]

—is a 5HT$_3$-receptor antagonist.

—is highly effective in treating **nausea and vomiting associated with chemotherapy**.

4. Ketanserin

—is a specific 5HT$_2$-receptor antagonist; also antagonizes α-adrenergic, H$_1$, and dopamine receptors.

—is an investigational drug that has been found to lower blood pressure in experimentally induced hypertension.

III. Ergots

A. Structure

—include a wide variety of compounds sharing the tetracyclic ergoline nucleus that are produced by the fungi *Claviceps purpurea*. These agents have a strong structural similarity to the neurotransmitters norepinephrine, dopamine, and serotonin.

1. Amine ergot alkaloids

—include **ergonovine, methysergide, lysergic acid** and **LSD,** and **methylergonovine**.

2. Peptide ergot alkaloids

–include **ergotamine, ergocristine, bromocriptine,** and **pergolide** [Permax].

B. Mechanism of action

–display varying degrees of agonist or antagonist activity in three receptor types: α-adrenoceptors, dopamine receptors, and serotonin receptors.

–pharmacologic application is determined by the relative affinity and efficacy of the individual agents for these receptor systems. Many agents exhibit partial agonist activities and therefore can cause either stimulatory or inhibitory effects.

C. Pharmacologic properties (Table 5.2)

–may be administered parenterally, rectally, sublingually, as inhalants, or orally, and vary widely in their intestinal absorption. Amine alkaloids are slowly and relatively poorly absorbed; the peptide alkaloids are completely absorbed.

–are extensively metabolized to compounds of varying activity and half-life.

D. Therapeutic uses

1. Postpartum hemorrhage

–**ergonovine** [Ergotrate] and **methylergonovine** [Methergine], the most uterine-selective agents, cause prolonged and forceful **contraction of uterine smooth muscle.**

–should not be used to induce labor.

–uterine sensitivity varies with hormonal status; uterus at term most sensitive.

2. Migraine

a. **Ergotamine** [Ergomar, Ergostat] is the preferred drug for relief of acute attack.

–major effect is **cerebral vasoconstriction;** reverses the rebound vasodilation that is the probable cause of pain.

Table 5.2. Pharmacologic Properties of Ergots

Drug	Receptor	Target Tissue and Response	Therapeutic Uses	Toxicity
Ergonovine	α-Adrenoceptor agonist	Uterine smooth muscle contraction	Postpartum hemorrhage	Hypertension, nausea
Ergotamine	α-Adrenoceptor agonist, 5HT-receptor agonist	Vascular smooth muscle; vasoconstriction	Acute migraine attacks	Nausea, diarrhea
Methysergide	5HT-Receptor antagonist	Vascular smooth muscle; prevent initial vasoconstriction	Migraine prophylaxis	Fibroblastic changes
Bromocriptine, pergolide	Dopamine agonists	Breast, uterus, pituitary; suppress lactation and decrease growth hormone levels	Hyperprolactinemia, amenorrhea, acromegaly	Dose-related effects, ranging from nausea to parkinsonian-like symptoms

–acts as a central 5HT-receptor and α-adrenoceptor agonist.
–is most effective if administered in the early (prodromal) stages of attack to reverse rebound vasodilation.
–is frequently **combined with caffeine,** which probably increases absorption.
–produces long-lasting and cumulative effects; weekly dosage must be strictly limited.

   b. Methysergide [Sansert] is used for **prophylaxis of migraine**.
–acts as serotonin-receptor antagonist and inhibits initial vasoconstriction in the early stages of migraine.
–is effective in 60% of patients for prophylaxis of migraine; ineffective after onset of attack.
–cumulative toxicity requires drug-free periods of 3–4 weeks every 6 months.

   c. Propranolol is also an effective agent for prophylaxis of migraine.

3. Hyperprolactinemia
–**bromocriptine mesylate** [Parlodel] and **pergolide** [Permax], dopaminergic agonists, cause specific **inhibition of prolactin secretion** (elevated prolactin secretion can induce infertility and amenorrhea in women and galactorrhea in men and women).
–are used to treat prolactin-secreting tumors of the pituitary, to counteract central dopaminergic antagonists, and to suppress normal lactation.
–are used as adjuncts to agents such as **levodopa** in the management of **Parkinson's disease** (not a prolactin-lowering effect).
–reduce growth hormone secretion.

4. Diagnosis of variant angina
–**ergonovine** produces a diagnostic vasoconstriction of coronary arteries that are prone to vasospasm, as in variant angina. Administered IV during angiography.

E. Adverse effects

1. Most serious is **prolonged vasospasm;** can lead to gangrene and is most frequently caused by **ergotamine** and **ergonovine**.

2. Most common is **gastrointestinal disturbances**.

3. Methysergide toxicity produces retroperitoneal fibroplasia and coronary and endocardial fibrosis, as well as CNS stimulation and hallucinations.

IV. Kinins

A. Biosynthesis
–kinins are found in the circulation and tissues as larger-molecular-weight precursors, **kininogens**. Specific serine proteases called **kallikreins** convert kininogens to the active kinins. Kallikreins are activated by Hageman factor, trypsin, and kinins.
–the major kinins are a group of three peptides with potent actions as vasodilators.

1. Bradykinin

–has the following amino acid sequence: Arg-Pro-Pro-Gly-Phe-Ser-Pro-Phe-Arg.

2. Lysyl-bradykinin (kallidin) has additional lysine residue on the *N*-terminus of the bradykinin.

3. Methionyl-lysyl-bradykinin has additional methionine and lysine dipeptide on *N*-terminus of bradykinin.

B. Actions

–effects mediated by specific bradykinin receptors (**B-receptors**).

–produce vasodilation by relaxation of precapillary arteriolar smooth muscle (10 times more potent than **histamine**), as well as vasoconstriction of capacitance vessels; these combined effects cause a rapid but transient fall in blood pressure.

–stimulate gastrointestinal smooth muscle.

–may play a role in the inflammatory process.

–activate peripheral nerve endings that sense pain.

C. Therapeutic uses

–agents that alter kinin release are under investigation for treatment of **inflammation**.

–**aprotinin** [Trasylol] inhibits kallikreins and thus the formation of kinins.

V. Eicosanoids

–are a large group of autacoids with potent effects on virtually every tissue in the body; are derived from metabolism of 20-carbon, unsaturated fatty acids (**eicosanoic acids**).

–are collectively called eicosanoids and include the prostaglandins, thromboxanes, leukotrienes, hydroperoxyeicosatetraenoic acids (**HPETEs**), and hydroxyeicosatetraenoic acids (**HETEs**).

A. Biosynthesis (Figure 5.2)

1. Arachidonic acid, the most common precursor of the eicosanoids, is formed by two pathways:

a. Phospholipase A_2-mediated production from membrane phospholipids; inhibited by glucocorticoids.

b. Phospholipase C in concert with diglyceride lipase can also produce free arachidonate.

2. Eicosanoids are synthesized by two pathways:

a. The **prostaglandin H synthase (cyclooxygenase) pathway** produces **thromboxane,** the primary prostaglandins (**prostaglandin E,** or PGE; **prostaglandin F,** or PGF; and **prostaglandin D,** or PGD), and **prostacyclin (PGI_2).**

b. The **lipoxygenase pathway** produces the HPETEs, HETEs, and the leukotrienes.

c. Additional metabolites of the HPETEs, hepoxilins and lipoxins, have been identified but their biological role is unclear.

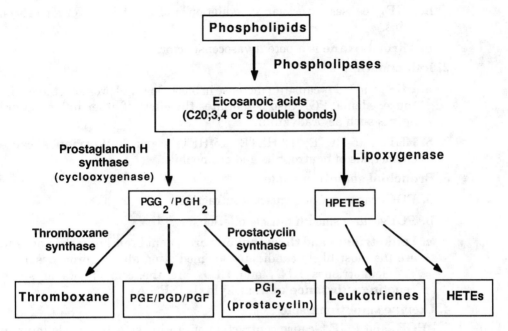

Figure 5.2. Biosynthesis of eicosanoids.

3. The eicosanoids all have short plasma half-lives (typically 0.5–5 minutes). Most catabolism occurs in the lung.

   a. Prostaglandins are metabolized by prostaglandin 15-OH dehydrogenase (PDGH) to 15-keto metabolites, which are excreted in the urine.

   b. **Thromboxane A$_2$ (TxA$_2$)** is rapidly hydrated to the less active TxB$_2$.

   c. **PGI$_2$** is hydrolyzed to 6-keto-PGF$_{1\alpha}$.

4. Various eicosanoids are synthesized throughout the body; synthesis can be very tissue-specific:

   a. **PGI$_2$** is synthesized in endothelial and vascular smooth muscle cells.

   b. **Thromboxane** synthesis occurs primarily in platelets.

   c. **HPETEs, HETEs,** and the **leukotrienes** are synthesized predominantly in mast cells, white blood cells, airway epithelium, and platelets.

B. Actions

–there is no universal mediator of eicosanoid action. A separate cell-surface receptor may mediate the activities of each class of metabolite. Virtually all of the known second-messenger systems have been implicated in the action of the eicosanoids, including stimulation or inhibition of cAMP and cGMP and alterations in Ca^{2+} flux.

1. Vascular smooth muscle

   a. **PGE$_2$** and **PGI$_2$** are potent vasodilators in most vascular beds. **PGE$_2$** also antagonizes the effects of vasoconstrictor substances such as norepinephrine.

b. PGF$_{2\alpha}$ causes arteriolar vasodilation and constriction of superficial veins.

c. Thromboxane is a potent vasoconstrictor.

2. Inflammation

a. PGE$_2$ and **PGI$_2$** cause an increase in blood flow and promote, but do not cause, edema. PGE also potentiates the effect of other inflammatory agents such as bradykinin.

b. HETEs (5-HETE, 12-HETE, 15-HETE) and **leukotrienes** cause chemotaxis of neutrophils and eosinophils.

3. Bronchial smooth muscle

a. PGFs cause smooth muscle contraction.

b. PGEs cause smooth muscle dilation.

c. Leukotrienes and **thromboxane** are potent bronchoconstrictors and are the most likely candidates for mediating allergic bronchospasm. The leukotrienes **LTC$_4$** and **LTD$_4$** are the components of **slow-reacting substance of anaphylaxis (SRS-A)**.

4. Uterine smooth muscle

–**PGE$_2$** and **PGF$_{2\alpha}$** cause contraction of uterine smooth muscle in pregnant women. The nonpregnant uterus has a more variable response to prostaglandins; **PGF$_{2\alpha}$** causes contraction and **PGE$_2$** causes relaxation.

5. Gastrointestinal tract

a. PGE$_2$ and **PGF$_{2\alpha}$** increase the rate of longitudinal contraction in the gut and decrease transit time.

b. The **leukotrienes** are potent stimulators of gastrointestinal smooth muscle.

c. PGE$_2$ and **PGI$_2$** inhibit acid and pepsinogen secretion in the stomach. In addition, prostaglandins increase mucus, water, and electrolyte secretion in the stomach and the intestine.

6. Blood

a. TxA$_2$ is a potent inducer of platelet aggregation.

b. PGI$_2$ and **PGE$_2$** inhibit platelet aggregation.

c. PGEs induce erythropoiesis by stimulating the renal release of erythropoietin.

d. 5-HPETE stimulates release of histamine; **PGI$_2$** and **PGD** inhibit histamine release.

C. Therapeutic uses

1. Induction of labor at term

–is produced by infusion of **PGF$_{2\alpha}$ (carboprost tromethamine)** [Hemabate] and **PGE$_2$ (dinoprostone)** [Prostin E].

2. Therapeutic abortion

–infusion of **carboprost tromethamine** or administration of vaginal suppositories containing **dinoprostone** is effective in inducing abortion in the second trimester.

3. Maintenance of ductus arteriosus

–is produced by **PGE₁** [Prostin VR] infusion; will maintain patency of the ductus arteriosus, which may be desirable before surgery.

4. Treatment of peptic ulcer

–**misoprostol** [Cytotec], a methylated derivative of PGE₁, is approved for use in patients taking high doses of nonsteroidal anti-inflammatory drugs (NSAIDs).

D. Adverse effects

–include local pain and irritation, bronchospasm, and gastrointestinal disturbances, including nausea, vomiting, cramping, and diarrhea.

E. Pharmacologic inhibition of eicosanoid synthesis

1. **Phospholipase A₂**-mediated release of eicosanoic precursors, such as arachidonic acid, is inhibited by glucocorticoids (induce synthesis of a protein called lipocortin, which may mediate this inhibition).

2. **Aspirin** and most NSAIDs inhibit prostaglandin G (**PGG**) and prostaglandin H (**PGH**) by their actions on the cyclooxygenase pathway. **Aspirin** can increase the synthesis of eicosanoids through the lipoxygenase pathway, perhaps by increasing substrate concentration.

3. **Eicosatetraenoic acid** is an arachidonic acid analog that inhibits both cyclooxygenase and lipoxygenase activity.

4. Imidazole derivatives such as **dazoxiben** appear to inhibit thromboxane synthase preferentially.

5. **Tranylcypromine** has some specificity in inhibiting prostacyclin synthase.

VI. Nonsteroidal Anti-inflammatory Drugs (NSAIDs)

A. Overview

1. The inflammatory response is complex, involving the immune system and the influence of various endogenous agents, including prostaglandins, bradykinin, histamine, chemotactic factors, and superoxide free radicals formed by the action of lysosomal enzymes.

2. **Aspirin,** other salicylates, and newer drugs with diverse structures are referred to as **NSAIDs** to distinguish them from the anti-inflammatory glucocorticoids. NSAIDs are used to **suppress the symptoms of inflammation associated with rheumatic disease.** Some are also used to relieve pain (analgesic action) and fever (antipyretic action).

B. Mechanism of action

1. Anti-inflammatory effect

–is due to irreversible inhibition of the enzyme prostaglandin H synthase (cyclooxygenase), which converts arachidonic acid to **prostaglandins,** and to **TxA₂** and **prostacyclin.**

–have no effect on lipoxygenase and therefore do not inhibit production of leukotrienes.

–additional mechanisms may include interference with the potentiative action of other mediators of inflammation (bradykinin, histamine, serotonin), modulation of T-cell function, stabilization of lysosomal membranes, and inhibition of chemotaxis.

2. Analgesic effect

–is thought to be related to peripheral inhibition of prostaglandin production, but also may be due to inhibition of pain stimuli at a subcortical site.

–prevent potentiating action of prostaglandins on endogenous mediators of peripheral nerve stimulation (e.g., bradykinin).

3. Antipyretic effect

–is believed to be related to inhibition of pyrogen (interleukin-1)–induced production of prostaglandins in the hypothalamus and the "resetting" of the thermoregulatory system, leading to vasodilatation and increased heat loss.

C. Therapeutic uses

1. Inflammation

–are first-line drugs used to arrest inflammation and the accompanying pain of rheumatic and nonrheumatic diseases, including **rheumatoid arthritis, juvenile arthritis, osteoarthritis, psoriatic arthritis, ankylosing spondylitis, Reiter's syndrome,** and **dysmenorrhea**.

–do not significantly reverse the progress of rheumatic disease, but rather slow destruction of cartilage and bone and allow patients increased mobility and use of their joints.

–are administered chronically in doses well above those used for analgesia and antipyresis and, at those dosages, are more likely to cause adverse drug effects. Drug selection is generally dictated by the patient's ability to tolerate adverse effects.

–anti-inflammatory effects may develop only after several weeks of treatment.

2. Analgesia

–**alleviate mild-to-moderate pain.** Are less effective than opioids and more effective against pain associated with integumental structures (pain of muscular and vascular origin, arthritis, and bursitis) than with that associated with the viscera.

3. Antipyresis

–**reduce elevated body temperature** with little effect on normal body temperature.

4. Miscellaneous uses

–**aspirin reduces formation of thrombi** and is used prophylactically to reduce recurrent transient ischemia, unstable angina, and the incidence of thrombosis after coronary artery bypass grafts.

D. Aspirin (acetylsalicylic acid) and nonacetylated salicylates

–include **sodium salicylate, magnesium salicylate, choline salicylate, sodium thiosalicylate,** and **salsalate**.

1. Pharmacologic properties

−are weak organic acids; **aspirin** pK_a = 3.5.

−are rapidly absorbed from the intestine as well as from the stomach, where the low pH favors absorption. Rate of absorption is increased with rapidly dissolving (buffered) or predissolved (effervescent) dosage forms.

−are hydrolyzed rapidly by plasma and tissue esterases to acetic acid and the active metabolite **salicylic acid**. Salicylic acid is more slowly oxidized to **gentisic acid** and conjugated with glycine to **salicyluric acid** and to ether and ester glucuronides.

−have a $t_{1/2}$ of 3–6 hours after acute administration. Chronic administration of high doses (to treat arthritis) or toxic overdose increases the $t_{1/2}$ to 15–30 hours because the enzymes for glycine and glucuronide conjugation become saturated.

−unmetabolized salicylates are excreted by the kidney. If the urine pH is increased above 8, clearance is increased approximately fourfold as a result of decreased reabsorption of the ionized salicylate from the tubules.

2. Therapeutic uses

−are used to treat **rheumatoid arthritis, juvenile arthritis,** and **osteoarthritis,** as well as other inflammatory disorders.

3. Adverse effects

a. Gastrointestinal effects

−are the most common adverse effects of high-dose **aspirin** use (70% of patients); may include nausea, vomiting, diarrhea or constipation, dyspepsia, epigastric pain, bleeding, and ulceration (primarily gastric).

−are thought to be due to a direct chemical effect on gastric cells or a decrease in the production and cytoprotective activity of prostaglandins, which leads to gastric tissue susceptibility to damage by hydrochloric acid.

−may contraindicate **aspirin** use in patients with active ulcer. Aspirin may be taken with prostaglandins to reduce gastric damage.

−substitution of enteric-coated or timed-release preparations, or the use of **nonacetylated salicylates,** may decrease gastric irritation. Gastric irritation is not prevented by using buffered tablets.

b. Hypersensitivity (intolerance)

−is relatively **common with the use of aspirin** (0.3% of patients); results in rash, bronchospasm, rhinitis, edema, or an anaphylactic reaction with shock, which may be life-threatening. Incidence is highest in patients with asthma, nasal polyps, recurrent rhinitis, or urticaria. Aspirin should be avoided in such patients.

−**cross-hypersensitivity** may exist **to** other **NSAIDs** and to the yellow dye tartrazine used in many pharmaceutical preparations.

−is not associated with **sodium salicylate** or **magnesium salicylate**.

−use of **aspirin** and other **salicylates** to control fever during viral infections (influenza and chicken pox) in children and adolescents is associated with an increased incidence of **Reye's syndrome,** an illness characterized by vomiting, hepatic disturbances, and encephalopathy, which has a 35% mortality rate. **Acetaminophen** is recommended as a substitute for children with **fever of unknown etiology**.

c. Miscellaneous adverse effects and contraindications

   —occasionally **decrease glomerular filtration rate,** particularly in patients with renal insufficiency.

   —occasionally produce **mild hepatitis,** usually asymptomatic, particularly in patients with systemic lupus erythematosus, juvenile or adult rheumatoid arthritis, or rheumatic fever.

   —**prolong bleeding time. Aspirin** irreversibly inhibits platelet prostaglandin H synthase (**cyclooxygenase**) and **TxA$_2$** production to suppress platelet adhesion and aggregation. Is contraindicated in patients with bleeding disorders, such as hypothrombinemia, hemophilia, hepatic disease, and vitamin K deficiency, and should be avoided in patients receiving anticoagulants such as **coumarin** and **heparin**.

   —are not recommended during pregnancy; may induce **postpartum hemorrhage** and lead to **premature closure of fetal ductus arteriosus**.

4. Drug interactions

   a. Action of anticoagulants may be enhanced by their displacement by **aspirin** from binding sites on serum albumin. Aspirin also displaces **tolbutamide, phenytoin,** and other drugs from their plasma protein–binding sites.

   b. Hypoglycemic action of **sulfonylureas** may be enhanced by displacement from their binding sites on serum albumin or inhibition of their renal tubular secretion by **aspirin.**

   c. Usual analgesic doses of **aspirin** (< 2 g/day) decrease renal excretion of **sodium urate** and antagonize the uricosuric effect of **sulfinpyrazone** and **probenecid**; **aspirin** is contraindicated in patients with gout taking uricosuric agents.

   d. Antacids may alter absorption of **aspirin.**

   e. Aspirin competes for tubular reabsorption with **penicillin G** and prolongs its half-life.

   f. Corticosteroids increase renal clearance of **salicylates**.

   g. Alcohol may increase gastrointestinal bleeding when taken with **aspirin**.

5. Toxicity

   a. In adults, **salicylism** (tinnitus, hearing loss, vertigo) occurs as initial sign of toxicity after **aspirin** or **salicylate overdose or poisoning**.

   b. In children, the common signs of toxicity include **hyperventilation** and **acidosis,** with accompanying lethargy and hyperpnea.

   c. Disturbance of acid-base balance results in **metabolic acidosis** in infants and young children and **compensated respiratory alkalosis** in older children and adults. **Salicylate toxicity** initially increases the medullary response to carbon dioxide, with resulting hyperventilation and respiratory alkalosis. In infants and young children, increases in lactic acid and ketone body production result in a metabolic acidosis. With increased severity of toxicity, respiratory depression occurs with accompanying respiratory acidosis.

d. Uncoupling of oxidative phosphorylation by **aspirin** results in **hyperthermia** and **hypoglycemia,** particularly in infants and young children. Nausea, vomiting, tachycardia, hyperpnea, dehydration, and coma may develop.

e. Treatment includes correction of acid-base disturbances, replacement of electrolytes and fluids, cooling, alkalinization of urine with bicarbonate to reduce salicylate reabsorption, forced diuresis, and gastric lavage or emesis.

E. Other nonsteroidal anti-inflammatory drugs

–like **aspirin,** are used for **inflammation** associated with rheumatic and nonrheumatic diseases.

–are absorbed rapidly after oral administration. Extensively bound to plasma proteins, especially albumin. Cause drug interactions due to displacement of other agents, particularly anticoagulants, from serum albumin; are similar to those seen with **aspirin**.

–are metabolized in the liver and excreted by the kidney; half-lives vary greatly (from 1–45 hr, with most between 10–20 hr). Required frequency of administration may influence drug choice because of possible problems with compliance.

–commonly produce **gastrointestinal disturbances.** Demonstrate **cross-sensitivity with aspirin** and with each other. Other adverse effects, such as **hypersensitivity,** are generally the same as for **aspirin;** cautions and contraindications are similar.

–are associated with non–dose-related instances of acute renal failure and nephrotic syndrome. May lead to renal toxicity in combination with angiotensin-converting enzyme (ACE) inhibitors. **Indomethacin, meclofenamate,** and **tolmetin** are generally more toxic than other NSAIDs.

1. Diflunisal [Dolobid]

–is a fluoridated salicylic acid derivative that is not metabolized to salicylic acid.

–has little antipyretic activity.

2. Ibuprofen [Motrin, Advil], naproxen [Naprosyn], fenoprofen [Nalfon], and ketoprofen [Orudis]

–are propionic acid derivatives.

–no reported interaction of **ibuprofen** or **ketoprofen** with anticoagulants; **fenoprofen** has been reported to induce **nephrotoxic syndrome**.

3. Sulindac [Clinoril] and tolmetin [Tolectin]

–are pyrrole acetic acid derivatives. **Sulindac** is a prodrug that is oxidized to a sulfone and then to the active sulfide, which has a relatively long $t_{1/2}$ (16 hours) due to enterohepatic cycling.

–**tolmetin** has minimal effect on platelet aggregation; is associated with a higher incidence of anaphylaxis than other NSAIDs; has relatively short $t_{1/2}$ (1 hour).

4. Indomethacin [Indocin]

–is the drug of choice for treatment of **ankylosing spondylitis** and **Reiter's syndrome**; is also used for acute gouty arthritis.

–is used also for management of **patent ductus arteriosus** in premature infants (otherwise not used in children); inhibits production of prostacyclins that prevent closure of duct.

–is not recommended as a simple analgesic or antipyretic because of the potential for severe adverse effects.

–bleeding, ulceration, and other adverse effects are more likely with **indomethacin** than most other NSAIDs. Headache is a common adverse effect; tinnitus, dizziness, or confusion also occasionally occur.

5. Piroxicam [Feldene]

–is an oxicam derivative.

–has $t_{1/2}$ of 45 hours.

–like **aspirin** and **indomethacin, bleeding** and **ulceration** are more likely than for other NSAIDs.

6. Meclofenamate [Meclomen] and mefenamic acid [Ponstel]

–are anthranilic acid derivatives; have $t_{1/2}$ of 2 hours.

7. Phenylbutazone [Azolid, Butazolidin]

–is a pyrazolone derivative.

–is metabolized to the active **oxyphenbutazone** and to a uricosuric compound.

–presents significant risk of **blood dyscrasias,** including agranulocytosis and aplastic anemia; no reported interaction with anticoagulants.

–is used when response to other drugs is inadequate.

8. Other NSAIDs

–include **flurbiprofen** [Ansaid], **diclofenac** [Voltaren], and **etodolac** [Lodine]. **Flurbiprofen** is also available for topical ophthalmic use.

F. Other anti-inflammatory drugs

–are used in the more advanced stages of some **rheumatoid diseases.**

1. Aurothioglucose [Solganal], gold sodium thiomalate [Myochrysine], and auranofin [Ridaura]

–are gold compounds that may **retard destruction of bone and joints** by an unknown mechanism.

–have long latency.

–**aurothioglucose** and **gold sodium thiomalate** are administered intramuscularly. **Auranofin** is administered orally and is 95% bound to plasma proteins.

–can produce **serious gastrointestinal disturbances, dermatitis,** and **mucous membrane lesions**. Less common effects include hematologic disorders such as aplastic anemia and proteinuria with occasional nephrotic syndrome.

2. Penicillamine [Cuprimine, Depen]
–is a chelating drug (will chelate gold) that is a metabolite of **penicillin**.
–has **immunosuppressant activity,** but mechanism of action is unknown.
–has long latency.
–incidence of severe adverse effects is high; are similar to those of the gold compounds.

3. Methotrexate [Rheumatrex]
–is an antineoplastic drug used for **rheumatoid arthritis** that does not respond to NSAIDs.
–commonly produces **hepatotoxicity.**

4. Chloroquine and hydrochloroquine [Plaquenil]
–are **antimalarial drugs.**
–have immunosuppressant activity, but mechanism is unknown.

5. Adrenocorticosteroids

G. Nonopioid analgesics and antipyretics

1. Overview
–**aspirin, NSAIDs, acetaminophen,** and **phenacetin** are useful for the treatment of mild-to-moderate pain associated with integumental structures, including **pain of muscles and joints, postpartum pain, and headache**.
–have **antipyretic activity** and, except for acetaminophen, have anti-inflammatory activity at higher doses.
–act by unknown mechanism. Peripherally mediated analgesic activity and centrally mediated antipyretic activity are correlated with inhibition of prostaglandin synthesis (except for **acetaminophen**).

2. Acetaminophen
–unlike aspirin and other NSAIDs, does not displace other drugs from plasma proteins, causes minimal gastric irritation, has little effect on platelet adhesion and aggregation, and does not block the effect of uricosuric drugs on uric acid secretion.
–has no significant anti-inflammatory or antiuricosuric activity.
–is administered orally and is rapidly absorbed. Metabolized by hepatic microsomal enzymes to sulfate and glucuronide.
–is a **substitute for aspirin** to treat mild-to-moderate pain for selected patients who are intolerant to aspirin, have history of peptic ulcer or hemophilia, are using anticoagulants or a uricosuric drug to manage gout, or are at risk for Reye's syndrome.
–overdose results in accumulation of a minor metabolite, *N*-acetyl-*p*-benzoquinone, which is responsible for hepatotoxicity. When enzymes for glucuronide and sulfate conjugation of acetaminophen and the reactive metabolite become saturated, an alternative glutathione conjugation

pathway (cytochrome P-450 dependent) becomes more important. If hepatic glutathione is depleted, the reactive metabolite accumulates and may cause hepatic damage by interaction with cellular macromolecules, such as DNA and RNA. Overdose is treated by emesis or gastric lavage and oral administration within 1 day of *N*-acetylcysteine to neutralize the metabolite.

3. Phenacetin

    —is structurally related to **acetaminophen** and is an analgesic/antipyretic that can no longer be prescribed but is still available OTC.

    —use is associated with the development of **renal failure**.

VII. Drugs Used for Gout

A. Gout

    —is a familial disease characterized by recurrent hyperuricemia and arthritis with severe pain; is caused by **deposits of uric acid** (the end-product of purine metabolism) in joints, cartilage, and the kidney.

    1. Acute gout is treated with NSAIDs, particularly **indomethacin,** or with **colchicine**.

    2. Chronic gout is treated with the uricosuric agents **probenecid** or **sulfinpyrazone,** which increase the elimination of uric acid, or **allopurinol,** which inhibits uric acid production.

B. Colchicine

    —is an alkaloid with anti-inflammatory properties; used for relief of inflammation and pain in **acute gouty arthritis**. Reduction of inflammation and relief from pain occurs 12–24 hours after oral administration.

    —mechanism of action in acute gout is unclear. Prevents polymerization of tubulin into microtubules and inhibits leukocyte migration and phagocytosis. Also inhibits cell mitosis.

    —adverse effects after oral administration, which occur in 80% of patients at a dose near that necessary to relieve gout, include **nausea, vomiting, abdominal pain,** and particularly **diarrhea**. IV administration reduces the risk of gastrointestinal disturbances and provides faster relief (6–12 hr), but increases the risk of sloughing of skin and subcutaneous tissue. Higher doses may, rarely, result in liver damage and blood dyscrasias.

C. Indomethacin [Indocin] and phenylbutazone [Azolid, Butazolidin]

    1. Indomethacin is preferred to the more disease-specific **colchicine** because of diarrhea associated with the use of colchicine.

    2. Phenylbutazone is used only for short-term treatment (< 3 days) because of associated **toxicity**.

D. NSAIDs (such as naproxen and sulindac)

    —are increasingly being used as substitutes for colchicine for treatment of **acute gouty arthritis**.

E. Probenecid [Benemid] and sulfinpyrazone [Anturane]

    —are organic acids that reduce urate levels by acting at the anionic transport site in the renal tubule to prevent reabsorption of uric acid.

    —are used for **chronic gout,** often in **combination** with **colchicine**.

−undergoes rapid oral absorption.

−inhibit excretion of other drugs that are actively secreted by renal tubules, including **penicillin,** NSAIDs, cephalosporins, and **methotrexate**. Dose reduction of these drugs may be warranted.

−increased urinary concentration of uric acid may result in formation of urate stones (**urolithiasis**). Risk is decreased with ingestion of large volumes of fluid or alkalinization of urine with potassium citrate.

−low doses of uricosuric agents and salicylates inhibit uric acid secretion. Aspirin is contraindicated in gout.

−common adverse effects include **gastrointestinal disturbances** and **dermatitis**; rarely, cause blood dyscrasias.

F. Allopurinol [Lopurin, Zyloprim]

−is used to treat **chronic, tophaceous gout** because it reduces the size of established tophi; **colchicine** is administered concomitantly during the first week of therapy to prevent gouty arthritis.

−inhibits the synthesis of uric acid by inhibiting **xanthine oxidase,** an enzyme that converts hypoxanthine to xanthine and xanthine to uric acid. **Allopurinol** is metabolized by xanthine oxidase to alloxanthine, which also inhibits xanthine oxidase. Also inhibits de novo purine synthesis.

−commonly produces **gastrointestinal disturbances** and **dermatitis**. More rarely causes hypersensitivity, including fever, hepatic dysfunction, and blood dyscrasias. Should be used with caution in patients with liver disease or bone marrow depression.

VIII. Immunosuppressive Agents

A. Inhibition of immune response

1. Nonspecific inhibition

−**azathioprine, cyclophosphamide,** and **methotrexate** suppress immune function by their cytotoxic action achieved through a variety of mechanisms, particularly by inhibition of DNA synthesis. Generally, immunosuppressive activity is achieved at nearly toxic doses.

2. Specific inhibition

−**glucocorticoids and cyclosporine** inhibit activation or actions of certain cells of the immune system and are generally less toxic than the nonspecific agents.

3. Suppression of the immune system increases the risk of opportunistic viral, bacterial, and fungal infections.

4. Development of tolerance

−to overcome an allergic reaction, small quantities of antigen are administered gradually to develop tolerance, most probably as a result of induction of IgG antibodies to neutralize a subsequent IgE reaction with allergen.

B. Use of immunosuppressive agents

−are used to treat syndromes or diseases that reflect **imbalances in the immune system,** including rheumatoid arthritis, systemic lupus erythematosus, inflammatory bowel disease, chronic active hepatitis, lipoid nephrosis, Goodpasture's syndrome, and autoimmune hemolytic anemia.

−are also used to **prevent allograft rejection,** which results when cytotoxic T lymphocytes develop in response to incompatible transplanted organs.

C. Individual agents

1. Glucocorticoids

−are thought to interfere with the cell cycle of activated lymphoid cells.
−are used for a wide variety of immunologically mediated diseases.
−are important agents in suppressing allograft rejection. Often used in **combination with** either **cyclosporine** or a cytotoxic agent.

2. Cyclosporine [Sandimmune]

−is a potent immunosuppressive cyclic polypeptide that binds to cyclophilins and inhibits T-helper cell activation and production of interleukin-2.
−has variable absorption from the gastrointestinal tract (20%–50%). Doses must be established after monitoring blood. Biphasic $t_{1/2}$, with terminal phase from 10–25 hours. Is metabolized in the liver and eliminated primarily in bile.
−main use is in **acute and chronic suppression of organ rejection in transplants** of kidney, liver, and heart. Generally used in combination with glucocorticoids.
−causes **nephrotoxicity** in 25%–75% of patients, with reduction in glomerular filtration and renal plasma flow; **hypertension** in 30% of patients; **neurotoxicity** (tremor and seizures) in 5%–50% of patients; and **hirsutism** and **gingival hyperplasia** in 10%–30% of patients.
−is synergistically nephrotoxic with other drugs affecting kidney function. Inhibition of hepatic microsomal enzymes elevates plasma concentration; induction of drug-metabolizing enzymes enhances clearance.

3. FK-506

−is an investigational antibiotic with immunosuppressive properties similar to **cyclosporine,** which may cause less toxicity.

4. Azathioprine [Imuran]

−is a cytotoxic agent that suppresses T-cell activity to a greater degree than B-cell activity. Also inhibits proliferation of promyelocytes in the marrow. Is S-phase–specific.
−is metabolized to **mercaptopurine,** which is also immunosuppressive.
−is most effective when given just after immunologic challenge. May enhance antibody response if given prior to challenge. Not effective on established responses.
−can be administered orally. Is eliminated mainly by metabolic degradation by **xanthine oxidase.** Dose reduction is necessary when administered with **allopurinol,** which reduces xanthine oxidase activity.
−is used with **prednisone** in **transplantation procedures** and some diseases of the immune system, including **systemic lupus erythematosus** and **rheumatoid arthritis**.
−major adverse effect is **bone marrow suppression.** At higher doses, occasional nausea and vomiting, gastrointestinal disturbances, and hepatic dysfunction occur.

5. Cyclophosphamide [Cytoxan, Neosar]

−is an alkylating agent developed as an anticancer drug.

−suppresses B lymphocytes to a greater degree than T cells.

−is the drug of choice in the treatment of **Wegener's granulomatosis**. Is also employed in severe cases of **rheumatoid arthritis** and other autoimmune disorders.

−causes adverse effects that include **cystitis** and **cardiomyopathy.**

6. Methotrexate [Folex, Mexate]

−is an anticancer agent that has immunosuppressive action.

−inhibits replication and function of T cells and possibly B cells.

−has been used for **graft rejection** and for autoimmune and inflammatory diseases.

−also has proven beneficial in the treatment of **severe psoriasis** refractory to other agents.

−**hepatotoxicity** is the major adverse effect.

Review Test

Directions: Each of the numbered items or incomplete statements in this section is followed by answers or by completions of the statement. Select the **one** lettered answer or completion that is **best** in each case.

1. Which of the following statements best describes a characteristic of the antimigraine agent ergotamine?

(A) It promotes vasodilatation
(B) It is useful in reducing premature contractions of the uterus
(C) It acts as a 5HT-receptor antagonist
(D) It acts as an α-adrenoceptor agonist

2. Which of the following statements concerning autacoids is true?

(A) Terfenadine is an H_2-receptor antagonist that does not cross the blood–brain barrier
(B) Diphenhydramine will inhibit the flare and itch of the triple response
(C) Gastric secretion is enhanced by H_2-receptor antagonists such as pyrilamine
(D) Ranitidine can be used to treat nasal congestion

3. A patient receiving warfarin develops rheumatoid arthritis. Which one of the following drugs would be contraindicated?

(A) Aspirin
(B) Tolmetin
(C) Aurothioglucose
(D) Ibuprofen

4. Which of the following phrases correctly defines prostacyclin?

(A) A potent endogenous vasoconstrictor
(B) Decreases cAMP in platelets
(C) A stable analogue of serotonin (5HT)
(D) Synthesized by the endothelial cells from PGH_2

5. Which of the following statements about prostaglandin biosynthesis is true?

(A) Glucocorticoids specifically inhibit thromboxane synthase
(B) Aspirin inhibits both thromboxane and leukotriene synthesis
(C) Sodium salicylate causes irreversible acylation of prostaglandin H synthase
(D) Glucocorticoids inhibit both thromboxane and leukotriene synthesis

6. Which of the following characteristics is associated with cyclosporine?

(A) Is a selective immunosuppressive agent
(B) Is often used to treat rheumatoid arthritis
(C) Is often ototoxic
(D) Is used to develop tolerance to antigens

7. Which of the following statements about ergots is correct?

(A) Methysergide is used to induce labor
(B) Ergotamine is a potent arterial dilator
(C) Bromocriptine is used to inhibit lactation because it is a dopamine agonist
(D) Ergot is a contaminant of German wine

8. Which of the following is characteristic of cromolyn?

(A) Inhibits reaginic antibody (IgE) synthesis
(B) Is a competitive antagonist of the H_1-receptor
(C) Stimulates β-adrenoceptors of mast cells
(D) Inhibits allergen-induced release of mast cell contents

9. Which of the following is a common mechanism shared by all NSAIDs?

(A) Inhibition of histamine release by inhibiting mast cell degranulation
(B) Inhibition of arachidonate release from the
plasma membrane by inhibiting phospho-
lipases
(C) Inhibition of the formation of leukotrienes
by inhibiting lipoxygenase
(D) Inhibition of the production of prostaglandins and thromboxanes from arachidonic
acid through the inhibition of prostaglandin H synthase

10. Which of the following agents may be used
to treat acute gout?

(A) Probenecid
(B) Indomethacin
(C) Acetylsalicylic acid
(D) Acetaminophen

11. Which of the following agents could be used
to treat inflammation in patients failing to respond to salicylates?

(A) Probenecid
(B) Sulfinpyrazone
(C) Acetaminophen
(D) Phenylbutazone

12. All of the following statements concerning
astemizole are correct EXCEPT

(A) Competitive inhibitor of the histamine H_1-
receptor
(B) Used as a prophylactic for treating aller-
gies
(C) Has little anticholinergic effect
(D) Readily penetrates blood–brain barrier

13. All of the following are characteristics of
phentermine EXCEPT

(A) Potent histamine H_1-receptor antagonist
(B) Amphetamine derivative
(C) Stimulates the release of catecholamines
(D) Reduces food-seeking behavior

Directions: The group of items in this section consists of lettered options followed by a set of numbered items. For each item, select the **one** lettered option that is most closely associated with it.
Each lettered option may be selected once, more than once, or not at all.

Questions 14–24
Match each characteristic or therapeutic use
with the drug most closely associated with it.

(A) Thromboxane A_2
(B) Carboprost tromethamine
(C) PGE_1
(D) Indomethacin
(E) Ondansetron
(F) Ergonovine
(G) Ergotamine
(H) Pergolide
(I) Methysergide
(J) Sumatriptan
(K) Cyproheptadine

14. A 5HT-receptor agonist that causes vasoconstriction of vessels in the carotid circulation

15. Used to treat adverse effects of carcinoid
tumor

16. Produces intense and sustained uterine
contraction

17. Used for prophylaxis of migraine

18. A 5HT-antagonist used for acute attacks of
migraine

19. A 5HT-antagonist useful for treating nausea and vomiting

20. Stimulates the platelet-release reaction

21. Used to induce first- and second-trimester
abortions

22. Stimulates gastric production of bicarbonate and mucus

23. Reversibly inhibits cyclooxygenase

24. A dopaminergic agonist at both D_1 and D_2
dopamine-receptors

Answers and Explanations

1–D. Ergotamine actions are mediated by agonist actions at both serotonin (5HT) receptors and α-adrenoceptors. Ergotamine causes vasoconstriction and is contraindicated during pregnancy.

2–B. Terfenadine is a potent H_1-receptor antagonist; its poor CNS penetration reduces sedative effects. Ranitidine is an H_2-receptor antagonist.

3–A. Aspirin will displace warfarin from plasma binding sites and can precipitate bleeding; the other agents appear not to cause this drug interaction.

4–D. Prostacyclin (PGI_2) is a potent vasodilator produced in endothelial and vascular smooth muscle cells. It has no effect on platelets.

5–D. Sodium salicylate does not cause acylation of prostaglandin H synthase but inhibits the enzyme by a different, reversible, mechanism. Glucocorticoids inhibit phospholipase A_2; aspirin does not diminish leukotriene synthesis.

6–A. Cyclosporine is a selective immunosuppressant that primarily affects cytotoxic T-lymphocytes. Nephrotoxicity rather than ototoxicity is a serious adverse effect of this drug. Cyclosporine is not used to treat rheumatoid arthritis nor to develop tolerance.

7–C. Bromocriptine is a potent dopamine agonist; prolactin-inhibiting factor is likely dopamine. Ergotamine is a potent vasoconstrictor; methysergide is useful in the prophylaxis of migraine.

8–D. Cromolyn does not affect histamine biosynthesis but impairs release of histamine and other autacoids from mast cells. It does not compete for histamine H_1- or H_2-receptors.

9–D. The common mechanism shared by all NSAIDs (nonsteroidal anti-inflammatory drugs) is inhibition of prostaglandin H synthase and the inhibition of inflammation. Additional mechanisms may also be involved, but they are less clearly defined, particularly regarding the action of NSAIDs as analgesics or antipyretic agents.

10–B. Indomethacin is particularly effective for the treatment of acute gout. Probenicid is effective for the chronic treatment of gout but is not used for acute attacks; aspirin can inhibit the anion transporter and cause further uricemia. Acetaminophen is a poor anti-inflammatory agent.

11–D. Phenylbutazone is used to treat inflammation when the response to other drugs is inadequate. Probenecid and sulfinpyrazone are used to prevent reabsorption of uric acid to treat gout. Acetaminophen has no significant anti-inflammatory activity.

12–D. Poor penetration across the blood–brain barrier and reduced anticholinergic actions reduce adverse effects with use of astemizole.

13–A. Phentermine is an amphetamine derivative that has no activity at the histamine H_1-receptor. It acts centrally to reduce food-seeking behavior.

14–J. Sumatriptan acts at the $5HT_{1D}$-receptor and causes relatively specific vasoconstriction in the carotid circulation, with minimal effects on other organs.

15–K. A potent H_1-receptor antagonist that also blocks both $5HT_1$- and $5HT_2$-receptors, cyproheptadine is used most frequently to limit diarrhea and spasms produced by serotonin-secreting carcinoid tumors.

16–F. Ergonovine causes prolonged and forceful contraction of uterine smooth muscle.

17–I. Methysergide is an effective agent for prophylaxis of migraines, but is ineffective after onset of attack. Cumulative toxicity requires "drug holidays" every 6 months.

18–G. Ergotamine is the preferred drug for relief of acute migraine attack.

19–E. Ondansetron is highly effective in treating nausea and vomiting associated with chemotherapy.

20–A. Thromboxane A_2 is a potent inducer of platelet aggregation.

21–B. Infusion of carboprost tromethamine is used to induce abortion; it can also be used to induce labor at term.

22–C. Prostaglandins increase mucus, water, and electrolyte secretion in the stomach and intestine. This accounts for the gastric protective action of these agents.

23–D. Indomethacin reversibly inhibits cyclooxygenase; in contrast, aspirin's action on the enzyme is irreversible.

24–H. Pergolide, a dopaminergic agonist, causes specific inhibition of prolactin secretion.

6

Drugs Used in Anemia and Disorders of Hemostasis

I. Drugs Used in the Treatment of Anemias

A. Iron deficiency anemias

1. Iron metabolism

a. Structure and storage of iron

- is an integral component of heme. As much as 70% of total body iron is found in **hemoglobin**. Heme iron is also an essential component of muscle **myoglobin** and of several enzymes, such as catalase, peroxidase, the cytochromes, and others.
- is stored in reticuloendothelial cells, hepatocytes, and intestinal cells as **ferritin** (a particle with a ferric hydroxide core and a surface layer of the protein apoferritin) and **hemosiderin** (aggregates of ferritin–apoferritin).

b. Absorption and transport

- heme iron is much more readily absorbed across the intestine than inorganic iron.
- inorganic iron in the **ferrous** state (Fe^{2+}) is much more readily absorbed than that in the **ferric** state (Fe^{3+}); gastric acid and ascorbic acid promote the absorption of ferrous iron.
- iron is actively transported across the intestinal cell and then oxidized to ferric iron and stored as ferritin or transported to other tissues.
- iron is transported in the plasma bound to the glycoprotein **transferrin;** cell-surface receptors bind the transferrin–iron complex, and the iron is delivered to the recipient cell by endocytosis.

c. Regulation

- except for menstruation and bleeding disorders, very little iron is lost from the body and no mechanism exists for increasing excretion. Therefore, iron storage is regulated at the level of **absorption**.
- **(1)** When plasma iron concentrations are low, ferritin synthesis and the number of transferrin receptors are increased, facilitating absorption.

(2) When iron stores are high, synthesis of ferritin and transferrin receptors decreases and additional absorption is inhibited.

2. Causes of iron deficiency anemia

a. Bleeding (approximately 30 mg of iron are lost in a normal menstrual cycle)

b. Dietary deficiencies

c. Malabsorption syndromes

d. Increased iron demands

3. Iron salt supplements

a. Oral agents

–several **ferrous iron salts** are available for oral use. All are essentially equivalent therapeutically if doses are adjusted according to iron content (gluconate, sulfate, and fumarate forms are 12%, 20%, and 33% iron by weight, respectively).

–approximately 25% of orally administered iron is absorbed; a typical daily dose is 100–200 mg iron/day.

–oral iron treatment may require 3–6 months to replenish body stores.

b. Parenteral agents

–a colloidal suspension of **ferrous hydroxide** and **dextran** can be administered by IV infusion or intramuscular injection.

–may be useful in patients with **iron absorption disorders** caused by inflammatory bowel disease, small-bowel resection, gastrectomy, or hereditary absorption defects.

–are indicated for patients with hypersensitivity reactions to oral iron salts.

–are useful in **severe anemic conditions** in which rapid correction of iron deficiency is desired.

–may be used to reduce toxic reactions on initiation of erythropoietin (epoeitin alfa) therapy in patients with renal disease.

c. Adverse and toxic effects

–produce gastrointestinal upset (nausea, cramps, constipation, and diarrhea).

–may cause hypersensitivity reactions (most common with parenteral administration), including bronchospasm, urticaria, and anaphylaxis.

–**fatal overdose** (1–10 grams) is possible; children are especially susceptible. **Deferoxamine** [Desferal], an iron chelating agent, is used to treat iron toxicity. Administered systemically or by gastric lavage, deferoxamine binds iron and promotes excretion.

B. Red cell deficiency anemias

1. Erythropoietin (EPO)

–is a **glycoprotein** produced by the peritubular cells in the kidney and is essential for normal reticulocyte production.

–**synthesis** is stimulated by hypoxia.

–is available as recombinant human EPO, **epoetin alfa** [Epogen, Eprex] for parenteral use (IV or subcutaneously).

2. Mechanism of action

–increases the rate of **stem-cell differentiation**.
–increases the rate of **mitosis** in red cell precursors, blast-forming units, and colony-forming cells.
–increases the **release of reticulocytes** from marrow.
–increases **hemoglobin synthesis**.
–requires adequate **stores of iron**.

3. Therapeutic uses

–is used to treat anemia in the following patients: **AIDS patients** treated with zidovudine (**AZT**), cancer patients undergoing **chemotherapy,** and patients in **renal failure;** all these conditions and treatments produce anemia.

4. Adverse and toxic effects

–include hypertension and seizures, probably caused by rapid expansion of blood volume.

C. Sideroblastic anemias

–are characterized by **decreased hemoglobin synthesis** and **intracellular accumulation of iron** in erythroid precursor cells.
–are often caused by agents that antagonize or deplete **pyridoxal phosphate**.
–are sometimes seen in alcoholics, in patients undergoing antituberculin therapy with **isoniazid** and **pyrazinamide,** and in certain inflammatory and malignant disorders.
–**hereditary sideroblastic anemia** is an X-linked trait.
–is treated with **pyridoxine** (vitamin B_6) administered orally (preferred route) or parenterally. **Pyridoxine** has variable efficacy with inherited forms of the disease.

D. Vitamin deficiency (megaloblastic) anemias

1. Vitamin B_{12}

a. Structure

(1) Vitamin B_{12} is a complex, **cobalt-containing molecule**. Various groups are covalently linked to the cobalt atom, forming the cobalamins. The endogenous cobalamins in humans are **methylcobalamin** and **5-deoxyadenosylcobalamin**.

(a) **Methylcobalamin** is a coenzyme essential for the production of methionine and *S*-adenosylmethionine from homocysteine and for the production of tetrahydrofolate from methyltetrahydrofolate.

(b) **Deoxyadenosylcobalamin** participates in the mitochondrial reaction that produces succinyl-CoA from methylmalonyl-CoA; vitamin B_{12} deficiency leads to the production of abnormal fatty acids.

(2) For pharmacologic use, vitamin B_{12} is supplied as the stable derivatives **cyanocobalamin** [Betalin, Redisol] or **hydroxocobalamin** [AlphaRedisol].

b. Transport and absorption
  - in the stomach, dietary vitamin B_{12} complexes with intrinsic factor, a peptide secreted by the parietal cells. The intrinsic factor–vitamin B_{12} complex is absorbed by active transport in the distal ileum.
  - vitamin B_{12} is transported in the plasma bound to the protein **transcobalamin II** and is taken up by and stored in hepatocytes.

c. Actions and pharmacologic properties
  - is essential for normal **DNA synthesis** and **fatty acid metabolism**. A deficiency results in impaired DNA replication, which is most apparent in tissues such as the gastrointestinal tract and erythroid precursors, which are actively dividing. The appearance of large macrocytic (megaloblastic) red cells in the blood is characteristic of this deficiency. Vitamin B_{12} **deficiency** can also result in irreversible neurologic disorders.
  - loss from the body is very slow (2 µg/day), and hepatic stores are sufficient for up to 5 years. **Vitamin B_{12}** is not synthesized by eukaryotic cells and is normally obtained from microbial synthesis.
  - parenteral administration is standard because the vast majority of situations requiring vitamin B_{12} replacement are due to malabsorption. Uncorrectable malabsorption requires lifelong treatment.
  - improvement in hemoglobin concentration is apparent in 7 days and normalizes in 1–2 months.

d. Therapeutic uses
  - is used to treat **pernicious anemia** (inadequate secretion of intrinsic factor with subsequent reduction in vitamin B_{12} absorption).
  - is used after partial or total **gastrectomy** to mitigate the loss or reduction of intrinsic factor synthesis.
  - is used to replace vitamin B_{12} in deficiency caused by **dysfunction of the distal ileum** with defective or absent absorption or the intrinsic factor–vitamin B_{12} complex.
  - is necessary in patients with **insufficient dietary intake** of vitamin B_{12} (occasionally seen in strict vegetarians).

e. Adverse effects
  - are minor and uncommon, even at large doses.

2. Folic acid (vitamin B_9) [Folvite]
  - is composed of three subunits: pteridine, *para*-aminobenzoic acid (PABA), and one to five glutamic acid residues.
  - typically occurs in the diet in a polyglutamate form, which must be converted to the mono-glutamyl form for absorption. Most folate is absorbed in the proximal portions of the small intestine and is transported to tissues bound to a plasma-binding protein.
  - its cofactors provide single carbon groups for transfer to various acceptors and are essential for the biosynthesis of purines and the pyrimidine **deoxythymidylate**. A deficiency in **folic acid** results in impaired DNA synthesis; mitotically active tissues such as erythroid tissues are markedly affected.
  - catabolism and excretion is more rapid than that of vitamin B_{12}; hepatic reserves are sufficient for only 1–3 months.

–is usually administered orally.

–is used to correct **dietary insufficiency** (commonly observed in the elderly), as a supplement during **pregnancy and lactation,** and in cases of rapid cell turnover such as **hemolytic anemia**.

II. Drugs Used in Hemostatic Disorders

A. Anticoagulants

1. Heparin [Calciparine, others]

a. Structure

–is a polymeric mixture of sulfated mucopolysaccharides. Commercial heparin contains 8–15 repeats of D-glycosamine-L-iduronic acid and D-glucosamine-D-glucuronic acid. It is highly negatively charged at physiologic pH.

–is synthesized as a normal product of many tissues, including the lung, intestine, and liver. Commercial preparations are derived from bovine lung or porcine intestinal extracts.

b. Actions

(1) Increases the activity of **antithrombin III** by 1000–fold

–**antithrombin III** inhibits activated serine proteases in the clotting cascade, including IIa (thrombin), IXa, Xa, XIa, XIIa, and XIIIa.

–**heparin, antithrombin III,** and the clotting factors form a ternary complex. The clotting factor is inactivated, and intact heparin is released and recycled in a catalytic manner. Some evidence suggests additional anticlotting factors, such as heparin cofactor II, may also be activated by heparin.

(2) Has a **direct anticoagulant activity** (can inhibit clotting in vitro)

(3) Releases **lipoprotein lipase** from vascular beds, which accelerates postprandial clearing of lipoproteins from the plasma

c. Pharmacologic properties

–must be given parenterally (by slow infusion or deep subcutaneous injection); is not injected intramuscularly due to the potential for hematoma formation.

–$t_{1/2}$ is dose-dependent.

–is metabolized in the liver by heparinase to smaller-molecular-weight compounds, which are excreted in the urine.

d. Therapeutic uses

–provides preoperative prophylaxis against deep vein thrombosis.

–is administered following acute myocardial infarction.

–prevents pulmonary embolism in patients with established thrombosis.

–prevents clotting in extracorporeal circulation devices.

e. Adverse effects

–**bleeding** is a common adverse effect, especially in older women. An increased incidence of bleeding is also seen in patients with renal disease. **Protamine sulfate,** a highly positively charged mixture of peptides, can be administered IV if bleeding does not abate after cessation of **heparin** therapy.

–causes **thrombocytopenia** in 25% of patients and severe platelet reductions in 5% of patients; heparin may induce antiplatelet antibodies and may also induce platelet aggregation and lysis.

–can cause **hypersensitivity reactions,** including chills, fever, urticaria, and anaphylaxis.

–may produce **reversible alopecia**.

–**osteoporosis** and predisposition to fracture are seen with long-term use.

f. Contraindications and drug interactions

–is contraindicated in patients who are **bleeding** (internally or externally) and in patients with **hemophilia, thrombocytopenia, hypertension, or purpura**.

–is also contraindicated before and after brain, spinal cord, or eye surgery.

–extreme **caution** is advised in treatment of **pregnant women;** however, alternative agents (coumarin derivatives) are teratogenic.

–should not be administered with **aspirin** or other agents that interfere with platelet aggregation.

–positively-charged drugs, aminoglycosides, and some histamine-receptor antagonists can reduce the effectiveness of **heparin** therapy.

2. Coumarin derivatives

a. Structure

–are derived from 4-hydroxycoumarin and include **dicumarol, warfarin sodium** [Coumadin], and **phenprocoumon** [Liquamar]. Of these agents, **warfarin** has the best bioavailability and the least severe adverse effects.

b. Actions and pharmacologic properties

–indirectly interfere with γ-carboxylation of glutamate residues in clotting factors II (prothrombin), VII, IX, and X, which is coupled to the oxidation of vitamin K. Continued production of functional clotting factors requires replenishment of reduced vitamin K from the oxidized form; this reduction is catalyzed by vitamin K epoxide and is blocked by coumarin derivatives.

–**clotting factors** are still synthesized and cleaved to active forms but cannot bind Ca^{2+} and hence cannot bind to platelet membranes; clotting factors produced before coumarin therapy decline in concentration as a function of factor half-life. This causes a latency period of 36–48 hours before effects are seen.

(1) **Warfarin** administered orally has 100% bioavailability. Highly teratogenic and fetotoxic, with a $t_{1/2}$ of 2.5 days, warfarin is extensively (99%) bound to plasma albumin and can displace many other drugs from this site.

(2) **Dicumarol** is much less well absorbed; a $t_{1/2}$ of approximately 2–10 days increases the potential for bleeding episodes.

c. Therapeutic uses

–are similar to those of **heparin;** also include prophylaxis of venous thrombosis and of pulmonary embolism.

d. Adverse effects

–**bleeding** is a common adverse effect with oral anticoagulants; prothrombin times should be frequently monitored.

–**warfarin** causes **hemorrhagic infarction** in the breast, intestine, and fatty tissues; also readily crosses the placenta and can cause hemorrhage in the fetus. Causes defects in normal fetal bone formation; teratogenic potential is high.

e. Drug interactions

–**phenylbutazone** and **sulfinpyrazone,** both of which displace **warfarin** from albumin, inhibit metabolism of the more active warfarin stereoisomer and inhibit platelet function.

–**aspirin** and **salicylates** increase **warfarin** action by inhibiting platelet function.

–**antibiotics** decrease microbial vitamin K production in the intestine.

–**barbiturates** and **rifampin** decrease **warfarin** effectiveness by inducing microsomal enzymes.

–**oral contraceptives** decrease **warfarin** effectiveness by increasing plasma clotting factors and decreasing antithrombin III.

3. Indanedione derivatives

–**anisindione** [Miradon] has actions and uses similar to those of the coumarin derivatives.

–has longer duration of action than coumarin.

–commonly cause bleeding and dermatitis. **Anisindione** has the potential for serious adverse effects and is reserved for patients who cannot tolerate coumarin derivatives.

B. Hemostatic agents

1. Vitamin K$_1$ (phytonadione) and vitamin K$_2$ (menaquinone)

–**vitamin K$_2$** is found in human tissues and is the form synthesized by intestinal bacteria. **Vitamin K$_1$** is found in foodstuffs and is available for oral or parenteral use. Adequate bile salts are required for oral absorption.

–**vitamin K** is required for post-translational modification of clotting factors II, VII, IX, and X.

–administration to newborns reduces the incidence of **hypothrombinemia of the newborn,** especially common in premature infants.

–IV administration is typical for patients with **dietary deficiencies** and for replenishment of normal levels reduced by **antimicrobial therapy or surgery**.

–IV **vitamin K$_1$** is effective in reversing **bleeding episodes induced by oral hypoglycemic agents**.

2. Plasma fractions

–must be administered intravenously.

–are frequently prepared from blood or plasma pooled from multiple individuals and hence are associated with an increased risk of exposure to hepatitis and human immunodeficiency viruses.

a. **Plasma protein preparations**

   –include the following:

   (1) Lyophilized factor VIII concentrate

   (2) Cryoprecipitate (plasma protein fraction obtained from whole blood)

   (3) Concentrates of plasma (contain variable amounts of factors II, IX, X, and VII)

   (4) Lyophilized factor IX concentrates

b. **Therapeutic uses**

   –include the treatment of various congenital defects of hemostasis, including the following:

   (1) Hemophilia A (classic hemophilia, due to a deficiency in Factor VIII)

   (2) Hemophilia B (Christmas disease, due to a deficiency in Factor IX)

3. Other agents that increase clotting capacity

a. **Desmopressin acetate** [DDAVP, Stimate] increases factor VIII activity and can be used before minor surgeries in patients with **mild hemophilia A.**

b. **Danazol** is an impeded androgen that increases factor VIII activity.

4. Inhibitors of fibrinolysis

a. **Aminocaproic acid [Amicar]**

   –is a **synthetic agent** similar in structure to lysine.

   –competitively inhibits plasminogen activation.

   –is used as an **adjunct** in the **treatment of hemophilia,** for postsurgical bleeding, and in patients with hyperfibrinolysis.

b. **Tranexamic acid [Amstat, Cyklokapron]**

   –is a more potent analog of aminocaproic acid.

C. Antithrombotics

1. Aspirin and aspirin-like agents

   –**decrease thromboxane A$_2$ production** in platelets by inhibiting cyclooxygenase.

   –**reduce antithrombotic action** by decreasing endothelial cell synthesis of PGI$_2$, which also requires cyclooxygenase. Low doses may impair prostaglandin synthesis in platelets to a greater extent than in endothelial cells.

2. Dipyridamole [Persantine, Pyridamole]

   –**inhibits cellular uptake of adenosine,** which has vasodilating and antiaggregating activity.

   –use as an antithrombotic agent is limited to patients with **prosthetic heart valves.**

3. Sulfinpyrazone [Anturane, Aprazone]

   –has **antithrombotic activity** produced by an unknown mechanism.

   –has no advantage over **aspirin.**

4. Dextran 40 [Gentran 40, 10% LMD Rheomacrodex] and dextran 70, 75 [Gentran 75, Macrodex]

   –**impair fibrin polymerization and platelet function** in vivo by an unclear mechanism.
   –adverse effects include **respiratory distress, urticaria,** and (rarely) anaphylaxis.

D. Thrombolytics

   –fibrin clots are dissolved by the serine protease plasmin. Inactive plasminogen is converted to plasmin in vivo by peptides called **tissue plasminogen activators**.

1. Streptokinase [Kabikinase, Streptase]

   –is a nonenzyme protein that is isolated from streptococci, and binds to plasminogen to catalyze the conversion of plasminogen to active plasmin.
   –acts on both circulating and fibrin-bound plasminogen.
   –therapeutic uses include **acute pulmonary embolism, deep vein thrombosis,** and **reperfusion of occluded peripheral arteries**.
   –administration immediately after **myocardial infarction** tends to limit the extent of cardiac damage and may reduce the risk of mortality. Reperfusion after coronary occlusion is successful in 60%–75% of patients.
   –major adverse effect is **systemic bleeding**. Hypersensitivity may be observed in individuals with antistreptococcal antibodies.

2. Urokinase [Abbokinase]

   –is a protease originally isolated from urine; the drug is now prepared from cultured kidney cells.
   –activates circulating and fibrin-bound plasminogen.
   –has identical indications to **streptokinase;** is less antigenic than streptokinase and is indicated in patients sensitive to streptokinase.
   –**pro-urokinase,** an investigational prodrug, acts selectively on fibrin-bound plasminogen.

3. Tissue plasminogen activator (tPA), alteplase [Activase]

   –is an endogenous protease that preferentially activates plasminogen bound to fibrin. **Alteplase** is a recombinant human protein produced in bacteria.
   –is most specific to fibrin-bound plasminogen; local activation of plasmin reduces the incidence of systemic bleeding.
   –has a shorter $t_{1/2}$ than **urokinase** or **streptokinase,** thus limiting systemic adverse effects.

4. Anistreplase (APSAC) [Eminase]

   –is composed of an inactive catalytic core of plasminogen–streptokinase, which binds avidly to fibrin. After administration, deacylation slowly activates the complex, producing plasmin.
   –is not selective to clots and can produce a long-lasting hypocoagulable state.

Review Test

Directions: Each of the numbered items or incomplete statements in this section is followed by answers or by completions of the statement. Select the **one** lettered answer or completion that is **best** in each case.

1. Which of the following descriptions correctly applies to the action of vitamin K?

(A) Acts as a cofactor for post-translational activation of precursors of clotting factors
(B) Acts to increase the transcription of mRNA for clotting factors
(C) Is a hydrophilic molecule co-transported with glucose
(D) Is used to treat pernicious anemia

2. Which of the following statements correctly describes the mechanism of action of heparin?

(A) It is hydrolyzed by protamine
(B) It inhibits only the intrinsic coagulation cascade
(C) It increases the affinity of antithrombin III for thrombin
(D) It increases the amount of circulating antithrombin III

3. Which of the following statements about the anticoagulant dicumarol is correct?

(A) It is absorbed more readily than warfarin
(B) Its effects are reversed by protamine
(C) It is the anticoagulant of choice during pregnancy
(D) It interferes with post-translational modification of clotting factors

4. All of the following variables increase the production of red blood cells EXCEPT

(A) hypoxia
(B) recombinant erythropoietin
(C) anistreplase
(D) testosterone

5. Which of the following statements about thrombolytic agents is most correct?

(A) These agents interfere with activation of thrombin
(B) They increase the activity of plasmin
(C) They are useful when combined with aspirin in prophylaxis of cardiovascular disease
(D) They reduce inflammation in acute gouty attacks

Directions: The group of items in this section consists of lettered options followed by a set of numbered items. For each item, select the **one** lettered option that is most closely associated with it. Each lettered option may be selected once, more than once, or not at all.

Questions 6–11

Match each of the following characteristics with the drug that is most closely associated with it.

(A) Heparin
(B) Urokinase
(C) TPA
(D) Warfarin
(E) Protamine
(F) Aspirin

6. Acts by interfering with a vitamin K–dependent carboxylation

7. Preferentially acts to decrease tissue-bound fibrin

8. Highly negatively charged anticoagulant

9. Thrombolytic agent synthesized in the kidney

10. Heparin antidote

11. Reduces platelet aggregation by decreasing thromboxane synthesis

Answers and Explanations

1–A. Vitamin K is a lipophilic molecule that is a critical cofactor for the post-translational carboxylation of clotting factors. It would not be used to treat pernicious anemia, but can be used to reduce the effects of warfarin.

2–C. Heparin can block both the intrinsic and extrinsic coagulation pathways by increasing the affinity of antithrombin III for thrombin. Protamine is a heparin antagonist that acts on the basis of charge.

3–D. The actions of dicumarol inhibiting post-translational modification of clotting factors are not blocked by protamine. Dicumarol absorption is significantly lower and more variable than that of warfarin. The agent is highly teratogenic and therefore should not be used during pregnancy.

4–C. Anistreplase is a thrombolytic agent with no effect on erythropoiesis. Androgens cause a moderate increase in the production of red cells, but their use has been largely superseded with the introduction of recombinant erythropoietin; this hormone is induced by hypoxia.

5–B. All of the available antithrombotics act to increase the activity of plasmin. They are not useful prophylactically and have no effect on inflammation.

6–D. Warfarin indirectly interferes with γ-carboxylation of glutamate residues in certain clotting factors, which requires oxidized vitamin K.

7–C. TPA, or tissue plasminogen activator, is an endogenous protease that preferentially activates plasminogen bound to fibrin.

8–A. Heparin is highly negatively charged at physiologic pH.

9–B. Urokinase was originally isolated from urine but is now prepared from cultured kidney cells.

10–E. Protamine is administered IV if bleeding does not abate after cessation of heparin therapy.

11–F. Aspirin decreases thromboxane A_2 production in platelets by inhibiting cyclooxygenase.

7
Drugs Acting on the Gastrointestinal Tract

I. Emetics and Antiemetics

A. Vomiting reflex
—is a coordinated reflex controlled by a bilateral **vomiting center** in the dorsal portion of the lateral reticular formation in the medulla.

—pharmacologic intervention relies on inhibition of inputs or depression of the vomiting center. The vomiting center receives inputs from several sources:

1. **Chemoreceptor trigger zone (CTZ)**

2. **Vestibular nucleus**

3. **Peripheral afferents** from the pharynx, gastrointestinal tract, and genitals

4. **Psychic input** from the central nervous system (CNS)

B. Vertigo

1. **True (objective) vertigo**
   —is **hallucination of movement,** usually caused by a brain lesion or damage to cranial nerve VIII (cochlear nerve, CN VIII) or the labyrinthine system.
   —is also associated with **Ménière's disease**.

2. **Subjective vertigo**
   —is **presyncopal light-headedness** frequently caused by cochlear or vestibular ischemia.

3. **Drug-induced vertigo**
   —may be caused by toxicity to CN VIII, such as arises from the use of **aminoglycosides**.
   —may also be caused by the use of agents that produce orthostatic hypotension, such as **antihypertensives**.

C. Antiemetics
—are drugs useful in the **treatment of vomiting** associated with motion sickness and chemotherapy.

1. Cholinergic antagonists

– reduce excitability of labyrinthine receptors and depress conduction from the vestibular apparatus to the vomiting center.

– are used to treat **motion sickness** and in **preoperative situations**. They are not useful in treating nausea caused by chemotherapy.

– produce adverse effects that include drowsiness, dry mouth, and blurred vision. Transdermal delivery of **scopolamine** via a skin patch applied behind the ear [Transderm Scōp] decreases the incidence of adverse effects and produces relief for 72 hours.

2. Histamine₁ (H₁)-receptor antagonists

– include **diphenhydramine** [Benadryl], **meclizine** [Antivert, D-Vert, Bonine], **cyclizine** [Marezine], **dimenhydrinate,** and **promethazine** [Phenergan].

– most likely act by inhibiting cholinergic pathways of the vestibular apparatus by receptor "crossover."

– are used to treat **motion sickness, true vertigo,** and **nausea of pregnancy.**

– produce sedation and dry mouth.

3. Dopamine antagonists

a. Metoclopramide [Reglan]

– blocks receptors within the CTZ.

– increases the sensitivity of the gastrointestinal tract to the action of acetylcholine (**ACh**); this enhances gastrointestinal motility and gastric emptying and increases lower esophageal sphincter tone.

– high doses antagonize serotonin (5-HT₃)-receptors in the vomiting center and gastrointestinal tract.

– is used to treat **nausea due to chemotherapy** (caused by agents such as **cisplatin** and **doxorubicin**) and **narcotic-induced vomiting**.

– produces sedation, diarrhea, extrapyramidal effects and elevated prolactin secretion.

b. Phenothiazines and butyrophenones

– include **chlorpromazine** and **prochlorperazine** (phenothiazines) and **haloperidol** and **droperidol** (butyrophenones).

– block dopaminergic receptors in the CTZ and appear to inhibit peripheral transmission to the vomiting center.

– are used to treat **nausea due to chemotherapy** and **radiation therapy** and to control **postoperative nausea**.

– adverse effects (less pronounced with butyrophenones) include anticholinergic effects (drowsiness, dry mouth, and blurred vision), extrapyramidal effects, and orthostatic hypotension. These agents are contraindicated in Parkinson's disease because of their extrapyramidal effects.

4. Cannabinoids

– include **dronabinol** (Δ-9-tetrahydrocannabinol) [Marinol] and a synthetic derivative, **nabilone** [Cesamet].

– may act by inhibiting the vomiting center, but the mechanism is unclear.

– are used to control **nausea induced by chemotherapy**.

– are either administered as oral preparations or smoked as a cigarette.

　　　–produce sedation, psychoactive effects ("high"), dry mouth, and orthostatis hypotension.

5. Glucocorticoids

　　　–include **dexamethasone** and **betamethasone**.

　　　–can be effective as treatment for **vomiting caused by highly emetic agents**. High doses are given as an IV bolus or orally for **delayed nausea**, often combined with **metoclopramide, haloperidol,** or **diphenhydramine**.

　　　–cause adrenal suppression and metabolic disturbances.

6. Benzodiazepines

　　　–include **lorazepam** and **diazepam**.

　　　–act as anxiolytic agents to reduce **anticipatory emesis. Diazepam** is useful as treatment for **vertigo** and controls symptoms in **Ménière's disease** in 60%–70% of patients.

　　　–also cause anterograde amnesia, which lasts 4–6 hours.

7. Ondansetron [Zofran]

　　　–is a serotonin (5-HT$_3$)-receptor antagonist. Activation of these receptors in the CNS and gastrointestinal tract is a key component in triggering vomiting.

　　　–is more effective than **metoclopramide** against **nausea induced by high-dose cisplatin**.

　　　–is administered intravenously.

　　　–does not produce extrapyramidal effects.

8. Emetrol

　　　–is an over-the-counter (OTC) preparation containing a mixture of fructose, dextrose, and buffered orthophosphoric acid.

　　　–is used to treat **vomiting in infants** and **morning sickness**.

D. Emetics

　　–are agents that induce reflex vomiting.

1. Ipecac

　　　–is a mixture of alkaloids, including **emetine** and **cephaeline,** derived from the ipecacuanha plant.

　　　–**induces vomiting** by stimulating the CTZ and by causing gastrointestinal irritation and afferent input to the vomiting center.

　　　–is administered orally and is fast-acting, causing vomiting in 85% of patients within 20 minutes.

　　　–is useful for removing unabsorbed toxins from the stomach; is less effective if toxins have cleared the pylorus.

　　　–is contraindicated in the absence of the gag reflex or coma and following ingestion of caustic agents and petroleum distillates (which may cause severe aspiration pneumonitis if emesis is not carefully controlled).

　　　–cardiac toxicity caused by the **emetine** in **ipecac** is noted in abusers such as bulimics.

2. Apomorphine

　　　–is a dopamine agonist that directly stimulates the CTZ.

　　　–is administered parenterally and is much more toxic than **ipecac**. It can cause CNS and respiratory depression.

II. Anorexigenics

—are drugs that **decrease appetite or promote satiety**. They have been approved for the adjunct treatment of obesity.

—prolonged use may lead to physical or psychological dependence.

A. Amphetamine and methamphetamine

—act centrally and elevate the synaptic concentration of catecholamines and dopamine, producing a **reduction in food-seeking behavior**.

—produce **adverse effects,** including **CNS stimulation** (nervousness, irritability, and insomnia).

—have high risk of dependence and so are no longer agents of choice. Are contraindicated in pregnancy.

B. Amphetamine derivatives

—include **diethylpropion** [Tenuate, Tepanil], which has similar mechanism of action but reduced adverse effects compared to amphetamines.

—also include **phentermine** [Adipex-P, others], **benzphetamine** [Didrex], and **phendimetrazine** [Plegine, Prelu-2, Statobex].

C. Mazindol [Mazanor, Sanorex]

—is chemically related to tricyclic antidepressants and blocks neuronal reuptake of norepinephrine, dopamine, and serotonin. Dependence has not been reported.

D. Fenfluramine [Pondimin]

—in contrast to other anorexigenics, it **depresses the CNS**.

—stimulates the release of serotonin and blocks its reuptake.

—acts by **promoting satiety** rather than inhibiting food-seeking behavior.

—produces sedation and mild hallucinations; long-term use can cause physical dependence; withdrawal can cause depression.

E. Phenylpropanolamine [Accutrim, Dexatrim]

—acts primarily as a direct α-adrenoreceptor agonist.

—has poor lipid solubility, which limits CNS effects.

—may cause severe hypertension if recommended dosage is exceeded.

III. Agents Used for Upper Gastrointestinal Tract Disorders

A. Goal of therapy

—is to reduce gastric acid production, neutralize gastric H^+, or protect the walls of the stomach from the acid and pepsin released by the stomach and thus treat **peptic ulcers** and **reflux esophagitis**.

B. Antacids

—are weak bases that are taken orally and partially **neutralize gastric acid** and **reduce pepsin activity**.

—reduce the pain associated with ulcers and may promote healing. High doses are required for healing: 40 mEq of base seven times daily.

1. Prototype agents

a. Sodium bicarbonate

—is absorbed systemically and should not be used for long-term treatment.

—is contraindicated in hypertension due to its high sodium content.

b. Calcium carbonate

—is partially absorbed from the gastrointestinal tract, and so has some systemic effects. It should not be used for long-term treatment.

—may stimulate gastrin release and thereby cause rebound acid production.

—is contraindicated in patients with renal disease.

c. Magnesium hydroxide

—is not absorbed from the gastrointestinal tract and therefore produces no systemic effects. Can be used for long-term therapy.

—most frequent adverse effect is diarrhea.

d. Aluminum hydroxide

—is not absorbed from the gastrointestinal tract, and has no systemic effects.

—causes constipation.

e. Combination products

—include several preparations [Maalox, Mylanta II, and Gelusil] that combine **magnesium hydroxide** and **aluminum hydroxide** to achieve a balance between the agents' adverse effects on the bowel.

2. Drug interactions

—alter bioavailability of many drugs by the following mechanisms:

a. Increase in gastric pH produced by antacids decreases absorption of acidic drugs and increases absorption of basic drugs.

b. The **metal ion** in some preparations can **chelate other drugs** (e.g., **digoxin** and **tetracycline**) and **prevent** their **absorption**.

c. Renal effects of antacids increase excretion of acidic drugs and decrease excretion of basic drugs.

C. Inhibitors of gastric acid production

1. H$_2$-receptor antagonists

a. Mechanism of action

—act as competitive inhibitors of the H$_2$-receptor, resulting in a marked decrease in gastric acid secretion. Although other agents may induce acid secretion, histamine is the predominant final mediator that **stimulates parietal acid secretion**.

b. Therapeutic uses

—promote healing of **gastric and duodenal ulcers**.

—are used to treat **hypersecretory states**.

—act as **prophylaxis for recurrent ulcers** in patients at risk.

—other suggested used include control of reflux esophagitis and bile reflux gastritis and prevention of aspiration pneumonitis.

c. Selected drugs

(1) Cimetidine [Tagamet]

—with typical 300-mg dose, reduces acid secretion by approximately 70% for 4–5 hours, given 4 times daily (qid).

—is associated with low incidence of mild gastrointestinal upset, headache, and mental confusion, especially in the elderly. The major adverse effect is **thrombocytopenia**. Also acts as an androgen-receptor antagonist and can induce gynecomastia and impotence.

—is a competitive inhibitor of cytochrome P-450 mixed-function oxidase system. Can increase the half-life ($t_{1/2}$) of drugs that are metabolized by this system (e.g., **warfarin, theophylline, phenytoin,** and the benzodiazepines).

—decreases absorption of **ketoconazole**.

—bioavailability of **cimetidine** is decreased by antacids.

(2) Ranitidine [Zantac]

—is 5 to 10 times more potent than **cimetidine;** requires less frequent dosing schedule, twice daily (b.i.d.).

—does not bind to the androgen receptor; effects on drug metabolism are reduced compared to **cimetidine**.

—has low incidence of headache and cutaneous rash.

(3) Famotidine [Pepcid]

—is approximately twice as potent as **ranitidine** with a longer duration of action; is given once daily.

—produces adverse effects similar to those of **ranitidine,** but does not bind androgen receptors. Clinical experience is limited.

(4) Nizatidine [Axid]

—is as effective as **ranitidine** and may be administered once daily.

—may produce hepatotoxicity, but does not inhibit drug metabolism in the absence of liver damage; does not bind androgen receptors.

2. Cholinergic antagonists

—include **propantheline** [Pro-Banthine], **isopropamide** [Darbid, Ornade], and **scopolamine**.

—decrease ACh-stimulated secretion and motility in the gastrointestinal tract. Required doses produce systemic anticholinergic effects.

—are rarely used alone, but are useful as adjuncts in patients resistant to H_2-receptor antagonists.

3. Omeprazole [Losec]

—is a covalent, irreversible inhibitor of the H^+,K^+-ATPase proton pump in parietal cells, and thereby blocks transport of acid from the cell into the lumen. Reduces both stimulated and basal acid secretion.

—reduces gastric damage induced by nonsteroidal anti-inflammatory drug (NSAID) therapy.

—is useful in patients with **Zollinger-Ellison syndrome,** for **reflux esophagitis,** and **ulcers** refractory to H_2-receptor antagonists.

—produces headaches and gastrointestinal disturbances; reduction in acid production may permit bacterial overgrowth.

—has produced hypertrophy of antral gastrin-producing cells with long-term use in animals.

4. Misoprostol [Cytotec]

—is a congener of prostaglandin E_1 that acts on parietal cells to inhibit acid secretion and stimulate bicarbonate and mucus production.

—is approved for use in **patients taking NSAIDs who are at risk for gastric ulcers**.

—produces diarrhea and stimulation of uterine contraction.

D. Protective agents

1. Sucralfate [Carafate]

—is a complex polysaccharide complexed with aluminum hydroxide. Gastric pH is low enough to produce extensive crosslinking and polymerization of sucralfate.

—has a particular affinity for exposed proteins in the crater of **peptic ulcers;** protects ulcerated areas from further damage and promotes healing. It stimulates mucosal production of prostaglandins and inhibits pepsin.

—produces constipation and nausea.

2. Carbenoxolone

—is a synthetic derivative of glycyrrhizic acid, a natural product found in licorice root; is used widely in Europe.

—stimulates gastric production and secretion of a viscous gastric mucosal layer. Beneficial and adverse effects may be related to a mineralocorticoid-like activity; **spironolactone** blocks both therapeutic and undesired effects.

—causes edema, hypertension, and hypokalemia.

IV. Agents That Affect Motility

A. Metoclopramide [Reglan]

—is a dopaminergic antagonist. In the gastrointestinal tract dopamine is inhibitory; blockade of dopamine receptors allows stimulatory actions of ACh at muscarinic synapses to predominate.

—does not act as an agonist at the muscarinic receptor.

—increases lower esophageal tone, stimulates gastric emptying, and increases rate of transit through the small bowel.

—is used to treat **reflux esophagitis, gastric motor failure** and **diabetic gastroparesis;** is used before radiologic examination of the gastrointestinal tract.

—produces sedation, extrapyramidal effects, and increased prolactin secretion.

B. Calcium-channel blockers and nitrates

—include **nifedipine** [Procardia], **diltiazem** [Cardizem], and **isosorbide dinitrate**.

—may be used to control **esophageal spasm**.

V. Drugs Used to Dissolve Gallstones

A. Chenodiol [Chenix]

—is identical to chenodeoxycholic acid, a primary bile acid.

—reduces the concentration of cholesterol in bile by increasing the secretion of bile acids and decreasing the secretion of cholesterol into bile. It is effective only against cholesterol gallstones and is ineffective in dissolving radiopaque stones. Complete dissolution of gallstones occurs in about 14% of patients. Treatment requires 3 months–2 years for complete stone dissolution.

—is administered orally and is well absorbed through the gastrointestinal tract; should be taken with meals.

—requires functioning gallbladder.

—causes a high incidence (41%) of diarrhea in patients on high-dose therapy and increases low-density lipoprotein (LDL) cholesterol by 10%.

B. Ursodiol [Actigall]

—is ursodeoxycholic acid, a minor primary bile acid.

—reduces cholesterol secretion into bile with little change in the bile acid fraction.

—is an oral agent that also requires months to years for full effect.

—may be combined with sonic lithotripsy to dissolve gallstone fragments.

—has a lower incidence of diarrhea than **chenodiol** and produces no change in LDL cholesterol levels.

C. Monooctanoin

—is a monoglyceride derivative that is effective at dissolution of cholesterol stones.

—must be administered by infusion via the common bile duct.

D. Methyl ter-butyl ether (MTBE)

—is a solvent that directly dissolves cholesterol gallstones.

—is much more rapid in dissolving stones than **monooctanoin**.

—is infused directly into gallbladder or bile duct.

VI. Digestive Enzyme Replacements

—are preparations of semipurified enzymes, typically extracted from pig pancreas. They contain various mixtures of lipase, proteolytic enzymes such as trypsin, and amylase.

—include **pancrelipase** [Cotazym-S, Entolase, others] and **lactase** [Lactrase, Lactaid].

—are used to treat **exocrine pancreatic insufficiency, cystic fibrosis,** and **steatorrhea. Lactase** is useful in lactose-intolerant individuals.

—produce hyperuricemia, hyperuricosuria, allergic reactions, and gastrointestinal upset.

VII. Agents That Act on the Lower Gastrointestinal Tract

A. Laxatives

—act by promoting an increase in the fluid accumulated in the bowel. The increase in luminal volume stimulates peristaltic reflexes, which increase the transit rate and decrease the transit time of the bowel contents. The decrease in transit time reduces water reabsorption from the fecal mass.

1. Bulk-forming laxatives

—include **psyllium** [Metamucil, others], **methylcellulose** [Citrucel], and dietary fiber (10–15 g/day).

—are hydrophilic natural or semisynthetic polysaccharide or cellulose derivatives that are poorly absorbed from the bowel lumen and retain water in the bowel. The increased luminal mass stimulates peristalsis.

—are the treatment of choice for **chronic constipation**.

—produce laxation after 2–4 days; adequate hydration is required.

—cause minimal adverse effects.

2. Osmotic agents

—include salt-containing and salt-free agents.

a. Salt-containing agents

—include **magnesium sulfate, magnesium citrate, magnesium hydroxide, sodium phosphates,** and **mineral water**.

—are poorly absorbed ions that retain water in lumen by osmosis and cause a reflex increase in peristalsis.

—are taken orally. **Sodium phosphates** are also effective rectally. Onset of action occurs typically 3–6 hours after oral administration and 5–15 minutes after rectal administration. They require adequate hydration for effect.

—are used for **acute evacuation of the bowel** before surgery or diagnostic procedures or for **elimination of parasites** after anthelmintic administration.

—some systemic effects are possible with these agents, especially in cases of renal dysfunction; these effects include hypermagnesemia and hypernatremia.

b. Salt-free osmotic agents

—include **glycerin, lactulose** [Chronulac], and **polyethylene glycol-electrolyte solutions** [Colyte, GoLYTELY].

—may be administered rectally (**glycerin**) or orally (**lactulose**).

3. Irritant agents

—include diphenylmethane derivatives such as **phenolphthalein** and **bisacodyl** [Modane, Dulcolax], the anthraquinone derivatives **cascara sagrada** and **senna** [Senokot], and **castor oil**.

—decrease water absorption from bowel lumen and stimulate intestinal secretions. Increased luminal contents stimulate reflex peristalsis. Irritant action stimulates peristalsis directly.

—onset of action occurs in 6–12 hours; they require adequate hydration.

—chronic use may result in cathartic colon, a condition of colonic distention and development of laxative dependence. Diphenylmethane derivatives are reabsorbed via enterohepatic circulation and have increased risk of abuse or overdose.

4. Stool softeners

—include **docusate** [Modane, Surfak, Colace, others].

—have detergent action that facilitates mixing of water and fatty substances to increase luminal mass.

—are used to produce **short-term laxation** and to reduce straining at defecation. They are used to **prevent constipation;** are not effective in treating ongoing constipation.

5. Coating agents: mineral oil

—coats fecal contents and thereby inhibits absorption of water.

—decreases absorption of fat-soluble vitamins. Lipoid pneumonia can develop if mineral oil is aspirated.

B. Nonspecific antidiarrheals

—aim to decrease fecal water content by increasing solute absorption and decreasing intestinal secretion and motility. Increased transit time facilitates water reabsorption.

1. Opiates and other opioid-containing preparations

a. Opium tincture [Laudanum], camphorated opium tincture [Paregoric], and codeine

—act directly on opiate μ receptors to decrease transit rate, stimulate segmental (nonpropulsive) contraction, and inhibit longitudinal contraction. Also stimulate electrolyte absorption (mediated by opiate Δ receptors).

—produce nausea, sedation, and vomiting. High doses may be necessary to control refractory diarrhea, resulting in a potential for dependence.

b. Diphenoxylate [Di-Atro, Lomotil]

—is a synthetic **morphine** analog developed to dissociate between the constipating and other actions of morphine.

—is available as a combination product with **atropine** to reduce potential for abuse and to further reduce motility.

2. Loperamide [Imodium]

—is a derivative of **haloperidol** with reduced CNS activity and marked effects on the intestine. It binds to opiate receptors in the gastrointestinal tract. It is essentially free of CNS effects.

—produces constipation.

3. Anticholinergic agents

—include **atropine, scopolamine, methantheline** [Banthine], and **propantheline** [Pro-Banthine].

—inhibit colonic peristalsis by blocking the response of intestinal smooth muscle to cholinergic stimulation.

—are used to **reduce colonic cramping** and have little effect on diarrhea.

4. Adsorbents

—include **kaolin and pectin** [Donnagel, Parepectolin] and dietary fiber.

—act by adsorbing toxic compounds from intestinal water.

—are nontoxic but less effective than other agents.

5. Bismuth subsalicylate [Pepto-Bismol]

—binds toxins produced by *Vibrio cholerae* and *Escherichia coli*. The salicylate can be absorbed across the intestine.

—inhibits production of prostaglandins in the intestine and reduces secretion.

—is effective both for treatment and prophylaxis of **traveler's diarrhea**.

—produces adverse effects that include tinnitus.

6. Glucocorticoids

—stimulate sodium absorption in the jejunum, ileum, and colon; have relatively long latency (12–36 hours).

—are used to treat **refractory diarrhea** unresponsive to other agents and chronic inflammatory bowel disease (**Crohn's disease**).

—systemic adverse effects limit long-term use.

7. Oral rehydration solutions

–include **WHO solution** and **Infalyate**.

–are balanced salt solutions containing glucose, sucrose, or rice powder.

–increase water absorption from bowel lumen by increasing Na^+-substrate transport across intestinal epithelial cells.

–can remedy 99% of acute cases of **childhood diarrhea**.

C. Antidiarrheals for specific causes

1. Octreotide [Sandostatin]

–is a synthetic 8-amino acid analog of **somatostatin**.

–is used in cases of **severe diarrhea caused by excessive release of gastrointestinal tract hormones,** including gastrin, motilin, vasoactive intestinal polypeptide, glucagon, and others.

–must be administered parenterally.

2. Sulfasalazine [Azulfidine], mesalamine [Asacol], and olsalazine [Dipentum]

–have the following structures: **mesalamine** is 5-aminosalicyclic acid (5-ASA), which is the active agent; **olsalazine** is a dimer of this compound; and **sulfasalazine** is a combination of sulfapyridine and 5-ASA. 5-ASA acts within the colon to limit prostaglandin and leukotriene production.

–are most effective for treatment of **mild to moderate ulcerative colitis; olsalazine** is approved for maintenance of remission but not treatment of this disorder.

Review Test

Directions: Each of the numbered items or incomplete statements in this section is followed by answers or by completions of the statement. Select the **one** lettered answer or completion that is **best** in each case.

1. Which of the following statements about the use of antacids is true?

(A) Antacid salts complexed to sodium are useful for long-term treatment of ulcerative disease
(B) Antacids should be given immediately before cimetidine to reduce gastric irritation
(C) Antacids are sold OTC because they do not cause drug interactions
(D) Antacids are generally more effective in liquid than in solid form

2. Which of the following mechanisms contributes to the action of phenolphthalein as a laxative?

(A) Stimulation of vagal efferents to gastrointestinal smooth muscle
(B) Stimulation of intestinal opioid receptor
(C) Inhibition of Na^+,K^+-ATPase-dependent absorption of water
(D) Neutralization of stomach acid content

3. Which of the following classifications describes cimetidine?

(A) Gastrin receptor antagonist
(B) H_1-receptor antagonist
(C) H_2-receptor antagonist
(D) Antiemetic

4. Which of the following statements regarding omeprazole is correct?

(A) Is an antagonist of the H_2 receptor
(B) Directly inhibits acid production by the gastric mucosa
(C) Is inhibited by spironolactone
(D) Alters the composition of gallstones

5. Which of the following phrases best describes the action of metoclopramide?

(A) Is a dopaminergic agonist
(B) Decreases propulsive contraction in the bowel
(C) Increases lower esophageal tone
(D) Useful for prophylaxis of motion sickness

6. Which of the following statements about the mechanism of action of fenfuramide is correct?

(A) Decreases dopamine concentrations in the CNS
(B) Decreases synaptic serotonin concentration
(C) Acts to decrease food-seeking behavior
(D) Produces a feeling of satiety

Directions: The group of items in this section consists of lettered options followed by a set of numbered items. For each item, select the **one** lettered option that is most closely associated with it. Each lettered option may be selected once, more than once, or not at all.

Questions 7–12

Match each of the following characteristics or actions with the appropriate drug.

(A) Octreotide
(B) Loperamide
(C) Bismuth subsalicylate
(D) Sulfasalazine
(E) Diphenhydramine
(F) Cromolyn
(G) Famotidine
(H) Ephedrine

7. Antibiotic used to treat inflammatory bowel disease

8. A stable somatostatin analog

9. Binds bacterially produced toxins

10. An opiate agonist

11. An H_1-receptor antagonist

12. Blocks gastrin-stimulated gastric acid production

Answers and Explanations

1–D. Liquid formulations of antacids are generally more effective than solid forms. Sodium antacids are absorbed from the gastrointestinal tract and, therefore, produce systemic effects that contraindicate their long-term use. Antacids interact with many drugs, including cimetidine, by altering their bioavailability.

2–C. Irritant laxatives such as phenolphthalein act to increase secretion and decrease water absorption in the gastrointestinal tract.

3–C. Cimetidine is a first-generation H_2-receptor antagonist and has no effect as an antiemetic.

4–B. Omeprazole acts directly to inhibit the proton pump in the gastric mucosa. Carbenoxolone is inhibited by the action of spironolactone.

5–C. Metoclopramide is a dopamine-receptor antagonist that blocks the chemoreceptor trigger zone. It is useful against nausea produced by anticancer agents but is ineffective for motion sickness. It also is useful in reflux esophagitis because it increases the tone of the lower esophageal sphincter.

6–D. Fenfuramide acts to increase synaptic levels of serotonin, which causes a feeling of satiety.

7–D. Sulfasalazine is a combination of the sulfonamide sulfapyridine and the anti-inflammatory 5-aminosalicylic acid (5-ASA). It is used to treat inflammatory bowel disease.

8–A. Octreotide is a synthetic 8-amino acid analog of somatostatin used to treat severe diarrhea caused by excessive gastrointestinal tract hormones.

9–C. Bismuth subsalicylate [Pepto-Bismol] is effective for traveler's diarrhea because it binds toxins produced by *Vibrio cholerae* and *Escherichia coli*.

10–B. Loperamide is an antidiarrheal that is a derivative of haloperidol. It binds to opiate receptors in the gastrointestinal tract.

11–E. Diphenhydramine, an H_1-receptor antagonist, is used to treat motion sickness, vertigo, and the nausea of pregnancy.

12–G. Famotidine, an H_2-receptor antagonist, promotes healing of gastric and duodenal ulcers through its actions at H_2 receptors. It acts as a competitive inhibitor of the H_2 receptor, resulting in a marked decrease in gastric acid secretion.

8

Drugs Acting on the Pulmonary System

I. Introduction to Pulmonary Disorders

–in **asthma, chronic bronchitis,** and **rhinitis,** the effective diameter of the airways is decreased. The goals of therapy are to decrease airway resistance by increasing the diameter of the bronchi and decreasing mucus secretion or stagnation in the airways.

A. Asthma

–is characterized by **acute episodes of bronchoconstriction** caused by underlying airway inflammation. A hallmark of asthma is bronchial hyperreactivity to endogenous or exogenous stimuli. In asthmatics, the response to various stimuli is amplified by persistent inflammation.

1. **Antigenic stimuli** trigger release of mediators (leukotrienes, histamine, and many others) that cause a bronchospastic response, with smooth muscle contraction, mucus secretion, and recruitment of inflammatory cells such as eosinophils, basophils, and macrophages (**early-phase response**).

2. **Late-phase response** (which may occur in hours to days) is an inflammatory response; levels of histamine and other mediators released from inflammatory cells rise again and may induce bronchospasm and eventually fibrin and collagen deposition and tissue destruction.

3. **Nonantigenic stimuli** (cool air, exercise, nonoxidizing pollutants) can trigger nonspecific bronchoconstriction after early-phase sensitization.

B. Chronic bronchitis

–is characterized by **pulmonary obstruction** caused by excessive production of mucus due to hyperplasia and hyperfunctioning of mucus-secreting goblet cells.
–is often induced by an irritant.

C. Rhinitis

–is a **decrease in nasal airways** due to thickening of the mucosa and increased mucus secretion.
–may be caused by allergy, viruses, vasomotor abnormalities, or rhinitis medicamentosa.

II. Agents Used to Treat Asthma and Other Bronchial Disorders

A. Adrenergic agonists

—stimulate β_2-adrenoceptors, resulting in relaxation of bronchial smooth muscle. Inhibit release of mediators and stimulate mucociliary clearance.

—are useful for treatment of **acute bronchoconstriction of asthma**.

1. **Bitolterol [Tornalate], metaproterenol [Alupent, Metaprel], terbutaline [Brethine, Bricanyl], and albuterol [Proventil, Ventolin]**

   —are agents with enhanced β_2 receptor selectivity.

   —can be administered by inhalation (**bitolterol** is available only as an inhalant); sustained-release oral preparations increase duration of action up to 12 hours. **Terbutaline** may be injected subcutaneously for severe attacks.

   —long-term use for treatment of chronic asthma has been associated with diminished control, perhaps due to β-receptor down-regulation.

2. **Isoproterenol [Isuprel, Medihaler-Iso, Vapoiso]**

   —is a relatively nonselective β-receptor agonist and a potent bronchodilator.

   —is most effective in asthmatics when administered as an inhalant. Typically requires dosing every 1–2 hours during an acute attack; oral preparations are administered 4 times daily (qid).

3. **Epinephrine [Primatene Mist, Bronkaid Mist, others]**

   —is available over-the-counter (OTC) and acts as a β_1-, β_2-, and α_1-adrenoceptor agonist.

   —can be administered as an inhalant or subcutaneously; onset of action occurs within 5–10 minutes; duration is 60–90 minutes.

4. **Ephedrine [Broncolate, Primatene Tablets, others]**

   —is a relatively nonselective β- and α_1-adrenoceptor agonist that should be used rarely in the treatment of asthma. Some preparations combine **ephedrine** with a methylxanthine.

5. **Adverse effects of adrenergic agonists**

   —are based on receptor occupancy.

   —are minimized by inhalant delivery of the adrenergic agonists directly to the airways.

   a. **Epinephrine, ephedrine,** and **isoproterenol** have significant β_1-receptor activity and can cause cardiac effects: tachycardia, arrhythmias, and exacerbation of angina.

   b. The most common adverse effect of β_2-adrenoreceptor agonists is **skeletal muscle tremor**.

   c. **Adverse effects** of α-adrenoceptor agonists include vasoconstriction and hypertension.

   d. **Tachyphylaxis,** a blunting in the response to adrenergic agonists on repeated use, can be countered by switching to a different agonist or adding a methylxanthine or corticosteroid to the regimen.

B. Methylxanthines (Figure 8.1)

—for asthma, the most frequently administered methylxanthine is **theophylline** (1,3-dimethylxanthine). Additional members of this family include **theobromine** and **caffeine**.

—because of the limited solubility of **theophylline** in water, it is complexed as salts as in **aminophylline** and **oxtriphylline.**

1. Mechanism of action

—cause bronchodilation by action on the smooth muscles in the airways, most probably by acting as adenosine-receptor antagonists (adenosine causes bronchoconstriction and promotes release of histamine from mast cells). Additionally, these drugs may decrease entry and mobilization of cellular Ca^{2+} stores. **Theophylline** is effective in reducing the synergistic effect of adenosine and antigen stimulation on histamine release. However, **theophylline** analogs that lack adenosine antagonist activity maintain bronchodilator activity. **Theophylline** inhibits phosphodiesterase, but this effect requires very high doses and its contribution to bronchodilation remains to be established.

2. Pharmacologic effects

a. Respiratory system

—affect a number of physiologic systems, but are most useful in the treatment of asthma because of the following:

(1) Produce **rapid relaxation of bronchial smooth muscle**

(2) Decrease histamine release in response to reagenic (immunoglobulin E) stimulation

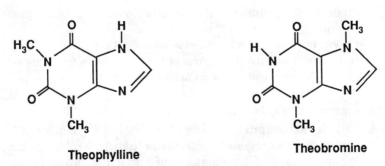

Figure 8.1. Structures of methylxanthines, including xanthine, caffeine, theophylline, and theobromine.

(3) **Stimulate ciliary transport of mucus**

(4) Improve respiratory performance by **improving the contractility of the diaphragm** and by stimulating the medullary respiratory center

b. **Effects on other systems**

(1) **Positive chronotropic and inotropic actions on the heart**

(2) **Pulmonary and peripheral vasodilation** but cerebral vasoconstriction

(3) An increase in alertness and cortical arousal at low doses; at high doses this can proceed to severe nervousness and seizures due to **medullary stimulation**

(4) Stimulation of **gastric acid** and **pepsinogen release**

(5) **Diuresis**

3. **Pharmacologic properties**

—are almost completely absorbed after oral administration.

—are readily permeable into all tissue compartments; cross the placenta and can enter breast milk.

—are metabolized extensively in the liver and are excreted by the kidney.

4. **Prototype drug: theophylline**

—is available in microcrystalline form for **inhalation** and as a **sustained-release preparation;** can be administered intravenously.

—has a very narrow therapeutic index; blood levels should be monitored upon initiation of therapy.

—has a variable half-life; $t_{1/2}$ is approximately 8–9 hours in adults but shorter in children. Clearance is affected by diet, drugs, and hepatic disease.

5. **Therapeutic uses**

—are used to treat **acute or chronic asthma** unresponsive to β-adrenoceptor agonists; can be administered prophylactically.

—are used to treat **chronic obstructive lung disease and emphysema**.

—are used to treat **apnea in pre-term infants** (based on stimulation of the central respiratory center); usually **caffeine** is the agent of choice for this therapy.

6. **Adverse effects**

—include arrhythmias, nervousness, vomiting, and gastrointestinal bleeding.

—may cause behavioral problems in children.

—combined use with $β_2$-adrenoceptor agonists is now suspected to be responsible for recent rises in asthma mortality.

C. **Muscarinic antagonists**

—include **ipratropium bromide** [Atrovent] and **atropine**.

—are competitive antagonists of acetylcholine (**ACh**) at the muscarinic receptor. They inhibit ACh-mediated constriction of bronchial airways. Anticholinergics also decrease vagal-stimulated mucus secretion.

−are somewhat variable in their effectiveness as bronchodilators in asthma but are useful in patients who are refractory to or intolerant of sympathomimetics or methylxanthines.

D. Cromolyn sodium [Intal]

−is disodium cromoglycate, a salt of very low solubility in aqueous solutions.

−by preventing influx of Ca^{2+}, inhibits the release of histamine and other autacoids (especially leukotrienes) from mast cells and thereby reduces bronchospasm. It does *not* cause relaxation of bronchial smooth muscle.

−is poorly absorbed. It must be administered by inhalation; it is available as a microparticulate powder or aerosol.

−is used prophylactically in **asthma;** does not reverse an established bronchospasm. It is the only antiasthmatic that inhibits both early- and late-phase responses.

−produces generally localized adverse effects, which include sore throat, cough, and dry mouth. May infrequently cause dermatitis, gastroenteritis, nausea, and headache.

1. **Ipratropium,** a quaternary amine that is poorly absorbed and does not cross the blood–brain barrier, is administered as an aerosol; its low systemic absorption limits adverse effects.

2. **Atropine** is readily absorbed into the systemic circulation; adverse effects include drowsiness, sedation, dry mouth, and blurred vision. This limits its use as an antiasthmatic.

E. Glucocorticoids

−include **beclomethasone** [Beclovent, Vanceril], **triamcinolone acetate** [Azmacort], and **flunisolide** [AeroBid].

−in some patients, produce a significant increase in airway diameter by an unclear mechanism. May act by attenuating prostaglandin and leukotriene synthesis via inhibition of the phospholipase A_2 reaction and by generally inhibiting immune response. They increase responsiveness to sympathomimetics and decrease mucus production.

−are available as oral, topical, and inhaled agents.

1. Use of **inhaled glucocorticoids** has increased as the role of inflammation in asthma has become better recognized. This method of administration reduces systemic absorption; the most common adverse effects to inhaled glucocorticoids are hoarseness and oral candidiasis.

2. **Topical glucocorticoids** are partially absorbed and can produce systemic effects, most seriously adrenal suppression.

3. Because of their systemic adverse effects, **oral glucocorticoids** are usually reserved for patients with severe refractory asthma.

F. Alpha₁-proteinase inhibitor [Prolastin]

−is used to treat **emphysema** caused by a deficiency in alpha₁-proteinase, a peptide that inhibits elastase. In patients with the deficiency, elastase destroys lung parenchyma.

−is administered by weekly IV injection to treat patients homozygous for this deficiency.

III. Drugs Used to Treat Rhinitis and Cough

A. Rhinitis

1. Characteristics of rhinitis

a. **Congestion** is caused by increased mucus production, vasodilation, and fluid accumulation in mucosal spaces.

b. **Mucus production, vasodilation,** and **parasympathetic stimulation** and **airway widening** are produced by inflammatory mediators (histamine, leukotrienes, prostaglandins, and kinins).

2. Selected drugs

a. **Antihistamines**

—are histamine$_1$ (H$_1$)-receptor antagonists, including **diphenhydramine, chlorpheniramine, cyproheptadine,** and **promethazine,** which decrease mucus secretion.

—reduce the parasympathetic tone of arterioles and decrease secretion through their anticholinergic activity. Anticholinergics might be more effective in rhinitis, but doses required produce systemic adverse effects. **Ipratropium** [Atrovent], a poorly absorbed ACh antagonist, is in trials for treatment of rhinitis.

b. **α-Adrenoceptor agonists**

—act as nasal decongestants.

—include **epinephrine** and **oxymetazoline,** which are administered as nasal aerosols; **phenylpropanolamine, pseudoephedrine,** and **xylometazoline,** which are administered orally; and **phenylephrine,** which may be administered orally or as a nasal aerosol.

—may be administered as **nasal aerosols** or as **oral agents**. Administration as an aerosol is characterized by rapid onset, few systemic effects, and an increased tendency to produce rebound nasal congestion. Oral administration results in longer duration of action, increased systemic effects, and less potential for rebound congestion and dependence.

—reduce airway resistance by constricting dilated arterioles in the nasal mucosa.

—produce adverse effects that include nervousness, tremor, insomnia, dizziness, and **rhinitis medicamentosa** (chronic mucosal inflammation due to prolonged use of topical vasoconstrictors, characterized by rebound congestion, tachyphylaxis, dependence, and eventual mucosal necrosis).

c. **Topical corticosteroids**

—include **beclomethasone** [Beconase, Vancenase] and **flunisolide** [Nasalide].

—are administered as nasal sprays to reduce systemic absorption and adverse effects.

—require 1–2 weeks for full effect.

d. **Cromolyn**

—an antiasthma agent, may also be used to treat rhinitis.

B. Cough

1. Characteristics of cough

−is produced by the cough reflex, which is integrated in the **cough center** in the medulla. The initial stimulus for cough probably arises in the bronchial mucosa, where irritation results in bronchoconstriction. "Cough" receptors, specialized stretch receptors in the trachea and bronchial tree, send vagal afferents to the cough center and trigger the cough reflex.

2. Selected drugs

a. Antitussive agents

(1) Codeine, hydrocodone, and hydromorphone

−are opiates that decrease sensitivity of the central cough center to peripheral stimuli and decrease mucosal secretions. Antitussive actions occur at doses lower than required for analgesia.

−produce constipation, nausea, and respiratory depression.

(2) Dextromethorphan

−is the *l*-isomer of an opioid; it is active as an antitussive but devoid of analgesic or addictive liability.

−is less constipating than **codeine**.

(3) Benzonatate [Tessalon]

−is a glycerol derivative chemically similar to **procaine**.

−reduces the activity of peripheral cough receptors and also appears to reduce the threshold of the central cough center.

(4) Diphenhydramine

−is an H_1-receptor antagonist; however, antitussive activity is probably not mediated at this receptor.

−acts centrally to decrease sensitivity of cough center to afferents.

b. Expectorants

−stimulate the production of a watery, less viscous mucus.

(1) Guaifenesin

−acts directly via the gastrointestinal tract to stimulate vagal reflex.

−near-emetic doses are required for beneficial effect; these doses are not attained in the typical OTC preparations.

(2) Terpin hydrate

−is a volatile oil derived from the eucalyptus tree; it may increase water content in mucus.

(3) Iodide

−has direct action on all secretory glands. Expectorant effect is accompanied by an increase in lacrimation, rhinorrhea, and salivation.

c. Mucolytics

(1) Acetylcysteine

−reduces viscosity of mucus and sputum by cleaving disulfide bonds.

−is delivered as an **inhalant**.

(2) Bromhexine

−acts to reduce mucus viscosity, probably by breaking down mucopolysaccharide fibers in mucus.

Review Test

Directions: Each of the numbered items or incomplete statements in this section is followed by answers or by completions of the statement. Select the **one** lettered answer or completion that is **best** in each case.

1. Which of the following agents is not indicated for the treatment of asthma?

(A) Theophylline
(B) Pseudoephedrine.
(C) Terbutaline
(D) Dextromethorphan

2. Which of the following statements about cough suppressants is true?

(A) Dextromethorphan acts centrally to inhibit the medullary cough center
(B) Rhinitis medicamentosa is a common adverse effect associated with prolonged use of dextromethorphan
(C) Hydrocodone acts peripherally to inhibit peripheral stretch receptors in bronchi
(D) Expectorants such as guaifenesin are proposed to act centrally to decrease the secretory activity of the respiratory tract

3. Which of the following statements regarding the pharmacokinetics of theophylline is correct?

(A) It is primarily metabolized by the kidney
(B) Its metabolism is dependent on age
(C) It is poorly absorbed after oral administration
(D) It has a wide therapeutic index

4. Which of the following statements correctly describes the action of theophylline?

(A) It stimulates cyclic AMP phosphodiesterase
(B) It is an adenosine-receptor antagonist
(C) It does not cross the blood–brain barrier
(D) It blocks the release of acetylcholine in the bronchial tree

5. Which of the following statements regarding opiate action is correct?

(A) It triggers a vagal reflex to suppress cough
(B) It can cause diarrhea
(C) Its expectorant action is caused by stimulation of mucus production
(D) It acts centrally to suppress the medullary cough center

6. Which of the following statements about the mechanism of action of ipratropium is correct?

(A) It acts centrally to decrease vagal ACh release
(B) It inhibits pulmonary ACh receptors
(C) It decreases mast cell release of histamine
(D) It blocks the action of histamine at H_1 receptors

Directions: The group of items in this section consists of lettered options followed by a set of numbered items. For each item, select the **one** lettered option that is most closely associated with it. Each lettered option may be selected once, more than once, or not at all.

Questions 7–14

Match each of the following characteristics or actions with the appropriate drug.

(A) Aminophylline
(B) Bitolterol
(C) Hydrocodone
(D) Oxymetazolone
(E) Beclomethasone
(F) Promethazine
(G) Cromolyn
(H) Ephedrine

7. A methylxanthine used to treat asthma

8. An opiate agonist

9. An H_1-receptor antagonist

10. A specific β_2-adrenoceptor agonist

11. An α-adrenoceptor agonist

12. A glucocorticoid that can be administered as an inhalant

13. Reduces histamine release from mast cells

14. A relatively nonselective adrenoceptor agonist

Answers and Explanations

1–C. Pseudoephedrine is used to treat rhinitis, and is not effective in treating asthma.

2–A. Dextromethorphan is a nonnarcotic antitussive that inhibits the cough center. Hydrocodone is an opiate analog that also acts centrally to suppress cough. Guaifenesin acts in the gut to decrease vagal efferents. Rhinitis medicamentosa is an adverse effect not related to cough suppressants.

3–B. Metabolism of theophylline is dependent on age; $t_{1/2}$ of the drug in children is much shorter than in adults. The methylxanthines are all well absorbed and are metabolized in the liver.

4–B. Theophylline may have several mechanisms of action, but its adenosine-receptor antagonist activity and the inhibition of phosphodiesterase are the best understood.

5–D. Opioids act centrally to decrease the sensitivity of the cough center; they also decrease propulsion in the bowel.

6–B. Ipratropium is an ACh-receptor antagonist and is poorly absorbed so most of its effect is in the lung. It does not cross the blood–brain barrier and does not block mediator release or H_1 receptors.

7–A. The methylxanthine most frequently administered to treat asthma is theophylline; because of its limited solubility in water, it is complexed as salts, as in aminophylline.

8–C. Hydrocone is an opiate agonist that is used to treat cough.

9–F. Promethazine is an antihistamine that treats rhinitis by decreasing mucus secretion.

10–B. Bitolterol is available as an inhalant to treat acute bronchoconstriction in asthma. It acts through its selective effects on β_2-adrenoceptors.

11–D. Oxymetazolone is an α-adrenoceptor agonist that is administered as a nasal aerosol to treat rhinitis.

12–E. Beclomethasone is administered as an inhalant to treat asthma. The use of inhaled glucocorticoids in asthma has increased as the role of inflammation in the disorder has become better recognized.

13–G. By preventing the influx of Ca^{2+}, cromolyn inhibits the release of histamine and other autacoids from mast cells, thereby reducing bronchospasm.

14–H. Ephedrine, a nonselective adrenoceptor agonist, is used rarely to treat asthma, but is sometimes administered in a combination with a methylxanthine.

9

Drugs Acting on the Endocrine System

I. The Hypothalamus

A. Agents affecting growth hormone

1. Growth hormone releasing hormone (GHRH)

–is an active peptide of 40 amino acids released by the hypothalamus.

–binds to specific membrane GHRH receptors on somatotrophs.

–rapidly elevates serum growth hormone (somatotropin) levels with high specificity.

–must be given intravenously (IV); peak response is achieved in about 1 hour.

–is used for **diagnostic evaluation of idiopathic growth hormone deficiency** and for characterization of pituitary responsiveness and growth hormone secretory capacity.

2. Somatotropin release-inhibiting hormone (SRIH, somatostatin)

–is a 14-amino acid peptide produced in the hypothalamus; it is also produced in other areas of the brain and by pancreatic D cells as well as by other cells in the gastrointestinal tract.

–binds to specific somatostatin receptors in target tissues.

–inhibits the release of growth hormone from the pituitary and the release of glucagon and insulin from the pancreas. Somatostatin also inhibits secretion of a number of gut peptides.

–must be administered IV; is rapidly cleared by the kidney.

–is used to treat severe diarrhea associated with **hypersecretory states,** such as **VIPomas,** and may be useful in the treatment of **acromegaly**.

–adverse effects include nausea, cramps, and increased gallstone formation.

–**octreotide** [Sandostatin] is a synthetic 8 amino acid peptide with potent somatostatin agonist activity.

B. Gonadotropin releasing hormone (GnRH) and analogs

–**endogenous GnRH** is a 10-amino acid peptide secreted from the hypothalamus. It binds to specific receptors on pituitary gonadotrophs.

—acute or pulsatile administration of GnRH agonists increases the synthesis and release of both **luteinizing hormone (LH)** and **follicle-stimulating hormone (FSH)**.

—chronic administration (2–4 weeks) inhibits release of both of these gonadotropins by causing a reduction in the number of GnRH receptors.

—adverse effects include a transient worsening of symptoms, hot flashes, and induction of ovarian cysts in the first months of chronic treatment.

1. **Gonadorelin acetate [Lutrepulse] and gonadorelin hydrochloride [Factrel]**

   —are synthetic peptides identical to endogenous GnRH.

   —are injected either subcutaneously or by IV infusion and possess a half-life ($t_{1/2}$) of approximately 10–20 minutes. Peak response is achieved 15 minutes after IV administration and 30–60 minutes after subcutaneous injection.

   —**induce ovulation** in women (pulsatile administration).

   —**increase spermatogenesis** in men (pulsatile administration).

   —treat primary **hypothalamic amenorrhea** (pulsatile administration).

   —cause pituitary inhibition (chronic administration); this is useful in treating **endometriosis, polycystic ovarian syndrome,** and some **sex hormone–dependent tumors** (e.g., prostatic cancers).

   —are used **to assess pituitary function in hypogonadotropic hypogonadism.**

2. **Leuprolide acetate [Leupron, Leupron Depot]**

   —is a synthetic 9-amino acid GnRH analog with increased potency.

   —is administered parenterally.

   —is used to treat **endometriosis** and to inhibit pituitary function in cases of **advanced prostatic cancer.**

3. **Nafarelin acetate [Synarel]**

   —is a synthetic decapeptide of GnRH administered as a nasal spray.

   —is used for the **management of endometriosis.**

C. **Prolactin releasing factor (PRF) and prolactin inhibiting factor (PIF)**

   —secretion of **prolactin** from the pituitary is controlled both by inhibition (mediated by PIF, which is probably dopamine) and stimulation (mediated by PRF).

   1. **PRF**

      a. Several peptides that increase the synthesis and release of prolactin have been identified in the hypothalamus and placenta; however, their physiologic role is unclear.

      b. Drugs that reduce CNS dopaminergic activity cause an increase in prolactin secretion, as will dopamine antagonists. These include:

         (1) **Antipsychotics,** including **chlorpromazine** [Thorazine, others] and **haloperidol** [Haldol]

         (2) **Antidepressants,** including **imipramine** [Janimine, Tofranil, others]

         (3) **Antianxiety agents,** including **diazepam** [Valium, others]

    c. Various hormones also stimulate prolactin secretion; these include tes-
tosterone, estrogen, thyrotropin releasing hormone (TRH), and vasoactive intestinal polypeptide (VIP).

    d. Drugs that promote prolactin secretion are used to treat lactation
failure.

2. PIF

    –PIF (dopamine) activity can be produced by a variety of dopamine
agonists, including **bromocriptine** [Parlodel] and **levodopa** [Dopar,
others].

    –therapeutic uses include inhibition of prolactin secretion in **amenor-
rhea, galactorrhea,** and **prolactin-secreting tumors;** also used to
correct **female infertility** secondary to hyperprolactinemia.

D. Corticotropin releasing hormone (CRH)

    –is a 41-amino acid peptide found in the hypothalamus; it has been chemi-
cally synthesized.

    –stimulates **adrenocorticotropic hormone** (ACTH) synthesis and release
in pituitary corticotrophs by binding to specific membrane receptors.

    –is subject to rapid proteolysis; must be given intravenously.

    –is used diagnostically in cases of ACTH deficiency or excess to **differ-
entiate between hypothalamic–hypophyseal or primary adrenal
disease**.

**E. Thyrotropin releasing hormone (TRH, protirelin) [Relefact TRH,
Thypinone]**

    –is a tripeptide (Glu-His-Pro) found in the hypothalamus and other locations
in the brain.

    –binds to specific membrane receptors and stimulates the secretion of
thyroid-stimulating hormone (TSH) from the pituitary and induces
prolactin secretion.

    –must be given IV; has a $t_{1/2}$ of approximately 5 minutes. Peak response is
achieved 20–30 minutes after administration.

    –is used for the **differential diagnosis of thyroid diseases;** is also used
in the diagnosis of acromegaly.

II. The Anterior Pituitary

**A. Growth hormone (GH, somatotropin) [Humatrope] and somatrem
[Protropin]**

1. Structure

    –is a 191-amino acid protein produced in the anterior pituitary. Secretion
is controlled by hypothalamic factors.

2. Actions and pharmacologic properties

    –effects are mediated by specific membrane receptors; intracellular mes-
sengers have not been identified.

    –major growth action is stimulation of somatomedin production in the
liver, kidney, and other tissues.

    –promotes protein synthesis and positive nitrogen balance.

    –causes lipolysis in adipose tissue and promotes lipid metabolism.

—initially produces an insulin-like effect on glucose transport. Ultimately antagonizes insulin action and can produce hyperglycemia and ketosis.
—is administered by intramuscular or subcutaneous injection. Peak blood levels are obtained in 2–4 hours; activity persists for 36 hours after administration due to the relatively long $t_{1/2}$ of somatomedins.

3. Therapeutic uses

—is used for replacement therapy in children with **growth hormone deficiency** prior to epiphyseal closure.
—stimulates growth in patients with **Turner's syndrome**.

4. Adverse effects and contraindications

—in 10%–30% of patients, anti-GH antibodies develop.
—is contraindicated in patients with closed epiphyses; however, recent studies have found beneficial effects on metabolism in elderly men.

B. Gonadotropins

1. Luteinizing hormone (LH) and follicle-stimulating hormone (FSH)

a. Structure

—are glycoproteins found in the anterior pituitary. LH, FSH, and TSH are all composed of an identical α subunit and a β subunit unique to each hormone.

b. Actions and pharmacologic properties

—activity is mediated by specific membrane receptors that cause an increase in intracellular cyclic AMP (cAMP).
—in women, LH increases estrogen production in the ovary and is required for progesterone production by the corpus luteum after ovulation. FSH is required for **normal development and maturation of the ovarian follicles**.
—in men, LH induces testosterone production by the interstitial (Leydig) cells of the testis. FHS acts on the testis to **stimulate spermatogenesis and the synthesis of androgen-binding protein**.

c. Therapeutic uses

—FSH and LH of pituitary origin are not used pharmacologically. Rather, the menopausal and chorionic gonadotropins described below are used as the source of biologically active peptides.

2. Human menopausal gonadotropins (hMG) and human chorionic gonadotropin (hCG)

a. hMG [Pergonal] is isolated from the urine of postmenopausal women and contains a mixture of LH and FSH.

b. hCG [Pregnyl, A.P.L., others] is produced by the placenta and can be isolated and purified from the urine of pregnant women. hCG is nearly identical in activity to LH but differs in sequence and in carbohydrate content.

c. hMG and **hCG** must be administered parenterally.

d. Therapeutic uses

—**hMG** is used in concert with **hCG** to **stimulate ovulation** in women with functioning ovaries; approximately 75% of women treated with these peptides ovulate.

–**hCG** can be used in both men and women to stimulate **gonadal ste-roidogenesis** in cases of **LH insufficiency**.

–**hCG** can be used to induce **external sexual maturation and sper-matogenesis** in men with secondary hypogonadism but may require months of treatment.

–in the absence of an anatomical block, **hCG** can also promote the de-scent of the testes in **cryptorchidism**.

e. **Adverse effects and contraindications**

–cause ovarian enlargement in about 20% of treated women.

–may cause a syndrome of ovarian hyperstimulation in up to 1% of pa-tients, resulting in ascites, hypovolemia, and shock.

C. **Thyroid-stimulating hormone (TSH) [Thytropar]**

–is a 211-amino acid glycoprotein with two subunits and is secreted from the anterior pituitary.

–stimulates the production and release of **triiodothyronine (T_3)** and **thy-roxine (T_4)** from the thyroid gland. The effect is mediated by stimulation of specific TSH receptors in the plasma membrane, thereby increasing in-tracellular cAMP.

–is available for intramuscular or subcutaneous injection.

–is used in concert with **radioiodine** in the treatment of some **metastatic thyroid carcinomas**.

–is used occasionally to **diagnose the cause of thyroid deficiency**.

D. **Adrenocorticotropic hormone (ACTH, corticotropin) [Acthar, oth-ers] and cosyntropin [Cortrosyn]**

1. **Structure**

–is a 39-amino acid peptide secreted from the anterior pituitary. The *N*-ter-minal 24-amino acid portion of the peptide has full biological activity.

–the *N*-terminal 13-amino acids of ACTH are identical to **α-melanocyte-stimulating hormone (α-MSH)**.

2. **Actions and pharmacologic properties**

–stimulates adrenocortical secretion of glucocorticoids and, to a lesser extent, mineralocorticoids and androgens. Effects are mediated by spe-cific membrane-bound ACTH receptors coupled to an increase in intra-cellular cAMP.

–excess ACTH levels may produce hyperpigmentation due to activity of the intrinsic α-MSH portion of the peptide.

–is available in both human and bovine purified preparations, as well as synthetic **1-24-ACTH** (cosyntropin).

–all preparations are administered parenterally.

3. **Therapeutic uses**

–is used in the evaluation of **primary or secondary hypoadrenalism**.

–may be used in special circumstances where an increase in glucocorti-coids is desired. However, the direct administration of steroids is usually preferred.

4. **Adverse effects and contraindications**

–are similar to those of glucocorticoids. Allergic reactions, acne, hirsutism, and amenorrhea have also been reported.

III. The Posterior Pituitary

A. Antidiuretic hormone (ADH, vasopressin)

1. Structure

–is a 9-amino acid peptide synthesized in the hypothalamus and stored in the posterior pituitary; is released in response to increasing plasma osmolarity or a fall in blood pressure.

2. Actions

–promotes water reabsorption in the collecting duct. The effect is mediated by two types of specific receptors: V_1, located in vascular smooth muscle and in the central nervous system, and V_2, located in renal tubules. V_1 **receptors** are probably coupled to increased inositide turnover; V_2 **receptors** are coupled to an increase in cAMP.
–causes vasoconstriction at higher doses.
–stimulates hepatic synthesis of coagulation factor VIII.

3. Pharmacologic properties

–several preparations of ADH are available:

a. Aqueous vasopressin [Pitressin], a short-acting preparation that acts on both V_1 and V_2 receptors, is administered parenterally and lasts 2–6 hours.

b. Vasopressin in oil, injected intramuscularly, lasts for 48–72 hours.

c. Lyressin [Diapid], a lysine-8-vasopressin analog, is used intranasally; remains effective for 4–6 hours.

d. Desmopressin acetate [DDAVP, Stimate] is a longer-lasting (10–20 hour) preparation administered intranasally or parenterally.

4. Therapeutic uses

a. Desmopressin is the most effective treatment for **severe diabetes insipidus** because its V_2 activity is 2000 times greater than its V_1 activity, but it is not effective in the nephrogenic form of the disease.

b. Vasopressin is useful in treating some types of gastrointestinal bleeding, specifically **esophageal variceal bleeding** and **bleeding caused by colonic diverticula**.

5. Adverse effects

–produce headache, nausea, cramps, and may cause constriction of coronary arteries.

6. Drug interactions

–**clofibrate** [Atromid-S] increases secretion of ADH from the pituitary and can be used to treat mild forms of diabetes insipidus.
–**chlorpropamide** [Diabinese, Glucamide] increases the sensitivity of the tubular cells to ADH.

B. Oxytocin [Pitocin, Syntocinon]

1. Structure

–is a 9-amino acid peptide synthesized in the hypothalamus and secreted by the posterior pituitary.
–differs from ADH by only two amino acids.

2. Actions and pharmacologic properties
—elicits milk production from the breast.
—stimulates contraction of uterine smooth muscle.
—is infused IV, administered intramuscularly, or delivered intranasally. Plasma $t_{1/2}$ is 5–10 minutes.

3. Therapeutic uses
—is used for **induction and maintenance of labor**.
—**stimulates milk ejection** from the breast.
—is sometimes used to control **postpartum uterine bleeding** (more readily controlled with ergot alkaloids).

4. Adverse effects and contraindications
—can produce hypertension and water intoxication.
—can cause uterine rupture and should not be used after uterine surgery or if signs of fetal distress are present.

IV. Drugs Acting on the Gonadal and Reproductive System

A. Estrogens

1. Structure

a. Natural estrogens (Figure 9.1)
—include **17-β-estradiol, estrone,** and **estriol,** which each contain 18 carbon atoms. The most potent natural estrogen is **17-β-estradiol**.
—are produced by the metabolism of cholesterol; **testosterone** is the immediate precursor of **estradiol**. Conversion of testosterone to **17-β-estradiol** is catalyzed by the enzyme aromatase.
—**estrone** and **estriol** are produced in the liver and other peripheral tissues from 17-β-estradiol and are frequently conjugated by esterification to sulfates.
—**equilin,** an estrone derivative, is a pharmacologically useful estrogen purified from horse urine.

b. Synthetic estrogens
—a variety have been produced. Frequently used synthetic estrogens include the steroidal agents **ethinyl estradiol** [Estinyl, Feminone, others] and **mestranol** and the nonsteroidal compounds **diethylstilbestrol (DES)** [Stilphostrol] and **dienestrol** [DV, Estraguard, Ortho Dienestrol].

2. Mechanism of action
—bind to specific intranuclear receptors. The hormone-receptor complex interacts with specific DNA sequences and alters the transcription rates of target genes. They may also affect the $t_{1/2}$ of specific messenger RNAs. These events lead to a change in the synthesis of specific proteins within a target cell.

3. Metabolism
—**17-β-estradiol** is extensively (98%) bound to sex steroid–binding globulin (SSBG) and to serum albumin.

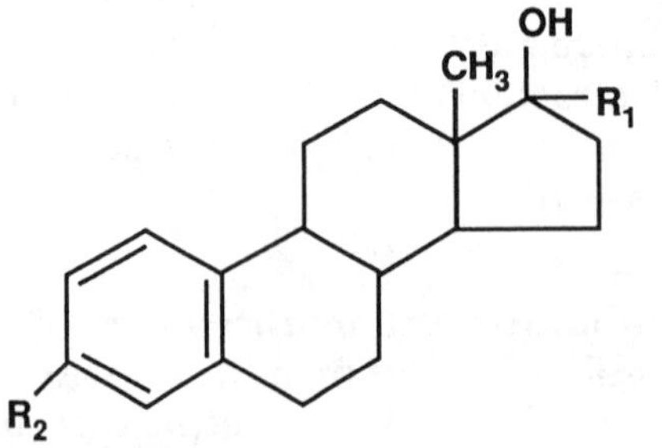

OH
CH₃
R₁
R₂

Estradiol
R₁: -H; R₂: -OH

Ethinyl estradiol
R₁: -C≡CH; R₂: -OH

Mestranol
R₁: -C≡CH; R₂: -OCH₃

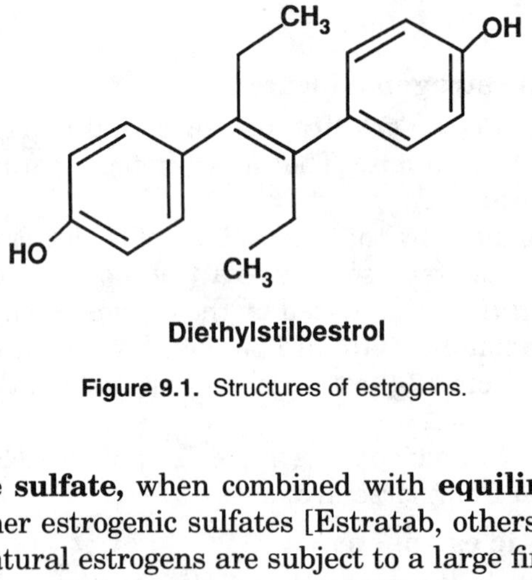

CH₃   OH

HO   CH₃

Diethylstilbestrol

Figure 9.1. Structures of estrogens.

—**estrone sulfate,** when combined with **equilin sulfate** [Premarin] or with other estrogenic sulfates [Estratab, others], is effective orally, but other natural estrogens are subject to a large first-pass effect. Synthetic estrogens may be administered orally, topically, transdermally, or by injection.

—all estrogens are extensively metabolized in the liver and conjugated with either glucuronic acid or sulfate, hydroxylated or *O*-methylated. Most metabolites are excreted in the urine, with approximately 10% undergoing enterohepatic circulation and eventual elimination in the feces.

4. Actions

a. Growth and development

—are required for the **development and maturation of female internal and external genitalia,** growth of the breasts, linear bone growth at puberty, and closure of the epiphyses. Typical female distribution of subcutaneous fat and pubic and axillary hair is also influenced by estrogens.

–are required in the uterus for **growth of myometrium** and for **growth and development of the endometrial lining**. Continuous exposure leads to endometrial hyperplasia and bleeding.

b. Menstrual cycle

–are required for **ovarian follicular development** and regulation of the menstrual cycle.

c. Systemic metabolism

–promote a positive nitrogen balance, increase triglycerides, and tend to decrease serum cholesterol by decreasing low-density lipoprotein (LDL) and increasing high-density lipoprotein (HDL) concentrations.

–decrease total serum proteins but increase levels of transferrin, steroid and thyroid–binding globulins, plasminogen, fibrinogen, and coagulation factors II, VII, VIII, IX, and X. Antithrombin III levels are decreased.

–decrease bone resorption with little effect on bone formation.

d. Influence libido and mood

5. Therapeutic uses

a. Hypogonadism

–are used for estrogen replacement therapy in ovarian failure or after castration.

b. Menstrual abnormalities

c. Postmenopausal therapy

–improves hot flashes, sweating, and atrophic vaginitis.

–slows rate of bone loss.

–are usually administered in a cyclical manner to avoid long periods of continuous exposure.

–concomitant use with a progestin reduces the incidence of endometrial carcinoma.

–transdermal delivery of **ethinyl estradiol** using a skin patch [Estraderm] is effective and long-lasting in treating postmenopausal symptoms.

d. Oral contraception

e. Androgen-dependent prostatic tumors are effectively treated by **DES**.

6. Adverse effects and contraindications

–are associated with nausea, headaches, hypertension, cholestasis, and gallbladder disease.

–present an increased risk (15 times) of **endometrial cancer** that is dose- and duration-dependent. Risk is reduced by periodic withdrawal of estrogen therapy and replacement by progestin treatment.

–estrogen therapy is the major cause of postmenopausal bleeding and may mask bleeding due to endometrial cancer.

–**DES** is associated with **adenocarcinoma of the vagina;** incidence in women exposed in utero to **DES** is 1:1000; genital malformation is much more common.

–are contraindicated in the presence of estrogen-dependent or estrogen-responsive carcinoma, liver disease, or thromboembolic disease.

B. **Progestins**

1. **Structure**

   - the most important natural progestin is **progesterone,** which is synthesized by the ovaries, testes, and adrenals.
   - synthetic progestins include the 19-nor compounds, such as **norethindrone** [Norlutin, others], **norgestrel** [Ovrette], and **levonorgestrel** [Norplant]. All of these agents are potent oral progestins derived from testosterone; some have androgenic activity (Figure 9.2).
   - several synthetic derivatives of progesterone have progestin activity, including **megestrol** [Megace], **medroxyprogesterone acetate** [Amen, Provera, others], and **hydroxyprogesterone caproate** [Delalutin, others].

2. **Actions and pharmacologic properties**

   - bind to an intranuclear receptor that causes transcription of target genes. Progestins slow the mitotic activity of the estrogen-stimulated uterus, cause vascularization of the endometrium, and induce a more glandular appearance and function.
   - slightly decrease triglycerides and HDL; slightly increase LDL, depending on preparation and dose. Also increase lipoprotein lipase.
   - increase basal and stimulated insulin secretion.

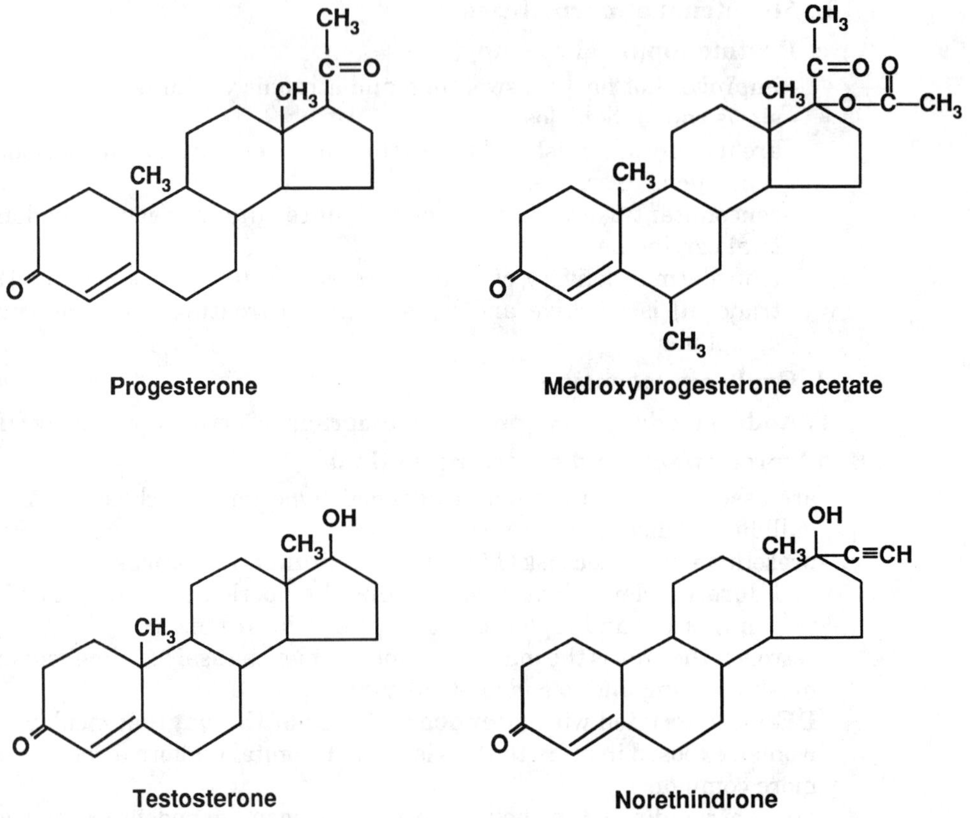

Progesterone

Medroxyprogesterone acetate

Testosterone

Norethindrone

Figure 9.2. Structures of androgens.

      −**progesterone** is extensively bound to corticosteroid-binding globulin in the plasma and is not administered orally due to rapid hepatic metabolism.

      −are eliminated by hydroxylation to **pregnanediol** and conjugation with glucuronic acid and subsequent urinary excretion.

3. Therapeutic uses

      −**oral contraception,** alone or combined with estrogens

      −treatment of **endometrial cancer**

      −control of **abnormal uterine bleeding**

      −**delay of menstruation** for surgical or postoperative reasons

      −diagnostically to evaluate endometrial function in **amenorrhea**

C. Hormonal contraceptives

1. Oral contraceptives

      −represent the primary use of estrogens and progestins.

a. Types of oral contraceptives

(1) Combination pills

      −contain mixtures of estrogens and a progestin. The estrogen component (20–50 μg/day) is either **ethinyl estradiol** or **mestranol** (mestranol is metabolized to ethinyl estradiol); a 19-nor progestin (0.05–2.5 mg/day), such as **norethindrone, norgestrel, levonorgestrel, norethindrone acetate,** or **ethynodiol diacetate,** is combined with one of the estrogens.

      −reduce the level and cyclicity of both LH and FSH, resulting in a failure to ovulate.

      −are typically taken continuously for 21 days followed by a 7-day withdrawal (or placebo) period to induce menses.

      −also affect the genital tract in ways that are unfavorable for conception: thickening cervical mucus, speeding ovum transport through the fallopian tubes, and making the endometrium less favorable for implantation.

(2) Progestin-only preparations ("mini pills")

      −contain **norethindrone** [Micronor, Nor-Q.D.] or **norgestrel** [Ovrette].

      −are taken daily on a continuous schedule.

      −do not completely suppress ovulation, resulting in irregular fertile periods.

      −mechanism of contraception is unclear but is likely due to formation of a relatively atrophic endometrium (which impairs implantation) and a viscous cervical mucus.

b. Adverse effects

(1) Cardiovascular

      −are associated with a twofold to fourfold increase in morbidity and mortality due to myocardial infarction.

      −the incidence of hypertension is 3–6 times higher among women taking oral contraceptives.

      −produce a marked increase (up to 50%) in triglyceride levels, depending on the relative doses of estrogens and progestins in the individual preparation.

—the risk of cardiovascular complications increases markedly in women over age 35 and in women who smoke.

(2) **Thromboembolic disease**

—the risk of stroke is 2–10 times higher in individuals taking oral contraceptives.

—estrogens increase levels of fibrinogen and coagulation factors II, VII, VIII, IX, and X while decreasing concentrations of antithrombin III.

(3) **Genitourinary tract**

—may reduce the incidence of ovarian and endometrial cancers.

(4) **Hepatobiliary system**

—increase incidence of gallbladder disease and gallstones.

(5) **Other adverse effects**

—include weight gain, edema, breast tenderness, headache, mood alteration, breakthrough bleeding, and amenorrhea on discontinuation.

c. **Contraindications**

—are contraindicated in cardiovascular disease, thromboembolic disease, estrogen-dependent or estrogen-responsive cancer, impaired liver function, undiagnosed bleeding, or migraine.

2. Subcutaneous progestin implants

—**levonorgestrel** encapsulated in Silastic tubing [Norplant] may be placed under the skin of the forearm, providing effective contraception for up to 5 years. Actual effectiveness is superior to that of combination oral contraceptives.

—adverse effects are dominated by menstrual irregularities.

—the relative risk of thromboembolic disease has not been established.

3. Intramuscular progestin injections

—**medroxyprogesterone acetate** [Depo-Provera] may be injected intramuscularly every 3 months.

—is effective as a contraceptive but safety has not been well established.

4. Postcoital oral contraceptives

—100 μg of **ethinyl estradiol** with 1 mg of **norgestrel,** taken twice 12 hours apart, has been found very effective if taken within 72 hours of coitus.

—2500 μg of **ethinyl estradiol,** taken twice daily for 5 days, is similarly effective.

—the use of **DES** in this circumstance is no longer approved.

—nausea and vomiting are common and can be severe. The risk of cancer in female offspring precludes this treatment if pregnancy is suspected.

D. Antiestrogens

—interfere with the binding of estrogen with its specific receptor. This class of compounds is distinguished from progestins and androgens, which also possess physiologic antiestrogenic activity.

1. Clomiphene [Clomid, Milophene, Serophene] and tamoxifen [Nolvadex]

—are nonsteroidal agents.

—bind competitively to the estrogen receptor and may also reduce levels of some mitogens. In some tissues, these agents exert a partial agonist activity.

—eventually reduce the number of functional receptors available for endogenous estrogens and diminish estrogen action both along the hypothalamic–hypophyseal axis and in peripheral tissues.

—are used to treat **infertility due to anovulation (clomiphene)** and **estrogen-dependent tumors of the breast (tamoxifen)**.

—may cause ovarian enlargement, hot flashes, nausea, and vomiting.

2. Danazol (Danocrine]

—is a testosterone derivative with antiandrogen activity.

—inhibits several of the enzymes involved in steroidogenesis; also inhibits gonadotropin release in both men and women.

—is used to treat **endometriosis** and **fibrocystic disease of the breast**.

—may cause edema, masculinization (deepening of the voice and decreased breast size) in some women, headache, and hepatocellular disease.

—is contraindicated in pregnant women or in patients with hepatic disease.

E. Androgens and anabolic steroids

1. Testosterone

—is synthesized primarily in the Leydig cells of the testis under the influence of LH. Many tissues contain the enzyme 5-α-reductase, which converts testosterone to the more potent metabolite **5-α-dihydrotestosterone.**

—is extensively bound (98%), mostly to SSBG and also to albumin.

2. Synthetic androgens

—the 17-substituted testosterone esters (**testosterone propionate** [Testex], **testosterone enanthate** [Andryl, Delatestryl, others], **and testosterone cypionate** [Andro-Cyp, others]) are administered by injection, usually as a depot in oil.

—17-alkyl testosterone derivatives include **methyltestosterone** [Metandren, Android, others], **fluoxymesterone** [Halotestin, others], **oxymetholone** [Anadrol, Anapolon], and **stanozolol** [Winstrol]. Absorption of these agents is greatest if administered sublingually, thus avoiding the large hepatic first-pass effect.

—**nandrolone** [Androlone, Deca-Durabolin, others] is a parenterally delivered testosterone derivative with the highest anabolic:androgenic ratio.

3. Actions

—form a complex with a specific intracellular receptor and interact with specific genes to modulate differentiation, development, and growth.

a. Androgenic actions

—differentiation and development of Wolffian structures, including the epididymis, seminal vesicles, prostate, and penis

—development and maintenance of male secondary sexual characteristics

b. Anabolic actions

—acceleration of epiphyseal closure; linear growth at puberty

–increase in muscle mass, positive nitrogen balance
–behavioral effects include aggressiveness and increased libido

4. **Uses**

a. **Prepubertal and postpubertal hypogonadism**

–promotes linear growth and sexual maturation and maintains male secondary sexual characteristics, libido, and potency.

b. **Anemia**

–stimulates secretion of erythropoeitin; has largely been supplanted by recombinant erythropoeitin (**epoetin**).

c. **Estrogen-dependent breast cancers**

d. **Illicit use by athletes**

–large doses increase the extent and rate of muscle formation; may increase the intensity of training.

5. **Adverse effects and contraindications**

–produce decreased testicular function, edema, and altered plasma lipids (increased LDL and decreased HDL levels).
–cause masculinization in women.
–increase plasma fibrinolytic activity, causing severe bleeding with concomitant anticoagulant therapy.
–17-alkyl substituted androgens (but not testosterone ester preparations) are associated with increases in hepatic enzymes, hyperbilirubinemia, and cholestasis, which may result in jaundice. Long-term use is associated with liver tumors.
–are contraindicated in pregnant women and patients with carcinoma of the prostate or hepatic, renal, or cardiovascular disease.

F. **Antiandrogens**

–are agents that impair the action or synthesis of endogenous androgens.

1. **Spironolactone [Aldactone]**

–completely antagonizes the binding of both androgen and aldosterone at their respective receptors; also decreases the activity of the steroidogenic enzyme 17-hydroxylase.
–is used as a **diuretic** and to treat **hirsutism** in women (usually in combination with **estrogen**).

2. **Flutamide [Eulexin]**

–is a potent antiandrogen and competitive androgen-receptor antagonist.
–treats **prostatic carcinoma** and is highly efficacious when combined with chronic GnRH agonist therapy.
–may cause gynecomastia and gastrointestinal disturbances.

3. **Ketoconazole [Nizoral]**

–is an antifungal agent that blocks multiple P-450–dependent steps in steroidogenesis.
–can be used in the treatment of **precocious puberty** and **hirsutism**.

4. **Cyproterone and cyproterone acetate**

–are potent investigational progestins with marked antiandrogen activity.

−treat **hirsutism** in women and **decrease sexual drive** in men. May also be useful in treating precocious puberty.

V. The Adrenal Cortex

A. Corticosteroids

1. Natural adrenocortical steroids

a. **Glucocorticoids** are synthesized under the control of ACTH (Figure 9.3). **Cortisol** (hydrocortisone) is the predominant natural glucocorticoid in humans. The 3-keto and 11-hydroxyl groups are important for biological activity.

b. The major **mineralocorticoid** of the adrenal cortex is **aldosterone**. 11-Deoxycorticosterone, an aldosterone precursor, has both mineralocorticoid and glucocorticoid activity.

c. The adrenals also synthesize various androgens, predominantly **dehydroepiandrosterone** and **androstenedione**.

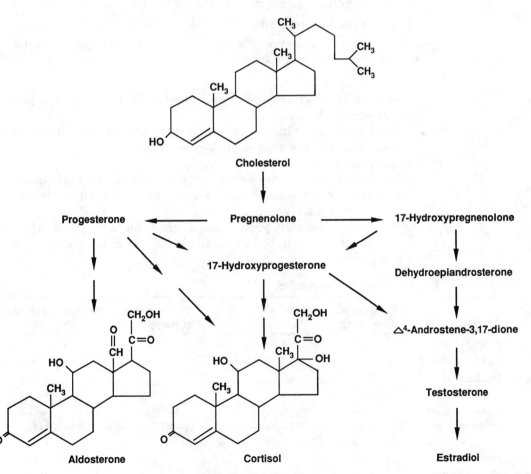

Figure 9.3. Biosynthesis of adrenal steroids.

2. Synthetic adrenocortical steroids

-a wide array of steroid compounds with various ratios of mineralocorticoid to glucocorticoid properties have been synthesized. The most important of these are listed in Table 9.1.

-**cortisone acetate** [Cortone] and **prednisone** [Meticorten, others] are 11-keto steroids that are converted to 11-hydroxyl groups by the liver to give **cortisol** and **prednisolone,** respectively.

-a C_1-C_2 double bond, as in **prednisolone** and **prednisone,** increases glucocorticoid activity without increasing mineralocorticoid activity.

-the addition of a 9-alpha-fluoro group (e.g., **dexamethasone** [Decadron, others] or **fludrocortisone** [Florinef]) increases activity.

-methylation or hydroxylation at the 16-alpha position abolishes mineralocorticoid activity with little effect on glucocorticoid potency.

3. Mechanism of action

-effects of mineralocorticoids and glucocorticoids are mediated by two separate and specific intracellular receptors. Natural and synthetic steroids enter cells rapidly and interact with these intracellular receptors. The resulting complexes modulate the transcription rate of specific genes and lead to an increase or decrease in the levels of specific proteins.

4. Actions of glucocorticoids

-affect virtually all tissues. Therapeutic actions and adverse effects are extensions of physiologic effects.

a. Physiologic effects

-are mediated by increased protein breakdown, leading to a **negative nitrogen balance**.

-**increase blood glucose levels** by stimulation of gluconeogenesis.

-**increase synthesis** of several **key enzymes** involved in glucose and amino acid metabolism.

-**increase plasma fatty acids and ketone body formation** via increased lipolysis and decreased glucose uptake into fat cells and redistribution of body fat.

-**increase kaliuresis** via increasing renal blood flow and GFR; increased protein metabolism results in release of intracellular potassium.

Table 9.1. Properties of Adrenocortical Steroids

Agent	Equivalent Dose (mg)	Metabolic Potency	Anti-inflammatory Potency	Sodium-retaining Potency
Cortisol	20	20	1	1
Cortisone	25	20	1	1
Prednisone	5	5	4	0.5
Prednisolone	5	5	4	0.5
Dexamethasone	0.75	1	30	0.05
Betamethasone	0.6	1.0–1.5	25–40	0.05
Triamcinolone	4	4	5	0.1
Aldosterone		0.3		3000
Fludrocortisone	0.01	0.1		125–250

–decrease intestinal absorption of Ca^{2+}.

–promote Na^+ and water retention.

b. Anti-inflammatory effects

–all of the **classic signs of inflammation** (erythema, swelling, soreness, and heat). Specific effects include:

(1) Inhibition of the antigenic response of macrophages and leukocytes

(2) Inhibition of vascular permeability by reduction of histamine release and the action of kinins

(3) Inhibition of arachidonic acid and **prostaglandin production** by inhibition of phospholipase A_2 and, perhaps, cyclooxygenase

c. Immunologic effects

–decrease circulating lymphocytes, monocytes, eosinophils, and basophils.

–increase circulating neutrophils.

–chronic therapy results in involution and atrophy of all lymphoid tissues.

d. Other effects

(1) Inhibition of plasma ACTH; can result in adrenal atrophy

(2) Inhibition of fibroblast growth and **collagen synthesis**

(3) Stimulation of acid and pepsin secretion in the stomach

(4) Altered CNS responses, influencing mood and sleep patterns

(5) Enhanced neuromuscular transmission

(6) Induction of surfactant production in the fetal lung at term

5. Actions of mineralocorticoids

–primarily affect the **kidney,** regulating salt and water balance and increasing sodium retention and potassium loss.

–**fludrocortisone** [Florinef] is the agent of choice for long-term treatment.

–adverse effects include sodium retention and hypokalemia, edema, and hypertension.

6. Pharmacologic properties

a. Plasma binding

–80% of circulating cortisol is bound to corticosteroid-binding globulin (CBG); 10% is bound to plasma albumin.

–some of the potent synthetic glucocorticoids, such as **dexamethasone,** do not bind to CBG, leaving all of the absorbed drug in a free state.

b. Both natural and synthetic steroids are excreted by the kidney following reduction and formation of glucuronides or sulfates.

c. All of the steroids listed in Table 9.1 (except **aldosterone**) may be administered orally. A variety of glucocorticoids, including **cortisol, prednisolone,** and **dexamethasone,** can be injected intramuscularly or subcutaneously. **Triamcinolone** [Aristocort, others], **dexamethasone, betamethasone** [Celestone, others], and **cortisol** can be applied topically. **Beclomethasone** [Beclovent, Beconase, others] is available as an inhalant.

d. Agents with the longest $t_{1/2}$ tend to be the most potent.

    (1) Short-acting agents such as **cortisol** are active for 8–12 hours.

    (2) Intermediate-acting agents such as **prednisolone** are active for 12–36 hours.

    (3) Long-acting agents such as **dexamethasone** are active for 39–54 hours.

e. Drug administration attempts to pattern the circadian rhythm: double dose in the morning, single dose in the afternoon.

f. Alternate-day therapy relieves clinical manifestations of the disease state while causing less severe suppression of the adrenal–hypothalamic–pituitary axis.

    —large doses of short-acting or intermediate-acting glucocorticoids are administered every other day.

g. Patients removed from long-term glucocorticoid therapy must be weaned off the drug over several days using progressively lower doses to allow recovery of adrenal responsiveness.

7. Therapeutic uses of glucocorticoids

a. Replacement therapy for primary or secondary insufficiency (Addison's disease); therapy usually requires the use of both a mineralocorticoid and a glucocorticoid.

b. Inflammation and immunosuppression

    —are used to treat the following disorders: rheumatoid arthritis, bursitis, lupus erythematosus, and other autoimmune diseases; asthma; nephrotic syndrome; ulcerative colitis; and ocular inflammation.

    —are also used in hypersensitivity and allergic reactions.

    —can reduce organ or graft rejection.

c. Sarcoidosis

d. Dermatologic disorders

e. Idiopathic nephrosis of children

f. Neuromuscular disorders, such as Bell's palsy

g. Shock

h. Adrenocortical hyperplasia

i. Stimulation of surfactant production and acceleration of lung maturation of the fetus

j. Neoplastic diseases, including adult and childhood leukemias

k. Diagnosis of Cushing's syndrome (dexamethasone suppression test)

8. Therapeutic uses of mineralocorticoids

    —replacement therapy to maintain electrolyte and fluid balance in hypoadrenalism

9. Adverse effects and contraindications

    —most of the adverse effects of glucocorticoids are exaggerated physiologic effects leading to a state of **iatrogenic Cushing's disease**.

    —certain glucocorticoids have mineralocorticoid activity, potentially causing sodium retention, potassium loss, and eventual hypokalemic, hypochloremic alkalosis.

—adverse effects include the following:

a. Adrenal suppression

b. Hyperglycemia and other metabolic disturbances

c. Osteoporosis

d. Peptic ulcer

e. Cataracts and increased intraocular pressure leading to glaucoma

f. Edema

g. Hypertension

h. Increased susceptibility to infection and poor wound healing

i. Muscle weakness and tissue loss

B. Adrenocortical antagonists

1. Mitotane (o,p′-DDD) [Lysodren]

—causes selective atrophy of the zona fasciculata and zona reticularis and can reduce plasma cortisol level in Cushing's syndrome produced by adrenal carcinoma.

—use is limited to **adrenal carcinomas** when other therapies are not feasible.

—severe adverse effects are not unusual and may include gastrointestinal distress, mental confusion, lethargy, and dermal toxicity.

2. Aminoglutethimide [Cytadren]

—blocks the conversion of cholesterol to pregnenolone and reduces adrenal production of aldosterone, cortisol, and androgens. The reduction in plasma cortisol triggers a compensatory increase in ACTH that antagonizes the effect of aminoglutethimide. ACTH release may be prevented by coadministration of a glucocorticoid such as **cortisol**.

—is useful in treating hyperadrenalism due to **adrenal carcinoma** or **congenital adrenal hyperplasia**.

—adverse effects include drowsiness, skin rashes, and nausea.

3. Metyrapone [Metopirone]

—blocks the activity of 11-hydroxylase, thereby reducing cortisol production.

—is used diagnostically to **assess adrenal and pituitary function**.

4. Trilostane [Modrastane]

—is a synthetic steroid with no intrinsic hormonal activity that interferes with steroidogenesis, thereby reducing cortisol and aldosterone levels.

—has been used to treat **hyperaldosteronism** and **refractory Cushing's syndrome**.

—causes mostly gastrointestinal adverse effects such as nausea, vomiting, and diarrhea.

VI. The Thyroid

A. Thyroid hormone receptor agonists

1. Synthesis of natural thyroid hormones

—are formed by iodination of tyrosine residues on the glycoprotein thyroglobulin. A tyrosine residue may be iodinated at one (monoiodotyrosine, MIT) or two (diiodotyrosine, DIT) positions. Two iodinated tyrosines are

then coupled to synthesize **triiodothyronine** (T_3; formed from one molecule each of MIT and DIT) or **thyroxine** (T_4; formed from two DIT molecules). T_4 synthesis exceeds T_3 synthesis by 10–20 times. Seventy-five percent of circulating T_3 is derived from deiodination of T_4.
  –biosynthesis is stimulated by TSH, which acts by a mechanism involving elevation of follicular cell cAMP.
  –I^- is a potent inhibitor of thyroid hormone release.

2. Thyroid hormone preparations

a. Levothyroxine sodium [Levothroid, Synthroid, others], a synthetic sodium salt of T_4, which maintains normal T_4 and T_3 levels

b. Liothyronine sodium [Cytomel], a synthetic sodium salt of T_3

c. Liotrix [Euthroid, Thyrolar], a 4:1 mixture of the above T_4:T_3 preparations

d. Thyroid USP [Armour Thyroid, Dathroid, others], prepared from dried and defatted animal thyroid glands and containing a mixture of T_4, T_3, MIT, and DIT
  –potency of this product can vary.
  –given the availability of synthetics, **thyroid USP** is not recommended for initial therapy.

e. Thyroglobulin [Proloid], prepared from porcine thyroid and containing thyroglobulin, T_3, and T_4, is not recommended for initial therapy.

3. Mechanism of action

  –interact with specific receptor proteins located in the nucleus of target cells and alter the synthesis rate of specific mRNAs, leading to increased production of specific proteins, including Na^+, K^+-ATPase. Increased ATP hydrolysis and oxygen consumption contribute to the effects of thyroid hormones on basal metabolic rate and thermogenesis. T_3 is 3–5 times more potent than T_4.

4. Pharmacologic properties

a. Greater than 99% of circulating T_4 is bound to plasma proteins; only 5%–10% of T_3 is protein-bound. The majority of T_3 and T_4 are bound to **thyroid-binding globulin (TBG)**. T_4 also binds to pre-albumin, and both T_4 and T_3 bind weakly to albumin.

b. T_3 has a $t_{1/2}$ of approximately 1 day; T_4 has a $t_{1/2}$ of approximately 5–7 days.

c. Levothyroxine sodium and **liothyronine sodium** can be administered orally or intravenously. Oral absorption rates range from 30%–65%. **Levothyroxine sodium** is preferred to **liothyronine** because it has better oral absorption, longer $t_{1/2}$, and favorable T_4:T_3 ratio.

d. Metabolism
  –T_3 and T_4 are inactivated by deiodination.
  –conjugation of T_3 and T_4 with glucuronic acid or sulfate occurs in the liver, and these metabolites are secreted in the bile.
  –some enterohepatic circulation of the metabolites occurs; 20%–40% of T_4 is eliminated in the feces.

5. Actions

  −are **essential for normal physical and mental development of the fetus**. Linear growth of the long bones, growth of the brain, and normal myelination are dependent on growth hormone. Hypothyroidism in infants leads to cretinism (myxedema with physical and mental retardation).
  −**increase** the **basal metabolic rate** and **blood sugar levels**. Increase synthesis of fatty acids; decrease plasma cholesterol and triglyceride levels.
  −**increase** the **heart rate** and **peripheral resistance**.
  −**inhibit TRH and TSH release** from the hypothalamus and pituitary, respectively.
  −exert **maintenance effects** on the CNS, reproductive tract, gastrointestinal tract, and musculature.

6. Therapeutic uses

  a. Primary, secondary, or tertiary hypothyroidism caused by:
   (1) Hashimoto's disease
   (2) Myxedema
   (3) Simple goiter (thyroid gland enlargement without hyperthyroidism)
   (4) Surgical ablation of the thyroid gland

  b. TSH-dependent carcinomas of the thyroid; may be treated with thyroid hormones if other therapies are not feasible.

7. Adverse effects

  −produce iatrogenic hyperthyroidism, nervousness, and headache.
  −induce arrhythmias, angina, or infarction in patients with underlying cardiovascular disease.
  −should be used cautiously in the elderly.

B. Antithyroid drugs

1. Thioamides

  −include **propylthiouracil (PTU)** and **methimazole** [Tapazole]; methimazole is approximately 10 times more potent than PTU.
  −interfere with several steps in the biosynthesis of thyroid hormones, including the organification and coupling of iodide.
  −remain active after oral administration; 50%–80% is absorbed.
  −have a $t_{1/2}$ of approximately 1–2 hours; are concentrated in the thyroid gland and inhibit thyroid hormone biosynthesis for 6–24 hours.
  −are eliminated in the urine as glucuronides.
  −treat hyperthyroidism from a variety of causes, including **Grave's disease** and **toxic goiter**. Thioamides are also used to **control hyperthyroidism prior to thyroid surgery**.
  −commonly cause skin rashes, headache, or nausea. May also induce leukopenia or agranulocytosis.

2. Anion inhibitors of thyroid function

  −include **thiocyanate, perchlorate,** and **fluoborate**.
  −are monovalent anions with a hydrated radius similar in size to that of iodide.

–competitively inhibit the transport of iodide by the thyroid gland.

–are limited by severe toxicities (including **fatal aplastic anemia**) to occasional **diagnostic use for thyroid function**.

3. Iodide

–in high intracellular concentrations, inhibits several steps in thyroid hormone biosynthesis, including iodide transport and organification (Wolff–Chaikoff effect).

–inhibits the release of thyroid hormone.

–is usually combined with a thioamide; rarely used as a sole therapy.

–is used prior to **thyroid surgery,** causing a firming of thyroid tissues and a decrease in thyroid vascularity, and in the treatment of **sporotrichosis**.

–may cause angioedema, skin rash, a metallic taste on administration, and hypersensitivity reactions.

4. Radioactive iodine ^{131}I [Iodotope]

–emits beta particles and X-rays and has a radioactive $t_{1/2}$ of approximately 8 days. ^{131}I is transported and concentrated in the thyroid like the nonradioactive isotope. High-energy radioiodine emissions are toxic to follicular cells.

–treats hyperthyroidism via **nonsurgical ablation of the thyroid gland** or reduction of hyperactive thyroid gland without damage to surrounding tissue.

–is helpful (in low doses) in the **diagnosis of hyperthyroidism, hypothyroidism, and goiter;** may be used to assess thyroid responsiveness.

–overdosage commonly induces hypothyroidism.

5. Oral cholecystographic agents

–include **ipodate** [Oragrafin] and **iopanoic acid** [Telepaque].

–cause a rapid reduction in serum T_3 and T_4. However, the release of iodine resulting from the metabolism of these drugs may stimulate thyroid hormone synthesis.

–are used singly or as adjuncts to thioamide in treating **hyperthyroidism**.

VII. The Pancreas and Glucose Homeostasis

A. Insulin

1. Structure and synthesis

–is a polypeptide hormone produced by the pancreatic β cell. Insulin consists of two chains, A and B, linked by two disulfide bridges.

–human insulin contains 51 amino acids. Bovine insulin differs from human insulin at three amino acid sites; porcine differs at only 1 amino acid.

–is stored as a complex with Zn^{2+}; two molecules of zinc complex six molecules of insulin.

–insulin synthesis and release are modulated by the following:

a. The most important stimulus is **glucose**. Amino acids, fatty acids, and ketone bodies also stimulate release.

b. The islets of Langerhans contains several cell types besides β cells that synthesize and release **peptide humoral agents** (including **glucagon** and **somatostatin**) that can modulate insulin secretion.

c. α-Adrenergic pathways inhibit secretion of insulin; this is the predominant inhibitory mechanism.

d. β-Adrenergic stimulation increases insulin release.

2. Mechanism of action

−binds to specific high-affinity receptors with tyrosine kinase activity located in the plasma membrane. The increase in glucose transport in muscle and adipose tissue is mediated by the recruitment of hexose transport molecules into the plasma membrane.

−alters the phosphorylation state of key metabolic enzymes, leading to enzymatic activation or inactivation.

−induces the transcription of several genes involved in increasing glucose catabolism and specifically inhibits transcription of other genes involved in gluconeogenesis.

3. Actions

−promotes systemic cellular K^+ uptake.

a. Liver

−inhibits **glucose production** and increases **glycolysis**.

−inhibits **glycogenolysis** and stimulates **glycogen synthesis**.

−increases **synthesis of triglycerides**.

−increases **protein synthesis**.

b. Muscle

−increases **glucose transport** and **glycolysis**.

−increases **glycogen deposition**.

−increases **protein synthesis**.

c. Adipose tissue

−increases **glucose transport**.

−increases **lipogenesis** and **lipoprotein lipase**.

−decreases **intracellular lipolysis**.

4. Pharmacologic properties

−possesses a $t_{1/2}$ of 5–10 minutes.

−is degraded by hepatic glutathione–insulin transhydrogenase, which reduces the disulfide linkages between the A and B chains, producing two biologically inactive peptides.

5. Insulin preparations (Table 9.2)

−are derived from three tissue sources: bovine, porcine, and human. Human insulin is prepared either by recombinant DNA techniques to produce the human peptide from altered bacteria [Humulin] or from semisynthetic conversion of porcine insulin to human insulin by altering the one differing amino acid [Novolin].

−are often mixed to control blood sugar levels: A single morning injection of a lente or ultralente form is typically supplemented with preprandial injections of a fast-acting product.

Table 9.2. Pharmacologic Properties of Agents Used for Long-Term Management
of Hyperglycemia

Agent	Route of Administration	Onset of Action	Duration of Action
Insulins			
Regular	Intramuscular, intravenous	15 min	5–7 hr
Semilente	Intramuscular	15 min	12–14 hr
Lente	Intramuscular	2 hr	24 hr
Isophane	Intramuscular	2 hr	24 hr
Ultralente	Intramuscular	4 hr	36 hr
Protamine–zinc	Intramuscular	4 hr	36 hr
Sulfonylureas			
Tolbutamide	Oral	20 min	6–10 hr
Acetohexamide	Oral	20 min	12–20 hr
Tolazamide	Oral	20 min	10–14 hr
Glipizide	Oral	30 min	16–24 hr
Glyburide	Oral	1–2 hr	24 hr
Chlorpropamide	Oral	1–2 hr	> 24 hr

    a. Fast-acting

       (1) Regular insulin is prepared from bovine, porcine [Iletin, others],
       or human insulin as a zinc-containing solution (typically ZnCl).

       (2) Semilente insulin is a suspension of a very fine insulin–zinc pre-
       cipitate.

    b. Intermediate-acting

       (1) Isophane insulin (NPH) is prepared by precipitating insulin–
       zinc complexes with protamine, a mixture of basic peptides.

       (2) Lente insulin is an amorphous insulin in larger precipitates than
       semilente products; onset is slower and the duration of action
       longer.

    c. Long-acting

       (1) Protamine–zinc insulin has a larger particle size than NPH in-
       sulin.

       (2) Ultralente insulin has a larger particle size than lente products.

6. Therapeutic uses

    –is used to treat all of the manifestations of hyperglycemia in both **type
    I (insulin-dependent) and type II (non-insulin-dependent) diabe-
    tes mellitus**. Most type II diabetics are treated with dietary changes and
    oral hypoglycemic agents. In serious cases of type II diabetes where these
    treatments are inadequate to control blood glucose levels, insulin may be
    required.

7. Adverse effects

    a. Hypoglycemia may occur from insulin overdose, insufficient caloric in-
    take, or strenuous exercise. Sequelae include tachycardia, sweating, and
    sympathetic and parasympathetic actions that can progress to coma.

b. Immune disorders
  (1) Production of anti-insulin antibodies
  (2) Hypersensitivity reactions (local urticaria and angioedema) to minor contaminants in preparations
  (3) Lipodystrophy or hypertrophy of subcutaneous fat at the injection site

B. Oral hypoglycemic agents (sulfonylureas)

1. Structure

  a. First-generation compounds include **tolbutamide** [Orinase, others], **acetohexamide** [Dymelor], **tolazamide** [Ronase, Tolinase], and **chlorpropamide** [Diabinese, Glucamide].

  b. Second-generation compounds include **glyburide** [DiaBeta, Micronase] and **glipizide** [Glucotrol] and are up to 200 times more potent than first-generation agents.

  c. All of the sulfonylureas are well absorbed after oral administration and bind to plasma proteins, notably albumin.

2. Mechanism of action

  −cause an **increase** in the **amount of insulin** secreted by the β cells in response to a glucose challenge. Sulfonylureas block K^+ channels in β cells, leading to depolarization and increased secretion.
  −**increase sensitivity to insulin,** perhaps by increasing the number of insulin receptors. However, sulfonylureas do not decrease the insulin requirements of patients with type I diabetes.
  −**decrease serum glucagon,** which opposes the action of insulin.

3. Pharmacologic properties (see Table 9.2)

  −pharmacologic failure with oral antidiabetic agents is common, initially affecting 15%–30% of patients and as many as 90% after 6–7 years of therapy.

  a. Short-acting agents
    −include **tolbutamide**.
    −are rapidly absorbed; absorption is not affected if taken with food.
    −as with all sulfonylureas, **hypoglycemia** is a potentially dangerous adverse effect. Other adverse effects include dermatologic disorders and gastrointestinal disturbances, including nausea and heartburn.

  b. Intermediate-acting agents
    (1) Acetohexamide
      −is rapidly absorbed.
      −is metabolized to hydrohexamide, which is biologically active and has $t_{1/2}$ of 6 hours.
      −has uricosuric properties, making it useful in diabetic patients with **gout**.
    (2) Tolazamide
      −is slowly absorbed.
      −exerts a **mild diuretic effect**.
    (3) Glipizide
      −is rapidly absorbed, but absorption can be delayed by food.
      −becomes highly protein-bound in the plasma.

(4) Glyburide

—is rapidly absorbed.

—inhibits hepatic glucose production.

—exerts a **mild diuretic effect**.

c. Long-acting agents

—include **chlorpropamide**.

—are rapidly absorbed.

—are extensively reabsorbed in the kidney; reabsorption is slowed under basic pH conditions.

—cause adverse effects more frequently than other sulfonylureas. Water retention is common, and alcohol consumption produces a **disulfiram-like reaction** in some patients.

—are contraindicated in elderly patients, in whom toxicities seem to be exacerbated.

4. Therapeutic uses

—are very useful in treating **type II diabetes mellitus** but are not effective against type I diabetes.

—should not be used in patients with renal or liver disease.

C. Agents that increase blood glucose (hyperglycemics)

1. Glucagon

a. Structure and synthesis

—is a **single-chain polypeptide** of 29 amino acids produced by the α cells of the pancreas.

—shares a structural homology with secretin, VIP, and gastric inhibitory peptide.

—**secretion** is **inhibited** by elevated plasma glucose, insulin, and somatostatin.

—**secretion** is **stimulated** by amino acids, sympathetic stimulation, and sympathetic secretion.

b. Actions and pharmacologic properties

—receptors are most abundant in the liver; response is coupled to an increase in cAMP.

—stimulates the use of glycogen stores and gluconeogenesis; in general, its actions oppose those of **insulin**.

—large doses produce a marked relaxation of smooth muscle.

—is extensively degraded in the liver and kidney and is also subject to hydrolysis in plasma. Plasma $t_{1/2}$ is approximately 3–5 minutes.

c. Therapeutic uses

—produces rescue from **hypoglycemic crisis**. Glucagon rapidly increases blood glucose in insulin-induced hypoglycemia if hepatic glycogen stores are adequate.

—provides **intestinal relaxation** prior to radiologic examination.

—causes β cell stimulation of insulin secretion; is used to **assess pancreatic reserves**.

d. Adverse effects

—are minimal; there is a low incidence of nausea and vomiting.

2. Diazoxide [Proglycem]
   −is a nondiuretic thiazide that promptly increases blood glucose levels by direct inhibition of insulin secretion.
   −is useful in cases of **insulinoma** or **leucine-sensitive hypoglycemia**.
   −may cause sodium retention, gastrointestinal irritation, and changes in circulating white blood cells.

VIII. The Calcium Homeostatic System

A. Calcium
   −is the major extracellular divalent cation, primarily (40%–50%) existing as free ionized Ca^{2+} (the biologically active fraction). Approximately 40% of serum Ca^{2+} is bound to plasma proteins, especially albumin, with the remaining 10% complexed to such anions as citrate.

B. Drugs affecting Ca^{2+} homeostasis

1. Parathyroid hormone (PTH)

a. Structure
   −is an 84-amino acid peptide secreted by the parathyroid glands in response to low serum ionized Ca^{2+}. Agents such as β-adrenoceptor agonists, which increase cAMP in the parathyroid gland, cause an increase in PTH secretion.

b. Actions and pharmacologic properties
   −activity in the kidney and probably in bone is mediated by specific PTH receptors, which are in turn coupled to an increase in cAMP. Significant quantities of cAMP are found in the urine after PTH stimulation.
   −in bone, PTH increases the number and activity of osteoclasts, resulting in a net increase in bone resorption.
   −in the kidney, PTH increases reabsorption of Ca^{2+} and Mg^{2+} and increases production of 1,25-$(OH)_2D_3$ from 25-$(OH)D_3$. PTH also decreases reabsorption of phosphate, bicarbonate, amino acids, sulfate, sodium, and chloride.
   −in the gastrointestinal tract, PTH increases intestinal absorption of Ca^{2+} indirectly through the increase in 1,25-$(OH)_2D_3$.
   −PTH is rapidly degraded ($t_{1/2}$ is 2–5 minutes) by renal and hepatic metabolism.

c. Uses
   −as a diagnostic agent to **distinguish pseudohypoparathyroidism from true hypoparathyroidism**.

2. Calcitonin

a. Structure
   −is a 32-amino acid peptide secreted by perifollicular cells of the parathyroid gland in response to elevated plasma Ca^{2+}. Gastrin, glucagon, cholecystokinin, and epinephrine can also increase calcitonin secretion.

b. Actions
   −antagonizes the actions of PTH through an independent mechanism:
   (1) Interacts with specific receptors on bone cells to decrease net reabsorption of Ca^{2+}. May also stimulate bone formation.
   (2) Increases renal excretion of Ca^{2+}, Na^+, and phosphate.

c. Pharmacologic properties

—**synthetic salmon calcitonin** [Calcimar, Miacalcin] differs from **human calcitonin** [Cibacalcin] at 16 of 32 amino acids and has a longer half-life.

—currently approved products are administered either subcutaneously or intramuscularly; nasal spray formulations are under investigation.

—decreases in plasma Ca^{2+} are seen in 2 hours and persist for 6–8 hours.

d. Therapeutic uses

—reduces hypercalcemia due to **Paget's disease, hyperparathyroidism, idiopathic juvenile hypercalcemia, vitamin D intoxication, osteolytic bone disorders,** and **osteoporosis.**

—patients frequently (20%) become refractory to chronic administration, possibly due to the production of anti-calcitonin antibodies (patients receiving salmon-derived preparations are especially vulnerable).

3. Vitamin D and vitamin D metabolites

a. Structure

—the calciferols, **vitamin D_3 (cholecalciferol)** and **vitamin D_2 (ergocalciferol),** are secosterol members of the steroid hormone family.

b. Synthesis

(1) Vitamin D_3

—is produced in the skin from cholesterol; this synthesis requires exposure to ultraviolet light.

(2) 25-(OH)D_3 (calcifediol) [Calderol]

—is produced in the liver by hydroxylation of vitamin D_3.

—is the most abundant calciferol metabolite in the plasma.

(3) 1,25-(OH)$_2D_3$ (calcitriol) [Rocaltrol, Calcijex]

—is produced in the kidney by further hydroxylation of 25-(OH)D_3 by 1-α-hydroxylase. Regulation of 1-α-hydroxylase activity determines the serum levels of **calcitriol.** Enzymatic activity is increased by PTH, estrogens, prolactin, and other agents and is decreased by 1,25-(OH)$_2D_3$ and phosphate (direct effect).

—is the most active metabolite of vitamin D.

(4) Vitamin D_2 (ergocalciferol) [Calciferol, Deltalin, Drisdol]

—is derived from plant metabolism of ergosterol and has a slightly different side-chain, which does not alter its biological effects in humans.

—is metabolized in the same manner as **vitamin D_3,** bypassing the need for ultraviolet light exposure.

(5) Dihydrotachysterol [DHT, Hytakerol]

—is a reduced form of ergosterol in which rotation of the A ring locates an hydroxyl group in the same position as the 1-OH group in 1,25-(OH)$_2D_3$.

c. Actions and pharmacologic properties (Table 9.3)

(1) Calcitriol increases plasma levels of both Ca^{2+} and phosphate by acting on several organ systems:

(a) Intestine: Increases Ca^{2+} absorption from the gastrointestinal tract

Table 9.3. Pharmacologic Properties of Vitamin D Preparations

Agent	Metabolic Route	Onset of Action	Half-life
Ergocalciferol	Hepatic, renal	10–14 days	30 days
Calcifediol	Renal	8–10 days	20 days
Dihydrotachysterol	Hepatic	8–10 days	15 days
Calcitriol		10 hr	15 hr

  (b) Bone: Mobilizes Ca^{2+} and phosphate, probably by stimulation of calcium flux out of osteoblasts
  (c) Kidney: Increases reabsorption of both Ca^{2+} and phosphate
(2) All vitamin D metabolites bind to a specific plasma-binding protein, vitamin D–binding protein (DBP).
(3) **Vitamin D, calcifediol, calcitriol,** and **dihydrotachysterol** are all administered orally; **DHT** and **calcitriol** may be administered parenterally.

  d. Therapeutic uses
    —are used to treat hypocalcemia caused by a number of diseases, including **vitamin D deficiency** (nutritional rickets), **hypoparathyroidism, renal disease, malabsorption,** and **osteoporosis.**

C. Secondary agents affecting Ca^{2+} homeostasis

  1. Diphosphonates
    —are analogs of pyrophosphate that reduce bone resorption, thereby reducing plasma Ca^{2+}; include **etidronate disodium** [Didronel].
    —bind directly to bone and retard the dissolution and formation of hydroxyapatite crystals.
    —are used orally to treat **Paget's disease** and **hypervitaminosis D,** but may require months of therapy before effects are seen.
    —cause inhibition of bone mineralization.

  2. Plicamycin (mithramycin) [Mithracin]
    —is a cytotoxic antibiotic that reduces bone resorption by impairing osteoclast function.
    —is used to treat **hypercalcemia due to Paget's disease or cancer.**

  3. Thiazide diuretics
    —reduce renal excretion of Ca^{2+} and incidence of kidney stone formation in patients with **idiopathic hypercalciuria.**

  4. Loop diuretics
    —agents such as **furosemide** increase renal excretion of Ca^{2+}.

  5. Glucocorticoids
    —increase bone resorption and reduce intestinal absorption of Ca^{2+} by interfering with $1,25\text{-}(OH)_2D_3$. Net effect is to reduce plasma Ca^{2+} levels.

  6. Estrogens
    —indirectly impair the action of PTH on bone and in the kidney.
    —are used in the treatment of **osteoporosis.**

7. Calcium supplements
    −are available in a variety of Ca^{2+} concentrations and in parenteral and oral formulations.
    −are useful as dietary supplements for the treatment or prevention of **osteoporosis** and for the immediate treatment of **acute hypocalcemia and hypocalcemic tetany**.
    −may cause hypercalcemia with chronic use.

Review Test

Directions: Each of the numbered items or incomplete statements in this section is followed by answers or by completions of the statement. Select the **one** lettered answer or completion that is **best** in each case.

1. Which of the following actions or properties is most closely associated with estradiol?

(A) Increases the production of thick cervical mucus
(B) Stimulates progesterone receptor biosynthesis in the uterus
(C) Is transported in the blood bound mainly to albumin
(D) Can be reversibly metabolized to testosterone

2. The sulfonylureas act to

(A) increase insulin secretion
(B) decrease glucocorticoid levels
(C) decrease tissue sensitivity to insulin
(D) decrease insulin $t_{1/2}$

3. Which of the following agents may be used to treat hypercalcemia?

(A) Furosemide
(B) Thiazides
(C) Vitamin D
(D) Parathyroid hormone (PTH)

4. Which of the following agents would be most effective in raising serum Ca^{2+} in a patient with impaired liver function?

(A) Ergosterol
(B) Dihydrotachysterol
(C) Calcitriol
(D) Cholecalciferol

5. Which of the following effects would result from chronic administration of leuprolide?

(A) Increased gonadotropin releasing hormone (GnRH) receptors
(B) Increased gonadotropin release
(C) Decreased gonadotropin release
(D) Reinitiation of menstrual cycles

6. Nandrolone esters may be useful adjuncts for the treatment of which one of the following conditions?

(A) Prostatic cancer
(B) Precocious puberty
(C) Threatened spontaneous abortion
(D) Hypogonadism

7. Which of the following is useful in treating hypocalcemia?

(A) Phosphate salts
(B) Vitamin D
(C) Glucocorticoids
(D) Loop diuretics

8. Which of the following is associated with an increase in the effectiveness of circulating insulin?

(A) Sulfonylureas
(B) Obesity
(C) Glucocorticoids
(D) Anti-insulin receptor antibodies

9. Dexamethasone has which of the following properties?

(A) Results in decreased leukotriene production
(B) Is effective immediately
(C) Is extensively bound to plasma proteins
(D) Is a cholinergic antagonist

10. Three formulations of insulin are indicated in each choice below. Which choice correctly ranks insulin, from quickest onset of action to slowest?

(A) Protamine–zinc insulin → regular insulin → lente insulin
(B) Ultralente insulin → lente insulin → regular insulin
(C) Regular insulin → isophane insulin → protamine–zinc insulin
(D) Isophane insulin → lente insulin → protamine–zinc insulin

11. Prednisone is more useful than cortisol for long-term immunosuppressive therapy because prednisone

(A) has greater metabolic effects
(B) has less mineralocorticoid activity
(C) is less likely to cause suppression of the pituitary–adrenal axis
(D) is more effective in patients with decreased liver function

12. Which of the following drugs has the most rapid onset of action?

(A) Calciferol
(B) Calcifediol
(C) Calcitriol
(D) Dihydrotachysterol
(E) Dehydrocholesterol

13. Tamoxifen is useful in the treatment of breast cancer because

(A) it has progestational activity that limits the growth-promoting effects of estrogens
(B) it blocks the binding of estrogen to estrogen receptors
(C) it decreases secretion of follicle-stimulating hormone (FSH)
(D) it enhances biliary excretion of estrogens

14. Which of the following agents decreases insulin secretion?

(A) β-Receptor agonists
(B) Leucine
(C) Sulfonylureas
(D) α-Receptor agonists

15. Hypoparathyroidism in the presence of renal disease is best treated with

(A) ergocalciferol
(B) cholecalciferol
(C) calciferol
(D) dihydrotachysterol

16. β-Adrenoceptor antagonists are useful adjuncts in the management of patients with hyperthyroidism because they

(A) reduce the secretion of T_3 and T_4
(B) help control the bradycardia associated with the disorder
(C) alleviate symptoms of hypercalcemia
(D) alleviate symptoms such as nervousness and weakness

17. Potential adverse effects of testosterone administration include all of the following EXCEPT

(A) precocious puberty
(B) virilization
(C) decreased sperm production
(D) hepatotoxicity

18. All of the following statements regarding estrogen therapy in postmenopausal women are true EXCEPT

(A) it may be useful to treat vasomotor symptoms
(B) it restores the loss of bone mass due to osteoporosis
(C) administration in a regimen including a progestin reduces the risk of endometrial carcinoma
(D) it is useful in the treatment of atrophic vaginitis

19. Adverse effects of chronic corticosteroid therapy include all of the following EXCEPT

(A) infection
(B) hypoglycemia
(C) suppression of the pituitary–adrenal axis
(D) increased rate of wound healing

20. All of the following glucocorticoids may be used as a topical treatment for a skin disease EXCEPT

(A) cortisol
(B) prednisone
(C) dexamethasone
(D) triamcinolone acetonide

21. All of the following statements about thyroid hormones are true EXCEPT

(A) secretion of the iodinated thyroid hormones is stimulated by thyroid-stimulating hormone
(B) iodinated thyroid hormones inhibit secretion of thyroid-stimulating hormone from the anterior pituitary gland
(C) thyroxine stimulates protein synthesis in target cells by interacting with a specific nuclear receptor
(D) methimazole is an antithyroid drug that inhibits the biosynthesis of thyroglobulin

22. Endometriosis may be treated with any of the following agents EXCEPT

(A) leuprolide
(B) a progestin
(C) danazol
(D) mestranol

23. Known adverse effects of combination oral contraceptives include all of the following EXCEPT

(A) hypertension
(B) benign liver tumors
(C) stroke
(D) uterine cancer

24. All of the following are adverse effects of glucocorticoid treatment EXCEPT

(A) osteoporosis
(B) negative nitrogen balance
(C) decreased ACTH secretion
(D) hypoglycemia

25. All of the following conditions are potential indications for use of glucocorticoid therapy EXCEPT

(A) hyperglycemia
(B) allergic reaction
(C) immunosuppression
(D) Addison's disease

Answers and Explanations

1–B. Estradiol stimulates progesterone receptor biosynthesis in the uterus. Progestins increase viscous mucus production. Estrogens are bound in the plasma with high affinity to sex steroid–binding globulin; the metabolism from testosterone to estrogen is irreversible.

2–A. Sulfonylureas increase the release of insulin from the pancreas. They also may cause an increase in insulin receptors, which increases tissue sensitivity to insulin. They do not slow insulin clearance and do not decrease glucocorticoid levels.

3–A. Thiazides and loop diuretics have opposite effects on Ca^{2+} excretion. Vitamin D and PTH both increase serum Ca^{2+}.

4–C. Calcitriol would be the most effective agent for hypocalcemia in a patient with impaired liver function. The liver provides the required 25-hydroxylation of DHT, cholecalciferol, and ergosterol.

5–C. Chronic administration of leuprolide decreases pituitary release of gonadotropins by reducing the number of GnRH receptors. This makes this mode of therapy useful for treating androgen-dependent tumors. Pulsatile administration increases pituitary release of gonadotropins.

6–D. Nandrolone is a potent androgen useful in the treatment of hypogonadism. It would be contraindicated in prostatic cancer and in precocious puberty and should not be used during pregnancy.

7–B. Vitamin D is the only agent listed that would increase serum Ca^{2+}. Phosphate salts would further decrease free Ca^{2+} levels, glucocorticoids diminish Ca^{2+} absorption, and loop diuretics increase Ca^{2+} excretion.

8–A. Oral hypoglycemic agents (sulfonylureas) increase tissue sensitivity to insulin. Obesity is associated with a reduction in insulin receptors and reduced insulin sensitivity; glucocorticoids increase plasma glucose and also decrease the number of insulin receptors. Antibodies to the insulin receptors block insulin action.

9–A. Part of the anti-inflammatory action of glucocorticoids can be attributed to inhibition of cytokine release. Dexamethasone, like all steroid hormones, acts by inducing the biosynthesis of new proteins. This process takes several hours to several days to produce desired results.

10–C. Large particles of insulin are the slowest to take effect.

11–B. The goal in the synthesis of prednisone is to reduce mineralocorticoid effects. Although potency may vary, prednisone will cause suppression of the pituitary–adrenal axis. Inactive prednisone is converted to the active agent prednisolone predominantly in the liver; thus decreased liver function would decrease its effectiveness.

12–C. Calcitriol requires no metabolism; all of the other agents must undergo at least one hydroxylation.

13–B. Tamoxifen is an estrogen-receptor antagonist. It does not have progestational activity nor does it alter estrogen secretion. Tamoxifen is currently under investigation to determine its effectiveness in the prophylaxis of breast cancer.

14–D. β-Receptor stimulation increases insulin release; α-receptor stimulation has the opposite effect. Leucine is a potent insulin secretagogue.

15–D. DHT (dihydrotachysterol) does not require 1-hydroxylation, a metabolic step that occurs in the kidney. All of the other compounds listed undergo this metabolism, which is compromised in renal disease.

16–D. Many of the symptoms of hyperthyroidism mimic the effects of catecholamine excess; these symptoms can be alleviated with β-adrenoceptor antagonists.

17–D. The 17-alkyl testosterones are associated with hepatotoxicity, but testosterone itself does not cause this adverse effect.

18–B. Estrogens decrease bone resorption, but do not increase bone formation. Their primary use in postmenopausal therapy is to improve vasomotor symptoms (i.e., hot flashes) and treat atrophic vaginitis.

19–D. Corticosteroid therapy can produce increased susceptibility to infection, poor wound healing, and hyperglycemia.

20–B. Prednisone must be metabolized to active agents in the liver, making it less useful as a topical agent. Cortisol, dexamethasone, and trimcinolone acetonide are all active topically.

21–D. Methimazole blocks the initial oxidation of iodine as well as the coupling of MIT and DIT into the mature hormone. It does not affect thyroglobulin synthesis.

22–D. Mestranol is a potent estrogen that would be contraindicated in this disorder. Chronic administration of leuprolide decreases luteinizing hormone (LH) levels and hence estradiol secretion, making it a useful treatment for endometriosis. Danazol and progestins also impede estrogen actions.

23–D. The incidence of uterine cancers is decreased in women using combination oral contraceptives. Hypertension, benign liver tumors, and stroke are associated with use of these agents.

24–D. Glucocorticoids do not produce hypoglycemia. They have various limiting adverse effects. These include renal suppression caused by inhibition of ACTH secretion and metabolic disturbances, including muscle wasting and osteoporosis.

25–A. Glucocorticoids promote gluconeogenesis and thereby increase blood glucose. Addison's disease requires both glucocorticoid and mineralocorticoid replacement.

10
Drugs Used in Treatment of Infectious Diseases

I. Infectious Disease Therapy

—is based on the principle of **selective toxicity**: Destroy the infecting organism without damage to the host by exploiting basic biochemical and physical differences between the two organisms.

—must take into consideration the following variables:

A. Choice of appropriate antibiotic

—drug of choice is usually the most active drug against the pathogen or the least toxic of several alternative drugs.

—base choice on sensitivity of the organism and the possibility of superinfection.

—must also determine whether bactericidal or bacteriostatic agent will be used.

B. Host determinants

—include history of drug reactions; site of infection; renal, hepatic, and immune status; age; pregnancy and lactation; metabolic abnormalities; preexisting organ dysfunction; and genetic factors.

C. Bacterial determinants

—include **intrinsic resistance,** escape from antibiotic effect, and **acquired resistance,** which can occur as a result of the following:

1. De novo chromosomal **mutations,** which occur at a frequency of $10^{-12}-10^{-5}$

2. Extrachromosomal **transfer** of drug-resistant genes

   a. **Transformation** (probably not clinically important)

   b. **Transduction** via R plasmids; asexual transfer of bacterial virus between bacteria of same species

   c. **Conjugation,** passage of genes from bacteria to bacteria via direct contact through sex pilus

–R-determinants containing genes for drug resistance combine with resistance transfer factors (RTFs), which have genes for conjugation, to form R factor or R plasmid. R factors may contain several genes, each of which confers resistance to a different drug.

–occurs primarily in gram-negative bacilli and is the principal mechanism of acquired resistance among enterobacteria.

d. Transpositions occur as a result of movement or "jumping" of **transposons** (stretches of DNA containing insertion sequences at each end) from plasmid to plasmid or plasmid to chromosome and back; this process is independent of bacterial recombination.

II. Antibacterials

A. Inhibitors of bacterial cell wall biosynthesis

1. Penicillins

a. Structure and mechanism of action

–are analogs of alanine dipeptide (Figure 10.1).

–consist of a thiazolidine ring attached to β-lactam ring. Integrity of β-lactam ring required for antibacterial activity. Modifications of R group side-chain (attached to β-lactam ring) alter pharmacologic properties and resistance to β-lactamase.

–inactivate transpeptidases and other **penicillin-binding proteins (PBPs)** and thus prevent crosslinking of peptidoglycan polymers of bacterial cell wall. Results in loss of rigidity and susceptibility to rupture. **Autolysins** are released from inhibition in presence of penicillin and further weaken cell wall.

–are bactericidal for growing cells. Gram-positive bacteria with thick external cell walls are particularly susceptible.

–major cause of resistance is production of β-**lactamases (penicillinases)**. Genes for β-lactamases can be transmitted during conjugation or as small plasmids (minus conjugation genes) via transduction. Common organisms capable of producing penicillinase include *Staphylococcus aureus, Escherichia coli, Pseudomonas aeruginosa, Neisseria gonorrhoeae,* and *Bacillus, Proteus,* and *Bacteroides* species.

b. Pharmacologic properties

–are absorbed rapidly after parenteral administration and are distributed throughout body fluids; penetrate the cerebrospinal fluid (CSF) and ocular fluid to a significant extent only during inflammation.

–most are excreted by the kidneys, predominantly via tubular secretion. Clearance can be slowed by administration of **probenecid**.

c. Selected drugs and their therapeutic uses (Table 10.1)
(1) Penicillin G and penicillin V

–are the most effective drugs for sensitive organisms.

–**penicillin G** is acid-labile, and only 30% of oral dose remains active. Is generally administered parenterally.

–**penicillin G benzathine** is administered intramuscularly; slow absorption yields prolonged circulating drug levels.

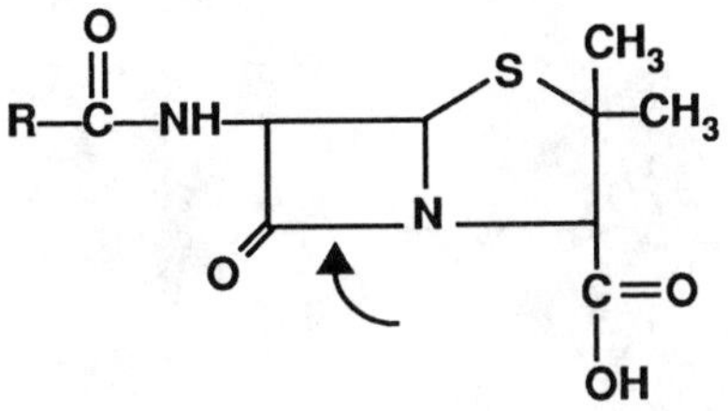

Penicillin nucleus

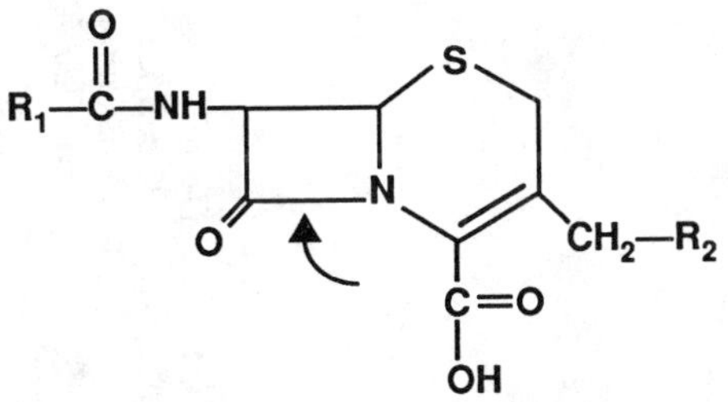

Cephalosporin nucleus

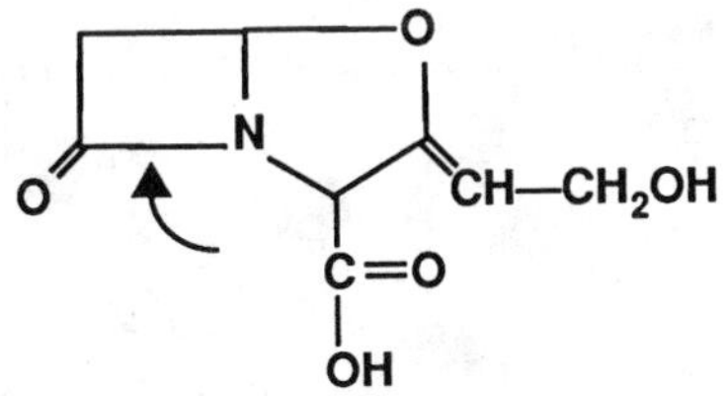

Clavulanic acid

Figure 10.1. Structures of penicillin, cephalosporin, and clavulanic acid nuclei. *Arrows* indicate bond attacked by β-lactamases.

–**penicillin V** can be administered orally.
–have half-life ($t_{1/2}$) of 30–60 minutes in normal patients and up to 10 hours in those with renal insufficiency.
–are used to treat infections with the following organisms.
(a) **Gram-positive cocci** (aerobic): Pneumococci, streptococci (except *S. faecalis*), and non-penicillinase-producing staphylococci
(b) **Gram-positive rods** (aerobic): *Bacillus* species
(c) **Gram-negative aerobes:** Gonococci (non-penicillinase-producing) and meningococci
(d) **Gram-negative rods** (aerobic): None
(e) **Anaerobes:** Most, except *Bacteroides fragilis*
(f) **Other:** *Treponema pallidum* (syphilis) and *Leptospira*
(g) Also **used prophylactically** for streptococcal infections, prevention of rheumatic fever recurrence, and surgical or dental procedures on patients with valvular heart disorders.

Table 10.1. Spectrum of Activity of Penicillins

Classification and Drugs	Gram-positive Cocci	Gram-positive Rods	Gram-negative Cocci	Gram-negative Rods	Anaerobes
Prototype					
Penicillin G, penicillin V	Most	*Bacillus*	Gonococci and meningococci*	None	Most (except *B. fragilis*)
Penicillinase-resistant					
Nafcillin, methicillin, oxacillin, cloxacillin, dicloxacillin	Staphylococci†	—	—	—	—
Extended-spectrum					
Ampicillin, amoxacillin, ampicillin/sulbactam, amoxacillin/clavulanic acid	Most penicillinase-producing staphylococci‡	*Bacillus*	Gonococci and meningococci†	*Salmonella, H. influenzae, Proteus,* and *E. coli*	—
Antipseudomonal					
Carbenicillin, ticarcillin, ticarcillin/clavulanic acid, mezlocillin, piperacillin	Less potent than prototypes	Less potent than prototypes	Less potent than prototypes	*H. influenzae, Proteus, E. coli, Salmonella, Pseudomonas, Enterobacter,* and *Klebsiella*	—
Other β-lactamase resistant					
Amdinocillin	None	None	Most	*E. coli, Enterobacter, Klebsiella, Shigella,* and *Salmonella*	—

*Non-penicillinase-producing
†Penicillinase-producing
‡Not effective against methicillin-resistant staphylococcal infections

   (2) Penicillinase-resistant penicillins
-   –are used predominantly for penicillinase-producing **staphylococcal infections**.
-   **(a)** Isoxazolyl derivatives (**oxacillin, cloxacillin,** and **dicloxacillin**) and **nafcillin** can be given orally.
-   **(b) Methicillin** [Staphcillin] is administered parenterally, but its use is declining because of the possibility of nephrotoxicity.
-   **(c) Nafcillin** [Nafcil, Unipen] is used parenterally for more serious infections.

   (3) Extended-spectrum penicillins
-   –are inactivated by β-lactamases.
-   –have greater activity than **penicillin G** against gram-negative bacteria.
-   –are used in combination with aminoglycosides in life-threatening situations.
-   **(a) Ampicillin [Amcil, Omnipen, Polycillin]**
    -   –is useful for infections caused by *Haemophilus influenzae* (non-penicillinase-producing), *Proteus mirabilis, E. coli,* and *Salmonella.*
    -   –has poor bioavailability from the gastrointestinal tract, but is usually administered orally.
-   **(b) Amoxicillin [Amoxil, others]**
    -   –is similar to **ampicillin** but has better oral absorption.
-   **(c) Carbenicillin [Geopen] and ticarcillin [Ticar]**
    -   –are quite effective against *Pseudomonas, Enterobacter,* and indole-positive *Proteus.*
-   **(d) Azlocillin [Azlin], mezlocillin [Mezlin], and piperacillin [Pipracil]**
    -   –have good activity against *Pseudomonas.* **Mezlocillin** and **piperacillin** are also effective against *Enterobacter* and many *Klebsiella.*

   (4) Clavulanic acid
-   –is structurally related to **penicillin** (see Figure 10.1), but has no antimicrobial properties of its own.
-   –irreversibly inhibits β-lactamase; when administered with penicillins, exposes penicillinase-producing organisms to therapeutic concentrations of **penicillin**.
-   –is used in combination products **amoxicillin/clavulanic acid** [Augmentin] and **ticarcillin/clavulanic acid** [Timentin] for oral and parenteral administration, respectively.

   (5) Sulbactam
-   –is a β-lactamase inhibitor structurally related to **penicillin**.
-   –is marketed in the combination product **ampicillin/sulbactam** [Unasyn].
-   –is used parenterally and provides coverage similar to that provided by amoxicillin/clavulanic acid [Augmentin].

   (6) Amdinocillin (mecillinam) [Coactin]
-   –has good activity against gram-negative organisms. Excellent activity against enterobacteria, including *E. coli, Enterobacter, Klebsiella, Shigella,* and *Salmonella.*

—has no synergy with aminoglycosides and is relatively resistant to β-lactamases.

—is administered parenterally.

d. Adverse effects

—cause hypersensitivity reactions in nearly 10% of cases. All types of reactions from simple rash to anaphylaxis can be observed within 2 minutes or up to 3 days following administration.

—other adverse effects result from direct irritation or pain on injection, cation (Na^+ or K^+) effects from large doses of the salt form of drugs, gastrointestinal upset, or superinfection.

2. Cephalosporins (Table 10.2)

a. Structure and mechanism of action

—consist of a 7-aminocephalosporanic acid nucleus and a β-lactam ring linked to a dihydrothiazine ring (see Figure 10.1). Substitutions at R_1 determine antibacterial activity. Substitutions at R_2 determine pharmacokinetics.

—have the same mechanism of action as penicillins: They inhibit transpeptidase.

b. Pharmacologic properties

—are widely distributed in body fluids; selected agents (**cefuroxime** [Zinacef], **moxalactam** [Moxam], **cefotaxime** [Claforan], and **ceftizoxime** [Cefizox]) penetrate CSF.

—are eliminated by renal secretion and filtration (except for **cefoperazone** [Cefobid], **ceftriaxone** [Rocephin], and **moxalactam,** which undergo significant biliary elimination). Probenecid slows secretion.

—some (**cephalothin** [Keflin, Seffin], **cephapirin** [Cefadyl], and **cefotaxime**) are metabolized by deacetylation.

—are relatively resistant to penicillinases but are sensitive to another class of β-lactamase, the **cephalosporinases** (genes are generally located on chromosomes as opposed to plasmids).

c. Selected drugs and therapeutic uses

(1) First-generation cephalosporins

—include **cephalothin, cephapirin, cephalexin** [Keflex], **cephradine** [Anspor, Velosef], **cefazolin** [Ancef, Kefzol], and **cefadroxil** [Duricef, Ultracef].

—have good activity against most gram-positive organisms and some gram-negative organisms. Used mainly for *E. coli, Klebsiella* infections, and for penicillin- and sulfonamide-resistant urinary tract infections. Also used prophylactically in various surgical procedures.

—half-lives range from 0.6–1.8 hours.

—**cephalothin, cephapirin,** and **cefazolin** are used parenterally; others can be administered orally.

—do not penetrate CSF.

(2) Second-generation cephalosporins

—include **cefamandole, cefoxitin** [Mefoxin], **cefaclor** [Ceclor], **cefuroxime, cefonicid** [Monocid], and **ceforanide** [Precef].

Table 10.2. Properties of Cephalosporins

Drugs and Route of Administration	Spectrum of Activity	Enters CNS	Resistance to β-Lactamase	
			Plasmid	Chromosomal
1st-generation Cephalothin (P)* Cephalexin (O)† Cephapirin (P) Cephradine (O) Cefadroxil (O) Cefazolin (P)	Gram-positive and some gram-negative organisms Use: *E. coli, Klebsiella, Proteus mirabilis,* penicillin- and sulfonamide-resistant UTI, surgical prophylaxis	No	Yes	No
2nd-generation Cefaclor (O) Cefamandole (P) Cefonicid (P) Ceforanide (P) Cefoxitin (P) Cefuroxime (P) Cefuroxime axetil (O)	Spectrum extends to *H. influenzae,* indole-positive *Proteus,* and anaerobes Use: UTI and surgical prophylaxis	No	Yes	Relatively
3rd-generation Ceftizoxime (P) Cefotaxime (P) Ceftriaxone (P) Ceftazidime (P) Cefoperazone (P) Cefixime (O)	Reduced gram-positive activity; *Pseudomonas* (cefoperazone and ceftazidime only), *N. gonorrhoeae, Enterobacter, Salmonella,* indole-positive *Proteus, Serratia, Providencia stuartii;* moderate anaerobe activity Use: Serious nosocomial infections (given with aminoglycosides)	Yes, especially ceftriaxone (but not cefoperazone)	Yes	Relatively (most)
Other agents Aztreonam Imipenem/cilastatin	Gram-negative organisms (no cross-sensitivity) Broad-spectrum use	Yes	Yes	Yes

*O = oral administration
†P = parenteral administration

—extend spectrum of the first generation to include *H. influenzae* and indole-positive *Proteus*.

—are used primarily in management of **urinary tract, bone, and soft-tissue infections,** and prophylactically in various surgical procedures.

—do not penetrate CSF.

—half-lives range from 0.8–4.4 hours.

—are administered parenterally except for **cefaclor** and **cefuroxime axetil** [Ceftin], the ester form of cefuroxime, which may be given orally.

(3) **Third-generation cephalosporins**

—include **cefotaxime, ceftizoxime, ceftazidime** [Fortaz, Tazidime], **cefixime** [Suprax], **cefoperazone,** and **moxalactam.**

—have somewhat reduced activity against gram-positive organisms, but enhanced activity against gram-negative organisms. Demonstrate high potency against *H. influenzae, N. gonorrhoeae, Enterobacter, Salmonella,* indole-positive *Proteus, Serratia,* and *Providencia stuartii,* and moderate activity against anaerobes. **Cefoperazone** and **ceftazidime** have excellent activity against *Pseudomonas aeruginosa.*

—most penetrate CSF to achieve therapeutically active concentrations. **Moxalactam** has particularly good CSF penetration, but use is limited because of possibility of bleeding disorders.

—have half-lives from 1.1–8.8 hours.

—are administered parenterally except for **cefixime.**

—are used primarily for serious **hospital-acquired gram-negative infections,** alone or in combination with an aminoglycoside.

d. **Adverse effects and drug interactions**

—most commonly cause **hypersensitivity reactions** (2%–5%); 5%–10% of penicillin-sensitive persons are also hypersensitive to cephalosporins.

—alcohol intolerance is seen with **cefoperazone, cefamandole** [Mandol], and **moxalactam.**

—may cause **bleeding disorders.**

—may be nephrotoxic when administered with diuretics. **Cephalothin** may be synergistically nephrotoxic with **gentamicin** or **tobramycin.**

3. **Other transpeptidase inhibitors**

a. **Aztreonam [Azactam]**

—is a naturally occurring monobactam lacking the thiazolidine ring that is highly resistant to β-lactamases.

—has good activity against gram-negative organisms, but lacks activity against anaerobes and gram-positive organisms; spectrum similar to aminoglycosides.

—demonstrates no cross-reactivity with penicillins or cephalosporins for hypersensitivity reactions.

—is administered parenterally.

—is useful for various types of infections caused by *E. coli, Klebsiella pneumoniae, H. influenzae, P. aeruginosa, Enterobacter* species, *Citrobacter* species, and *Proteus mirabilis.*

b. Imipenem

- –is a derivative of thienamycin that has a very broad spectrum of antibacterial activity.
- –is marketed in the combination product **imipenem/cilastatin** [Primaxin]; **cilastatin** is an inhibitor of renal dehydropeptidase I (which inactivates **imipenem**).
- –is relatively resistant to β-lactamase.
- –demonstrates no cross-resistance with other antibiotics.
- –is useful for infections caused by penicillinase-producing *S. aureus, E. coli, Klebsiella, Enterobacter,* and *H. influenzae,* among others.
- –requires dose reduction in presence of renal impairment.
- –patients allergic to **penicillin** may also have hypersensitivity to **imipenem**.

4. Other inhibitors of bacterial cell wall biosynthesis

  a. Vancomycin [Vancocin]

- –is a tricyclic glycopeptide that binds to preexisting peptidoglycan and prevents attachment of incoming moiety.
- –is active against gram-positive organisms. Resistant strains have been reported recently.
- –is synergistic with aminoglycosides but ototoxic and nephrotoxic; dose adjustment is required in renal impairment.
- –is excreted by the kidney; $t_{1/2}$ is approximately 6 hours.
- –is used in **serious methicillin-resistant staphylococcal infections** and in patients allergic to penicillins and cephalosporins.
- –penetrates the CSF only during inflammation.
- –is administered by slow IV infusion, except in the treatment of enterocolitis when it is given orally. Rapid infusion may cause anaphylactoid reactions and red neck syndrome.
- –demonstrates no cross-resistance with other antibiotics.

  b. Bacitracin

- –inhibits dephosphorylation and reuse of the phospholipid required for acceptance of *N*-acetylmuramic acid pentapeptide, the building block of the peptidoglycan complex.
- –is used topically in combination with neomycin and polymyxin for minor infections.

  c. Cycloserine [Seromycin]

- –is an amino acid analog that inhibits alanine racemase and the incorporation of alanine into the peptidoglycan pentapeptide.
- –is used only as a second-line drug for treatment of **mycobacterial infections**.

B. Inhibitors of bacterial protein synthesis

  1. Aminoglycosides

    a. Structure and mechanism of action

- –are amino sugars in glycosidic linkage to a hexose-aminocyclitol.
- –are polycations that require active uptake (gram-negative aerobes only).

—inhibit bacterial protein synthesis; are bacteriostatic.

—interact with S_{12} protein on 30S ribosomal subunit. This "freezes" the initiation complex and leads to a buildup of monosomes. Also causes translation errors.

—resistance generally results from bacterial enzymes that inactivate the drugs by addition of phosphoryl (*o*-phosphotransferases), acetyl (*o*-acetyltransferases), or adenylyl (*o*-adenylyltransferases) moieties. Resistance contained on plasmids transmitted by conjugation. Bacteria may carry genes for more than one modifying enzyme. Resistance also occurs as a result of decreased uptake of aminoglycosides.

b. Pharmacologic properties

—are not absorbed orally; must be administered parenterally.

—do not penetrate CSF.

—are excreted renally by glomerular filtration; $t_{1/2}$ in serum approximately 2–3 hours; $t_{1/2}$ in inner ear fluid approximately 10 hours.

c. Selected drugs and therapeutic uses

—are active against most gram-negative aerobic bacteria. Use is decreasing as a result of development of broader-spectrum **penicillins** and **cephalosporins** and other antibiotics that are less toxic.

(1) Streptomycin

—is currently used only for **plague** (*Yersinia pestis*), **severe cases of brucellosis,** and as an adjunct to treatment of recalcitrant **mycobacterial infections**.

(2) Gentamicin, tobramycin, and netilmicin

—are active against *Enterobacter,* indole-positive *Proteus, Pseudomonas, Klebsiella,* and *Serratia,* among other gram-negative organisms. Often used in combination with β-lactam antibiotic for serious infections where broad coverage is required.

(3) Amikacin

—is used in the treatment of **severe gram-negative infections,** especially those resistant to gentamicin or tobramycin.

(4) Neomycin

—is too toxic for parenteral use; is administered topically for minor **soft-tissue infections** (often in combination with **bacitracin** and **polymyxin**) or orally for **sterilizing the intestine** before bowel surgery.

d. Adverse effects

—are thought to result from interaction of aminoglycosides with polyphosphoinositides of host cell. Have narrow therapeutic index; may be necessary to monitor serum concentrations and individualize dose. Patients with impaired renal function, sepsis, or burns; those who are febrile or obese; elderly patients; and neonates are especially at risk.

—are **ototoxic,** either vestibular (**streptomycin, gentamicin** [Garamycin], and **tobramycin** [Nebcin]) or cochlear (**neomycin, kanamycin** [Kantrex], **amikacin** [Amikin], **gentamicin,** and **tobramycin**). Toxic effect more often seen in individuals with renal impairment. Damage may be permanent. Aminoglycosides should not be given with other ototoxic drugs (i.e., **ethacrynic acid** or **furosemide**). **Kanamycin** is the most ototoxic of the aminoglycosides.

—are **nephrotoxic;** produce acute tubular necrosis that leads to a reduction in glomerular filtration rate and rise in serum creatinine and blood urea nitrogen. Damage is usually reversible.

—produce neuromuscular blockade. Reduce acetylcholine (ACh) release from nerve terminals and decrease sensitivity of postsynaptic membrane to ACh.

—rarely cause hypersensitivity reactions except **neomycin,** which, when applied topically, can cause contact dermatitis in as many as 8% of patients.

2. Tetracyclines

a. Structure and mechanism of action

—are tetracyclic ring derivatives of naphthalene carboxamide. Various congeners have different degrees of hydrophilicity.

—**inhibit protein synthesis;** are **bacteriostatic.**

—bind to 30S subunit of bacterial ribosomes and prevent binding of aminoacyl tRNA. Inhibit eukaryotic protein synthesis at high concentrations.

—rely on two transport systems (one fast and one slow) for active uptake of the drug. Although tetracyclines can inhibit protein synthesis in mammalian cells, they rarely attain inhibitory concentrations in these cells because of lack of transport systems.

—resistance results from decreased ability to accumulate in the bacteria as a result of an active drug "export" system. Resistance genes are predominantly carried on plasmids but can be chromosomal. Resistance to one tetracycline generally confers resistance to all congeners and often to other antibiotics.

b. Pharmacologic properties

—are adequately absorbed from the gastrointestinal tract. Can also be administered parenterally. Absorption is impaired by stomach contents, especially milk and antacids, as a result of complex formation with ions, particularly magnesium, calcium, and aluminum. **Minocycline** [Monocid] and **doxycycline** [Vibramycin], which are highly lipophilic, are more readily absorbed and better transported by bacteria.

—are distributed throughout body fluids, and therapeutic concentrations can be achieved in the CSF.

—are extensively metabolized (except for **minocycline**); concentrated in liver and excreted into bile, leading to enterohepatic recirculation.

—are eliminated via renal (filtration) and biliary routes; $t_{1/2}$ approximately 6–16 hours (longer in renal failure). **Doxycycline** is excreted almost entirely via feces and, hence, is the safest tetracycline to administer to individuals with impaired renal function.

c. Spectrum and therapeutic uses

—are active against both gram-negative and gram-positive organisms, but use is declining because of increased resistance and development of safer drugs.

—are used predominantly for treatment of **rickettsial infections,** including Rocky Mountain spotted fever, typhus, and Q fever; also employed for infections caused by *Chlamydia* and *Mycoplasma*. May be useful for treatment of **inflammatory acne vulgaris**.

d. Adverse effects

—produce gastrointestinal upset, including nausea, vomiting, and diarrhea.

—at high doses, can cause hepatic damage, particularly in pregnant women. **Oxytetracycline** [Oxymycin, Terramycin] and **tetracycline** are the least hepatotoxic agents.

—when exposed to strong ultraviolet light, as in sunlight, can cause dermatologic reactions, especially with **demeclocycline** [Declomycin].

—can complex with calcium in bone. Children age 6 months to 5 years receiving tetracycline therapy can develop teeth discolorations. Can also retard bone growth in neonates.

—can cause superinfection by resistant staphylococci or *Clostridia* as a result of altered gut ecology; can be life-threatening (especially in patients with impaired immune systems).

3. Chloramphenicol

a. Structure and mechanism of action

—contains a nitrobenzene moiety and is a derivative of dichloroacetic acid.

—inhibits bacterial protein synthesis.

—binds to 50S ribosomal subunit and prevents peptide bond formation. High concentrations inhibit eukaryote protein synthesis. Mitochondrial protein synthesis is also affected.

—resistance results from production of an acetyltransferase capable of inactivating the drug, which is transmitted via R factor during conjugation.

b. Pharmacologic properties

—is absorbed well from the gastrointestinal tract. Can also be administered intravenously.

—is distributed throughout body fluids and therapeutic levels can be obtained in the CSF.

—is metabolized in the liver by glucuronyl transferase. Unmetabolized drug cleared by glomerular filtration; conjugates eliminated by tubular secretion; $t_{1/2}$ approximately 1.5–3.5 hours (longer in patients with decreased hepatic or renal function).

c. Therapeutic uses

—is used to treat most gram-negative organisms, many anaerobes, *Clostridia, Chlamydia, Mycoplasma,* and *Rickettsia*. However, because of the potential for severe and sometimes fatal adverse effects, use is limited to treatment of infections that cannot be treated with other drugs. These include **typhoid fever** (although resistance is increasingly a problem), **meningitis** due to *H. influenzae* in patients allergic to penicillins and the newer cephalosporins, and some instances of infections caused by **ampicillin-resistant strains**.

—may also be used for treatment of certain anaerobic infections of the brain (especially *Bacteroides fragilis*) in combination with **penicillin** and as an alternative to **tetracycline** in treatment of rickettsial disease.

d. Adverse effects

—causes dose-related **bone marrow suppression** resulting in pancytopenia that may lead to irreversible aplastic anemia. This effect has low incidence (1:30,000), but high mortality rate.

—causes **reticulocytopenia,** perhaps as a result of inhibition of mitochondrial protein synthesis.

—in neonates given large doses of **chloramphenicol, gray baby syndrome** occurs. Results from inadequacy of both cytochrome P-450 and glucuronic acid conjugation systems to detoxify the drug. Elevated plasma **chloramphenicol** levels cause a shocklike syndrome and reduction in peripheral circulation. High incidence (40%) of fatalities.

—also produces hypersensitivity reactions.

4. Erythromycin

a. Structure and mechanism of action

—is a macrolide antibiotic composed of a multimembered lactone ring attached to deoxysugars.

—inhibits protein synthesis by binding to 50S ribosomal subunit; restricts the size of the peptide synthesized.

b. Pharmacologic properties

—is inactivated by stomach acid and therefore is administered as an **enteric-coated tablet**. Absorption is reduced by gastric contents.

—**penetrates** into all **body fluids,** except CSF.

—can also be administered intravenously. A prodrug (erythromycin estolate) that is converted to active drug by bacteria is available. The estolate is more stable than erythromycin base and is not as affected by stomach contents.

—is **concentrated in the liver;** is excreted predominantly via the biliary route. Cautious use is advised in the presence of impaired hepatic function.

c. Therapeutic use

—is active against **gram-positive organisms**.

—can replace penicillin in penicillin-hypersensitive patients.

—is the most effective drug for Legionnaires' disease (*Legionella pneumophila*); also is useful for treatment of *Mycoplasma pneumoniae*.

d. Adverse effects

—rarely produces serious adverse effects; oral form of **erythromycin** may cause allergic cholestatic hepatitis, which is readily reversible by cessation of the drug.

−has high incidence of **thrombophlebitis** when administered intravenously.

5. Clindamycin [Cleocin]

−binds 50S ribosomal subunit and suppresses protein synthesis.

−can be administered orally and is well distributed throughout body fluids except for the CNS. Is largely protein bound and extensively metabolized in the liver. It is excreted in urine and bile.

−use is limited to alternative therapy for **abscesses associated with infections** caused by **anaerobes**.

−produces **diarrhea,** observed in up to 20% of individuals. Potential severe pseudomembranous colitis occurs as a result of superinfection by resistant *Clostridium*.

C. Inhibitors of bacterial metabolism

1. Sulfonamides

a. Structure and mechanism of action

−are structural analogs of *para*-aminobenzoic acid (PABA).

−inhibit synthesis of folic acid by competing with PABA at the level of dihydropteroate synthetase, which synthesizes **dihydropteric acid,** the penultimate molecule in the folic acid pathway.

−do not affect bacteria that can utilize preformed folic acid or mammalian cells (which *require* preformed folic acid). *Para*-amino group is required for activity.

−resistance generally develops as a result of altered enzyme amounts or affinity, which leads to the ability to synthesize folic acid in the presence of the drugs.

b. Pharmacologic properties

−most are well absorbed from the gastrointestinal tract and readily penetrate CSF.

−are extensively bound to plasma proteins.

−are metabolized to various degrees in the liver, usually by acetylation of the *para*-amino group. Acetylated derivatives are not active. Glucuronidation may also occur.

−are eliminated via the kidney, predominantly through filtration; $t_{1/2}$ ranges from 4–7 hours (longer in renal failure). Acetylated derivatives are poorly soluble in the acid pH of urine. Combination of different sulfonamides with varying solubilities helps overcome this problem.

c. Spectrum and therapeutic uses

−inhibit both gram-negative and gram-positive organisms, *Actinomyces, Chlamydia, Toxoplasma,* and plasmodia.

(1) **Short-acting agents** include **sulfisoxazole** [Gantrisin] and **sulfadiazine. Sulfisoxazole** is used mainly to treat **urinary tract infections**. Because it attains relatively high concentrations in the CSF, **sulfadiazine** is the best sulfonamide for the treatment of **meningitis**. Because of its relative insolubility and propensity to crystallize in the urine, **sulfadiazine** should be used with care; good hydration should be maintained.

(2) Sulfamethoxazole [Gantanol], an **intermediate-acting agent,** has a $t_{1/2}$ of approximately 12 hours. Half-life is similar to that of **trimethoprim,** which is an inhibitor of bacterial dihydrofolate reductase, the enzyme that converts dihydrofolic acid to tetrahydrofolic acid. Because **sulfamethoxazole** and **trimethoprim** inhibit two unrelated enzymes of the same metabolic pathway, they are synergistic and are marketed in the combination product **trimethoprim/sulfamethoxazole (co-trimoxazole)** [Bactrim, Septra], which is used for chronic and recurrent **urinary tract infections, bacterial prostatitis, gastrointestinal infections** (particularly shigellosis), and **traveler's diarrhea**. At high doses the combination is effective against *Pneumocystis carinii*. Resistance may occur, primarily as a result of reduced permeability; frequency of resistance to the combination is lower than to either agent alone.

(3) Long-acting sulfonamides include **sulfadoxine,** which is marketed in the combination **sulfadoxine/pyrimethamine** [Fansidar]. **Pyrimethamine** is an inhibitor of parasitic dihydrofolate reductase. The combination is used in the treatment of **malaria** caused by chloroquine-resistant *Plasmodium falciparum*. This combination also appears to be effective in treatment of **toxoplasmosis** and in prophylaxis and treatment of *P. carinii* **pneumonia** in patients with AIDS.

(4) Some **derivatives,** such as **sulfasalazine,** are poorly absorbed from the gastrointestinal tract and are used to treat **ulcerative colitis** and **regional enteritis**. Other agents, such as **sulfacetamide** and **silver sulfasalazine,** are employed for ophthalmic and topical uses.

d. Adverse effects

–produce hypersensitivity reactions (rashes, fever, eosinophilia) in approximately 3% of individuals receiving oral doses. Except for ophthalmic solutions and special preparations for burns, topical application is discouraged because of high incidence of local hypersensitivity.

–rarely cause **Stevens-Johnson syndrome,** an infrequent but fatal form of erythema multiforme associated with lesions of skin and mucous membranes.

–occasionally produce photosensitivity and serum sickness reactions.

–patients with glucose-6-phosphate dehydrogenase deficiency are more susceptible to adverse effects (manifested primarily as hemolytic aplastic anemia). Agranulocytosis and thrombocytopenia are observed infrequently.

–produce bilirubinemia in neonates.

–may potentiate the effects of other drugs, such as oral anticoagulants, sulfonylureas, and hydantoin anticonvulsants, possibly by displacement from albumin.

D. Inhibitors of bacterial events involving nucleic acids

1. Rifampin [Rifadin, Rimactane]

–is an RNA synthesis inhibitor.

−inhibits bacterial RNA polymerase by binding to β subunit of the polymerase.

−is absorbed from the gastrointestinal tract; widely distributed, including to CSF. Deacetylated in the liver (metabolite also active). Enhances metabolism of other drugs, such as anticoagulants, contraceptives, and corticosteroids.

−is active against most gram-positive organisms, *Neisseria* species, and mycobacteria. Used in combination with other drugs for treatment of most atypical mycobacteria (including *Mycobacterium leprae*). Resistance develops rapidly, and use for other bacterial infections is limited to treatment of meningococcal carriers.

−causes dermatitis and red-orange discoloration of feces, urine, tears, and sweat.

2. DNA-binding agents

a. Quinolones and nitrofurans

−include **nalidixic acid** [NegGram] and **cinoxacin** [Cinobac], which are quinolones, and the nitrofuran **nitrofurantoin** [Furadantin].

−cause DNA damage.

−are used as **urinary tract antiseptics** since therapeutic plasma levels are not achieved at nontoxic levels.

−**furazolidone,** a nitrofuran derivative, is useful for intestinal infections caused by *Salmonella, Shigella,* and *Giardia.*

b. 4-Quinolone derivatives

−include **norfloxacin** [Noroxin], **ciprofloxacin** [Cipro], **enoxacin,** and **ofloxacin**.

−inhibit bacterial DNA topoisomerase II (DNA gyrase). Gram-negative organisms appear to be more sensitive than gram-positive bacteria. Have poor activity against anaerobes and are generally bactericidal.

−are absorbed from the gastrointestinal tract; possess minimal adverse effects. May cause CNS stimulation.

−are eliminated primarily via renal route (secretion and filtration). Dose reduction is necessary in presence of compromised renal function.

−are useful against infections caused by *N. gonorrhoeae* or **methicillin-resistant staphylococci, and urinary tract infections** as well as a variety of other infections.

III. Antimycobacterial Agents (Table 10.3)

A. First-line drugs used in the treatment of tuberculosis

1. Isoniazid

a. Structure and mechanism of action

−is an analog of pyridoxine (vitamin B_6).

−inhibits synthesis of the mycobacterial cell wall.

b. Pharmacologic properties

−penetrates most body fluids and accumulates in caseated lesions. Enters host cells and has access to intracellular forms of mycobacteria.

−can be administered orally.

Table 10.3. Major Uses of Antibacterial and Antifungal Drugs

Drug	Major Organisms	Alternative Drugs
Penicillin	All aerobic gram-negative and gram-positive cocci (except penicillinase-producing and methicillin-resistant staphylococci, penicillinase-producing gonococci, and *Streptococcus faecalis*); *Leptospira*; *Treponema* (syphilis, yaws); all gram-positive anaerobes (peptococci, peptostreptococci, *Clostridia*) and gram-negative anaerobes (except *Bacteroides fragilis*)	Ampicillin or tetracycline, amoxicillin/clavulanic acid, ticarcillin/clavulanic acid, chloramphenicol, or erythromycin*
Penicillinase-resistant penicillins	Penicillinase-producing staphylococci	Vancomycin or cephalosporin
Vancomycin	Methicillin-resistant staphylococci	Trimethoprim/sulfamethoxazole
Ampicillin	*Streptococcus faecalis*	Penicillin and aminoglycoside or vancomycin
Aminoglycosides	Coliforms (*Escherichia coli, Klebsiella, Enterobacter, Serratia, Proteus, Providencia, Arizona*)	Third-generation cephalosporin, trimethoprim/sulfamethoxazole, or extended-spectrum penicillin*
Aminoglycoside and extended-spectrum penicillin	*Pseudomonas aeruginosa*	Third-generation cephalosporin
Tetracycline	*Brucella, Campylobacter, Yersinia pestis* (plague), *Francisella tularensis* (tularemia), *Vibrio, Pseudomonas pseudomallei and mallei, Borrelia* (relapsing fever), *Mycoplasma pneumoniae, chlamydiae,* and rickettsiae	Streptomycin, erythromycin, chloramphenicol, or trimethoprim/sulfamethoxazole
Chloramphenicol	*Salmonella, Haemophilus* species	Trimethoprim/sulfamethoxazole, ampicillin, or third-generation cephalosporin
Erythromycin	*Legionella* species	
Trimethoprim/ sulfamethoxazole	*Shigella*	
Sulfonamides	*Nocardia*	
Metronidazole	*Bacteroides fragilis*	
Isoniazid (and rifampin and/or ethambutol)	*Mycobacterium tuberculosis* and atypical *Mycobacterium* species	
Dapsone (and rifampin)	*Mycobacterium leprae*	
Amphotericin B	*Candida, Torulopsis,* coccidioidomycosis, histoplasmosis, aspergillosis, and mucormycosis	
Amphotericin B and flucytosine	*Cryptococcus neoformans*	
Ketoconazole	blastomycosis, paracoccidioidomycosis, and sporotrichosis	

*Choice of particular drug dependent on sensitivity of individual organism.

–is the most active drug against *Mycobacterium tuberculosis,* but it is not active against most atypical mycobacteria.

–demonstrates no cross-resistance with other first-line antitubercular drugs.

–is acetylated in the liver; acetylisoniazid is eliminated faster than isoniazid. Metabolism genetically determined; for fast acetylators $t_{1/2}$ is approximately 80 minutes; for slow acetylators, $t_{1/2}$ is approximately 180 minutes.

c. Therapeutic use

–is administered in combination with one and sometimes two other first-line drugs. Typical regimen includes isoniazid and rifampin for 1–3 months of intensive daily therapy followed by twice-weekly therapy for at least 9 months.

–is used alone for prophylaxis in family members.

d. Adverse effects

–can inhibit mammalian pyridoxal kinase; high serum concentrations may result in **peripheral neuropathy;** slow acetylators are more susceptible. Minimized by coadministration of pyridoxine.

–metabolites may be hepatotoxic; fast acetylators are more susceptible. **Hepatotoxicity** is observed in up to 3% of individuals over age 35.

–may produce allergic reactions.

–inhibits metabolism of other drugs, especially diphenylhydantoin.

2. Rifampin

–is administered orally in combination with isoniazid.

–demonstrates no cross-resistance with other antimycobacterial agents; resistance develops rapidly when used alone. Most atypical mycobacteria are sensitive.

–**ansamycin** is a rifampin derivative that has good activity against many atypical strains.

3. Ethambutol [Myambutol]

a. Structure and mechanism of action

–is a diaminodibutanol. Mechanism of action is unknown; specific for mycobacteria.

b. Pharmacologic properties

–is partially metabolized to aldehyde and acid in the liver. Substrate for alcohol dehydrogenase.

–is eliminated via the renal route by filtration and secretion; $t_{1/2}$ is 3–4 hours (longer in renal failure).

–demonstrates good CSF penetration.

c. Therapeutic use

–is administered orally in combination with **isoniazid** or **isoniazid** and **rifampin**.

–demonstrates no cross-resistance with other antimycobacterial agents; resistance develops rapidly when used alone.

–some atypical mycobacteria (*M. kansasii, M. avium*-intracellulare) are sensitive.

d. Adverse effects

−produces visual disturbances, resulting from reversible retrobulbar neuritis, and minor gastrointestinal disturbances. May have to adjust dose in renal failure.

4. Streptomycin

−is administered parenterally in combination with other antimycobacterial agents; may be part of three-drug regimens for resistant strains.
−is used in combination with rifampin to treat *M. ulcerans*.

B. Second-line drugs used in the treatment of tuberculosis

1. Pyrazinamide

−is an analog of nicotinamide.
−is administered orally and eliminated via renal glomeruli.
−is used in combination for treatment of resistant strains.
−is hepatotoxic.

2. *Para*-aminosalicylic acid

−is an analog of *para*-aminobenzoic acid; works like sulfonamides but only penetrates mycobacteria.
−is administered orally.
−produces gastrointestinal disturbances.

3. Ethionamide

−is a nicotinamide derivative.
−is orally administered.
−produces gastrointestinal disturbances and is hepatotoxic.

4. Cycloserine

−is an amino acid analog that inhibits cell wall biosynthesis.
−is orally administered and does not demonstrate cross-resistance with other effective antimycobacterial agents.
−causes central nervous system (CNS) toxicity; alcohol increases possibility of seizures.

5. Other agents

a. Parenterally administered agents include **minocycline, viomycin, kanamycin, amikacin,** and **capreomycin,** protein synthesis inhibitors.

b. Orally administered agents include **erythromycin, minocycline,** and **clofazimine**.

C. Drugs used in the treatment of infections caused by *Mycobacterium leprae* (leprosy)

1. Dapsone

−is structurally related to sulfonamides and inhibits folic acid biosynthesis.
−is more effective against *M. leprae* than against *M. tuberculosis*.
−is slowly absorbed from the gastrointestinal tract; $t_{1/2}$ is 10–50 hours.
−most (70%) is eliminated via the kidney.
−treatment may require several years to life; may be used in combination with **rifampin**. May be used to provide prophylaxis for family members.

Acedapsone is the repository form of dapsone. Inhibitory levels maintained for up to 3 months after intramuscular injection.

—produces hemolysis, methemoglobinemia, nausea, rash, and headache.

2. Rifampin

—is used in combination with **dapsone**.

3. Clofazimine [Lamprene]

—is used for **sulfone-resistant leprosy** or in patients intolerant to sulfones; may also be effective against atypical mycobacteria.

IV. Antifungal Agents (see Table 10.3)

A. Drugs that affect fungal membranes

1. Amphotericin B [Fungizone]

a. Structure and mechanism of action

—is an antibiotic that binds to ergosterol (a major component of fungal cell membranes) and alters membrane to allow leakage of cellular contents.

b. Pharmacologic properties

—is poorly absorbed from the gastrointestinal tract and so is administered intravenously; has poor penetration into the CNS.

—is eliminated predominantly through the biliary route. Binds to tissue membranes and serum lipoproteins.

—can be detected in urine for weeks after cessation of therapy.

c. Therapeutic uses

—is used to treat most severe fungal infections, including those caused by *Candida albicans, Histoplasma capsulatum, Cryptococcus neoformans, Coccidioides immitis, Blastomyces dermatitidis, Aspergillus* species, and *Sporothrix schenckii,* especially in immunocompromised patients.

—is the most effective antifungal agent and is usually the drug of choice for major systemic infections. **Liposome-encapsulated amphotericin B** is under investigation and appears to be less toxic.

—in some cases, combination therapy with **flucytosine** is advantageous.

d. Adverse effects

—are significant; causes **chills and fever** in 50% of patients and **impaired renal function** in 80%.

—also may produce anaphylaxis, thrombocytopenia, severe pain, and seizures.

2. Ketoconazole, miconazole, clotrimazole, and fluconazole

a. General properties

—are imidazole derivatives that block the synthesis of ergosterol by inhibiting the cytochrome P-450-mediated sterol 14α-demethylase.

—are broad-spectrum antifungals; also inhibit many gram-positive bacteria and some protozoa.

b. Ketoconazole [Nizoral]

—can be administered orally; elevation of gastric pH impairs absorption. It does not penetrate CSF.

–is extensively bound to plasma protein. It is metabolized in the liver by o-dealkylation and hydroxylation to inactive metabolites; $t_{1/2}$ is approximately 3 hours.

–most commonly causes **gastric upset** (3%–20% of patients). Itching, rashes, and headaches are observed in 1% of patients.

–rarely causes gynecomastia with breast pain in males and reversible liver dysfunction.

–is useful for treatment of **mucocutaneous candidiasis, histoplasmosis,** and **paracoccidioidomycosis** as well as dermatophyte infections.

c. Miconazole [Monistat]

–is available for IV administration, but this is associated with a high incidence of adverse effects (phlebitis, pruritus, nausea, and anemia). It is generally used only when amphotericin B is contraindicated.

–is available for topical application, which is associated with high incidence of burning and itching. Can be used for tinea pedis, ringworm, and cutaneous and vulvovaginal candidiasis.

d. Clotrimazole [Lotrimin, Mycelex] and terconazole [Terazol]

–are available for topical application and are useful for many dermatophyte infections.

e. Fluconazole [Diflucan]

–is available for IV or oral administration.

–is useful for oropharyngeal, isopharyngeal, and systemic **candidiasis**. Also used for acute and maintenance therapy of **cryptococcal meningitis.**

–has negligible effect on mammalian enzymes.

3. Nystatin

–is a polyene antibiotic similar in structure and mechanism of action to **amphotericin B.**

–is too toxic for systemic administration. Is not absorbed from the gastrointestinal tract; oral preparations can be used for infections of the mouth.

–is used primarily for *Candida* infections of the skin, mucous membranes, and intestinal tract. Sometimes used prophylactically with **tetracycline** to prevent superinfection of the intestine.

B. Other antifungal agents

1. Griseofulvin [Fulvicin, Grisactin]

–binds to microtubules and prevents spindle formation and mitosis in fungi. Also binds filament proteins such as keratin. The drug accumulates in skin, hair, and nails.

–is adequately absorbed after oral administration and is partially metabolized by the liver and slowly excreted in feces and urine.

–is administered as oral therapy for **dermatophyte infections**.

–is used for long-term therapy of **hair and nail infections**.

–is generally well-tolerated; rare CNS effects and hepatotoxicity occur.

2. Flucytosine [Ancobon]

  —is actively transported into fungal cells and is converted to **5-fluoro-uracil** and subsequently to **5-fluorodeoxyuridylic acid,** which is an inhibitor of pyrimidine and nucleic acid synthesis. Human cells lack the ability to convert large amounts of flucytosine to the uracil form.

  —is well-absorbed after oral administration; penetrates many tissues, including the CNS. The drug is not metabolized and is excreted by glomerular filtration.

  —is rarely used as a single drug, but often is used in **combination with other antifungal agents**.

  —resistance develops rapidly and limits its use. The major adverse effect is **depression of bone marrow function**.

3. Tolnaftate

  —is a thiocarbonate that is used topically for **dermatophyte infections**.

  —is frequently used for **tinea pedis;** it is ineffective against *Candida* infections.

V. Antiparasitic Drugs

A. Agents active against protozoal infections

1. Antimalarials

a. Malaria

  (1) Four major species of protozoal parasites infect humans: *Plasmodium vivax, P. ovale, P. malariae,* and *P. falciparum.*

  (2) In the primary state of infection, sporozoites are injected into the host by the mosquito. In this **preerythrocytic stage,** the sporozoites are resistant to drug therapy. The sporozoites migrate to the liver (**exoerythrocytic stage**) and then sporulate. The merozoites that emerge infect erythrocytes (**erythrocytic stage**), where asexual division leads to cell lysis and causes clinical symptoms. The merozoites released can reinfect other red blood cells, reinfect the liver, or differentiate into sexual forms (gametocytes) that can reproduce in the gut of the female mosquito.

  (3) *P. falciparum* differs from the other plasmodia in that the merozoites cannot reinfect the liver to produce a secondary exoerythrocytic stage. The lack of a tissue reservoir makes therapy somewhat easier for *P. falciparum* infections. However, this parasite rapidly develops resistance to therapy.

b. Therapy rationale

  (1) Chloroquine is used to treat the acute attack (erythrocytic stage). It is effective against all plasmodia except chloroquine-resistant *P. falciparum.* For the latter infections, **quinine sulfate** plus **pyrimethamine/sulfadoxine** [Fansidar] is used.

  (2) In prophylaxis, chloroquine is used to suppress erythrocytic forms during exposure; **primaquine** is added after exposure to treat exoerythrocytic forms. In regions with chloroquine-resistant strains, **mefloquine** is used for prophylaxis. Alternatively, **doxycycline** or **chloroquine** plus **pyrimethamine/sulfadoxine** can be used.

(3) **Primaquine** provides a radical cure (by removing residual exo-erythrocytic forms).

c. **Chloroquine, primaquine, quinine, and mefloquine**
(1) **Structure and mechanism of action**
   –have quinoline ring as part of structure. Are thought to exert their toxic effects by binding to DNA.
(2) **Chloroquine [Aralen]**
   –is absorbed from the gastrointestinal tract and tissues. Partly metabolized by liver; excreted by the kidney. Should not be administered intravenously.
   –is effective against erythrocytic forms of the parasite. Is used for control of acute, recurrent attacks, but is neither prophylactically nor radically curative. Many species of *P. falciparum* are resistant to chloroquine.
   –is also occasionally used in **rheumatoid arthritis** for anti-inflammatory action.
   –toxicity is generally limited to gastric upset, mild CNS disturbances, and yellowish discoloration of skin, nails, and mucous membranes. Reversible visual disturbances may occur. Irreversible retinopathy and ototoxicity are observed rarely with prolonged use.
(3) **Primaquine (8-aminoquinoline)**
   –is rapidly absorbed from the gastrointestinal tract and metabolized in the liver. Metabolites are quite active and may promote hemolysis. Glucose-6-phosphate dehydrogenase deficiency in African Americans and dark-skinned Caucasians may result in intravascular hemolysis.
   –is effective against the exoerythrocytic stage of the parasite life cycle. Also kills gametocytes.
   –is used for radical cure of relapsing malaria. It is the best available drug against *P. vivax*.
(4) **Quinine (cinchona alkaloid)**
   –is readily absorbed orally; liver metabolizes the drug, which is excreted by the kidney.
   –is active against the erythrocytic stage. Is useful for chloroquine-resistant *P. falciparum,* often in combination with **pyrimethamine/sulfadoxine** [Fansidar]. Resistance is uncommon. Also can inhibit growth of many unicellular organisms, including yeast and trypanosomes.
   –produces curare-like effects on skeletal muscle. Can impair function of cranial nerve VIII (**CN VIII**) and yield **loss of hearing and vision** (cinchonism). Is also a gastrointestinal irritant; produces CNS disturbances, renal damage, and rare hemolytic anemia.
(5) **Mefloquine [Lariam]**
   –is well absorbed from the gastrointestinal tract. Is bound to plasma proteins and tissues. Is excreted mainly in feces.
   –is generally well tolerated.
   –is useful for **chloroquine-resistant *P. falciparum;*** it is the only drug available that is effective against multiresistant strains.

—produces dose-related adverse effects; up to 60% of patients may develop dizziness, gastrointestinal and visual disturbances, and headache. CNS toxicity may occur.

d. Dihydrofolate reductase inhibitors

(1) Pyrimethamine (also trimethoprim)

—is well absorbed from the gastrointestinal tract; excreted in urine and in milk of nursing mothers.

—is used in combination with **sulfadoxine,** a sulfonamide with similar pharmacologic properties, in the combination product Fansidar.

—produces suppressive cure, more effective than **chloroguanide;** slow to clear parasites and clinical attacks; of little value in acute malaria.

—is associated with megaloblastic anemia and folate deficiency (at high doses).

(2) Chloroguanide [Progunil]

—is slowly but adequately absorbed from the gastrointestinal tract. Accumulates in erythrocytes; is bound to plasma proteins. Must be activated by metabolism. Synergistic with sulfonamides.

—is the least toxic antimalarial and has few adverse effects.

—is used to treat clinical symptoms. Not prophylactic against relapsing malaria; does not affect exoerythrocytic stage. Slow at abolishing clinical symptoms; resistance rapidly develops.

e. Antibacterial agents

(1) Sulfonamides and sulfones

—are particularly important in the prophylaxis of chloroquine-resistant strains; **dapsone** is occasionally used with **cycloguanide** or **chloroguanide** for suppression of *P. falciparum.*

(2) Tetracyclines (doxycycline)

—are sometimes used in combination with **quinine** against acute attack caused by multiresistant strains of plasmodia.

2. Agents active against amebiasis

a. Amebiasis

—major infecting organism is *Entamoeba histolytica,* which is ingested in cyst form, divides in the colon, and can invade the intestinal wall. It is excreted in the feces as cysts by asymptomatic carriers or as the less mature trophozoites by individuals with diarrhea.

b. Metronidazole [Flagyl]

—is a 5-nitroimidazole that acts on anaerobes by providing an electron sink, thereby depriving cells of reducing equivalents. May also inhibit DNA synthesis and alter DNA repair.

—is well absorbed from the gastrointestinal tract. High concentrations are achieved in the CNS. Nonresponders show poor accumulation of drug; $t_{1/2}$ approximately 8 hours. Metabolized by the liver; metabolites partially active. Eliminated via renal or hepatic routes.

—inhibits all forms of the parasite; 10% of asymptomatic carriers are resistant; does not completely suppress luminal infections.

—is used for **intestinal amebiasis** as well as for **amebic liver abscesses,** often in combination with **iodoquinol** (to eradicate luminal disease). Also active against *Giardia intestinalis* (formerly *G. lamblia*) and *Trichomonas vaginalis*. Shows activity against many anaerobic bacteria, including *Bacteroides* and *Clostridia*.

—produces adverse effects that include gastrointestinal irritation and mild, reversible CNS disturbances. Carcinogenic in rodents.

—**tinidazole,** another nitroimidazole marketed outside the United States, is similar in effectiveness to **metronidazole** and may be better tolerated.

c. Iodoquinol (diiodohydroxyquin) [Yodoxin]

—is active against both trophozoite and cyst forms, but mechanism is unknown.

—is poorly absorbed from the gastrointestinal tract; is excreted in urine and feces.

—produces adverse effects that include optic atrophy and visual defects and subacute myelo-optic neuropathy (**SMON syndrome**).

—is useful for **intestinal amebiasis;** is administered alone for asymptomatic carriers or in combination with **metronidazole** for active cases.

d. Paromomycin [Humatin]

—is useful for treatment of **mild** to **moderate infections** or in asymptomatic carriers in place of **iodoquinol;** it is not absorbed from the gastrointestinal tract. May be used for **luminal infections**.

e. Diloxanide furoate [Furamide]

—is directly amebicidal by an unknown mechanism.

—is orally absorbed and produces few adverse effects.

—is the preferred agent for treatment of **asymptomatic amebiasis**.

f. Emetine and dehydroemetine

—are protein synthesis inhibitors that are used only as alternative agents when **metronidazole** has failed. Are administered parenterally and are slowly metabolized.

—produce gastrointestinal irritation and cardiovascular effects, such as tachycardia, dyspnea, and electrocardiographic (ECG) abnormalities.

g. Chloroquine

—may be used after **emetine or dehydroemetine** therapy for treatment of **hepatic abscesses**.

3. Agents active against leishmaniasis

a. Stibogluconate sodium [Pentostam]

—is a pentavalent antimonial; mechanism of action is unknown.

—is administered parenterally; is cleared by the kidney.

—is effective against all *Leishmania;* therapy is a 10-day or 30-day course and may need to be repeated.

—produces gastrointestinal and ECG disturbances and allergic reactions; contraindicated in patients with cardiovascular, liver, or renal disease.

b. Pentamidine [Pentam]

　–acts by unknown mechanism.

　–is administered intramuscularly to treat *L. donovani* **infections** when antimonials have failed or are contraindicated.

　–produces adverse effects that include pain and allergic reaction at injection site and high incidence of renal toxicity (24%), liver abnormalities (10%), hypotension (10%), and hypoglycemia (10%).

c. Amphotericin B

　–has some activity against *L. braziliensis* and *L. mexicana*. Also used when antimonials are ineffective or contraindicated.

d. Allopurinol

　–is useful for *L. donovani* **infections** and infections resistant to traditional therapy. Metabolites are toxic to parasite.

4. Agents used in the treatment of trypanosomiasis

a. Nifurtimox [Lampit]

　–has mechanism similar to that of nitrofurans; causes DNA damage.

　–is well absorbed from the gastrointestinal tract, metabolized in the liver, and eliminated by the kidney.

　–is used to treat South American trypanosomiasis, caused by *Trypanosoma cruzi* (**Chagas' disease**).

　–produces anorexia and other gastrointestinal disturbances, as well as adverse CNS effects.

b. Suramin (Bayer 205) [Belganyl, Germanin, Naphuride]

　–has a complex dye structure. Mechanism of action is not defined; may exert effect by binding to cationic sites on proteins. Does not penetrate mammalian cells, but binds to serum protein, which can be taken up by the phagocytic cells of the reticuloendothelial system. Taken up by trypanosomes by endocytosis.

　–is administered by IV infusion; persists in the circulation for days. Does not enter CSF and is not metabolized.

　–is useful for treatment of **African trypanosomiasis,** or **sleeping sickness** (caused by *T. gambiense* or *T. rhodesiense*), in the hemolytic stage; is not effective against *T. cruzi*.

　–can cause severe adverse effects that include nausea, vomiting, and shock. Also may cause renal dysfunction.

c. Eflornithine hydrochloride

　–inhibits ornithine decarboxylase, an enzyme required for trypanosome growth.

　–is effective in **arousing comatose sleeping sickness patients** (the "resurrection drug").

　–must be administered IV.

d. Melarsoprol (mel B) [Arsobal]

　–is a trivalent arsenical that reacts with sulfhydryl groups in proteins.

　–is administered by IV infusion and enters CSF.

　–is useful in the treatment of the **meningoencephalitic stage of African trypanosomiasis,** especially that caused by *T. gambiense*.

  −produces hypertension, abdominal pain, and rashes. Potentially fatal effect is **reactive encephalopathy** (seen in 1%–5% of patients).
  −**tryparsamide,** also an arsenical, is used as alternative therapy for late trypanosomiasis with CNS involvement. It is useful in combination with **suramin**.

  ### e. Pentamidine
  −can be used as an alternative to **suramin** in the early stage of the disease.

  ## 5. Drug therapy for other protozoal infections

  ### a. Giardiasis
  −**quinacrine** is the drug of choice; **metronidazole** and **furazolidone** are suitable alternatives.

  ### b. *Pneumocystis carinii*
  −**trimethoprim/sulfamethoxazole** is effective; **pentamidine isethionate** or **aerosol pentamidine** is an alternative.

  ### c. Trichomoniasis
  −may be treated with **metronidazole**.

  ### d. Toxoplasmosis
  −is treated with **pyrimethamine** and **trisulfapyrimidines** (mixture of **sulfadiazine, sulfamerazine,** and **sulfamethazine**).

B. Agents active against metazoan infections (anthelmintics)

1. Agents effective against nematode (roundworm) infections

a. Mebendazole [Vermox]
  −is a benzimidazole carbamate that binds to parasite tubulin; also inhibits glucose uptake by nematodes. Resulting glycogen depletion immobilizes the parasite.
  −is poorly absorbed from the gastrointestinal tract; oral administration is effective for intestinal parasites but not tissue forms. Produces no systemic toxicity.
  −is recommended for treatment of **roundworm infections** caused by *Ascaris lumbricoides, Capillaria philippinensis, Enterobius vermicularis* (pinworm), *Necator americanus* (hookworm), and *Trichuris trichiura* (whipworm). Also recommended for infections caused by the cestodes *Echinococcus granulosus* and *E. multilocularis*.

b. Pyrantel pamoate [Antiminth]
  −selectively inhibits acetylcholinesterase (AChE) of the worm, resulting in paralysis; intestinal nematodes are flushed from the system.
  −is poorly absorbed from the gastrointestinal tract and most is excreted unchanged in the feces.
  −is useful for the treatment of infections caused by *A. lumbricoides, E. vermicularis, N. americanus* and, occasionally, *T. trichiura*.
  −causes minor gastrointestinal and neurologic disturbances.

c. Thiabendazole [Mintezol]
  −is a benzimidazole that may inhibit microtubule assembly or anaerobic metabolism of parasites.

–is absorbed from the gastrointestinal tract.

–is used primarily for **strongyloidiasis** (*Strongyloides stercoralis* infection), **trichostrongylus infections,** and **trichinosis**. Topical applications are used for treatment of **cutaneous larva migrans** (creeping eruption).

–produces adverse effects that include nausea, dizziness, malaise, malodorous sweat and urine, and disorientation.

d. Piperazine citrate [Antepar]

–blocks response to ACh; results in altered parasite membrane permeability and paralysis.

–is absorbed from gastrointestinal tract; adverse effects are minimal.

–provides effective treatment of **ascariasis** and **enterobiasis**.

2. Agents effective against cestode (tapeworm) and trematode (fluke) infections

a. Praziquantel [Biltricide]

–causes muscle contraction in the worm, which prevents effective positioning of the worm in the intestine. Mechanism is not known.

–is absorbed from the gastrointestinal tract and metabolized in the liver.

–is the most effective drug against all types of fluke infections; including blood fluke infections (**schistosomiasis**), intestinal and liver fluke infections, and lung fluke infections (**paragonimiasis**). It is also useful in the treatment of **tapeworm infections**.

–produces minor gastrointestinal and neurologic disturbances.

b. Niclosamide [Niclocide]

–inhibits glucose uptake, oxidative phosphorylation, and anaerobic metabolism of the parasite.

–is not absorbed from the gastrointestinal tract but is given orally; produces minimal adverse effects.

–is useful for treatment of tapeworm infections caused by *Taenia saginata, T. solium, Diphyllobothrium latum,* and *Hymenolepsis nana* (beef, pork, fish, and dwarf tapeworm, respectively).

c. Bithionol

–inhibits parasite respiration. Recommended for *Fasciola hepatica* (sheep liver fluke infection) and as an alternative to **praziquantel** for **acute paragonimiasis**.

VI. Antiviral Drugs

A. Inhibitors of early events in virus life cycle

1. Amantadine [Symmetrel]

–inhibits single-stranded RNA viruses after uncoating prior to transcription; may prevent release of nucleic acid into cell.

–is absorbed from the gastrointestinal tract and excreted by the kidneys; $t_{1/2}$ approximately 12 hours.

–is used to treat orthomyxovirus (**influenza A**) infections when administered within the first 48 hours of symptoms, and as prophylaxis during flu season. Does not suppress immune response to influenza A vaccine.

—causes mild CNS effects (insomnia, nervousness). Patients with history of epilepsy require close monitoring.

2. Arildone

—interacts with capsid proteins and inhibits uncoating of DNA and RNA viruses.

—demonstrates no cross-resistance with other antivirals.

—is used topically only, primarily for **herpetic lesions of the eye;** is too toxic for systemic use.

B. Inhibitors of viral synthesis

1. Pyrimidine analogs

—need to be converted to nucleoside triphosphate.

a. Idoxuridine (iododeoxyuridine, IDU) and trifluridine (trifluo-rothymidine, F$_3$Thd)

—replace thymidine in viral DNA and cause fraudulent base pairing; also inhibit viral DNA polymerase and enzymes in dTTP pathway.

—may produce toxicity, probably due to incorporation in host DNA.

—are used topically for **herpetic infections of the eye**.

b. Zidovudine (3'-azido-3'-deoxythymidine, AZT) [Retrovir]

—inhibits reverse transcriptase and also acts as a DNA chain terminator.

—is orally absorbed, metabolized in the liver, and cleared by renal tubular secretion; t$_{1/2}$ is approximately 30 minutes.

—penetrates CSF to some extent.

—**dose-limiting toxicities** are **granulocytopenia** and **anemia**.

—is used in the treatment of the RNA virus known as HIV, the causative agent in **AIDS**.

c. Zalcitabine (dideoxycytidine, ddC)

—inhibits HIV reverse transcriptase; is a DNA chain terminator.

—is undergoing trials for HIV treatment; **peripheral neuropathy** may limit use.

—may be useful in combination with **zidovudine** in the treatment of **AIDS**.

2. Purine analogs

—need to be converted to nucleoside triphosphate.

a. Vidarabine (adenine arabinoside, ara-A)

—inhibits viral DNA polymerase and ribonucleotide reductase to a greater extent than host enzymes.

—is administered IV to treat **herpes simplex encephalitis, herpes simplex infections in neonates,** and **varicella-zoster virus** in immunocompromised patients, and ophthalmically for **herpetic eye infections.**

—produces anorexia, nausea, rash, and CNS disturbances.

b. Acyclovir (9-[2-hydroxyethoxymethyl] guanine, acycloguanine) [Zovirax]

—requires viral thymidine kinase to be converted to monophosphate. Triphosphate form inhibits viral DNA polymerase; incorporated molecule is DNA chain terminator; does not eradicate latent virus.

—is orally absorbed and is eliminated via kidney; $t_{1/2}$ approximately 2–3 hours (longer in renal failure). Good CSF penetration.

—is active against **herpes simplex virus** types I and II, **Epstein-Barr virus, varicella-zoster virus,** and **cytomegalovirus (CMV);** chronic oral administration provides suppression of recurrent genital herpes and herpes zoster in immunocompromised patients, ophthalmic application is used to treat **herpes simplex dendritic keratitis,** and topical application is used for **mucocutaneous herpetic infections** in immunosuppressed patients.

—is cross-resistant with **idoxuridine,** but not usually with **vidarabine** or **trifluridine.**

—produces adverse effects that include nausea and vomiting (2.7%) on short-term administration; headache observed with chronic use.

c. Ganciclovir [Cytovene]

—is a deoxyguanosine analog that, as the triphosphate, inhibits replication of CMV.

—unconverted drug has a $t_{1/2}$ of approximately 3 hours; triphosphate has a longer half-life in cells.

—penetrates CNS. Administered IV; loading dose is followed by maintenance dose.

—is used to treat **CMV retinitis, colitis, or esophagitis** in immunocompromised patients.

—dose-limiting toxicity is **reversible neutropenia** and **thrombocytopenia.**

d. Didanosine (dideoxyinosine, ddI) [Videx]

—is a triphosphate recognized by HIV reverse transcriptase in place of either dATP or dGTP; is a DNA chain terminator.

—is available for treatment of **HIV infection;** may be less marrow-suppressive than **zidovudine.**

—dose-limiting toxicities are **pancreatitis** and **sensory peripheral neuropathy.**

—is not cross-resistant with **zidovudine.**

3. Other inhibitors

a. Ribavirin (1β-D-ribofuranosyl-2,4-triazol-3-carboxamide)

—inhibits inosine monophosphate dehydrogenase and viral DNA and RNA polymerases; mechanism not clear.

—is administered as an aerosol to treat **respiratory syncytial virus;** IV formulation is used outside U.S. for treatment of **Lassa fever.**

b. Foscarnet (trisodium phosphonoformate)

—inhibits viral DNA polymerase by binding to the pyrophosphate binding site.

—is not cross-resistant with most other antivirals.

—is being investigated for use against **HIV, CMV, and herpes simplex virus.**

c. Interferons

—are naturally occurring peptides that stimulate antiviral activity of the host. Single-stranded RNA viruses are the most sensitive.

–include **human interferon alpha-2a** [Roferon A] and **interferon alpha-2b** [Intron A].

–are used for **herpes zoster virus** in immunosuppressed patients, **AIDS-related Kaposi's sarcoma,** and **juvenile papilloma virus**. Some efficacy seen in the treatment of **hairy cell leukemia**. Effective in treatment of **chronic hepatitis B and C**.

–are inactivated in the gastrointestinal tract; adverse effects include chills, fever, and malaise. High-dose therapy limited by marrow suppression and neurotoxicity. Neutralizing antibodies may develop on extended use.

Review Test

Directions: Each of the numbered items or incomplete statements in this section is followed by answers or by completions of the statement. Select the **one** lettered answer or completion that is **best** in each case.

1. Trimethoprim/sulfamethoxazole might be best used for which one of the following conditions?

(A) *Pneumocystis carinii* infection
(B) *Leishmania* infection
(C) Herpes simplex infection
(D) Influenza A infection
(E) *Ascaris lumbricoides* infection

2. Which of the following phrases best describes the antibiotic action of clavulanic acid?

(A) Broad-spectrum antibiotic
(B) Inhibits transpeptidases
(C) Inhibits β-lactamases
(D) Folic acid analog

3. Which of the following antibacterials is susceptible to β-lactamases?

(A) Methicillin
(B) Vancomycin
(C) Ticarcillin
(D) Oxacillin
(E) Bacitracin

4. Which of the following agents would be appropriate therapy for *Mycobacterium tuberculosis*?

(A) Rifampin
(B) Isoniazid and chloramphenicol
(C) Ethambutol
(D) Isoniazid and rifampin
(E) Doxycycline

5. Important characteristics of erythromycin include which one of the following?

(A) Inhibition of protein synthesis by binding to 30S subunit and "freezing" initiation complex
(B) Good efficacy against *Mycoplasma* and *Legionella* infections
(C) Excretion in the urinary tract in unchanged form
(D) Association with high incidence of nephrotoxicity

6. Incorporation into DNA is an important aspect of the action of which of the following antiviral agents?

(A) Acyclovir
(B) Trifluridine
(C) Idoxuridine
(D) Zidovudine
(E) All of the above

7. Which one of the following agents interferes with folate synthesis?

(A) Dapsone
(B) Sulfamethoxazole
(C) *Para*-aminosalicylic acid
(D) Trimethoprim
(E) All of the above

8. Which one of the following agents would be effective therapy for a penicillinase-producing *Staphylococcus aureus* infection?

(A) Nafcillin
(B) Ampicillin
(C) Amoxicillin
(D) Azlocillin
(E) Piperacillin

9. Which one of the following agents would be useful in treating methicillin-resistant staphylococcal infections?

(A) Amantadine
(B) Piperacillin
(C) Isoniazid
(D) Vancomycin
(E) All of the above

10. Which one of the following drugs is effective in treating *Haemophilus influenzae* infections?

(A) Cephalexin
(B) Interferon
(C) Cefotaxime
(D) Methicillin

11. Probenecid alters the $t_{1/2}$ of which of the following agents?

(A) Gentamicin
(B) Erythromycin
(C) Rifampin
(D) Penicillin
(E) Doxycycline

12. Which one of the following drugs might be used in the treatment of nematode infection?

(A) Mebendazole
(B) Niclosamide
(C) Mefloquine
(D) Praziquantel
(E) Suramin

13. Which of the following is a characteristic of stibogluconate sodium?

(A) Is an effective agent against trypanosomiasis
(B) Can be safely given to patients with cardiovascular or renal disease
(C) Commonly causes discoloration of the teeth
(D) Is an effective agent against leishmaniasis

14. Which of the following is a characteristic of suramin?

(A) Is an effective antiviral agent
(B) Can be administered orally
(C) Penetrates mammalian cells well
(D) Can be used for African trypanosomiasis

Questions 15–17

Use the structure below to answer questions 15 through 17.

15. The structure is the basic building block for which of the following groups of drugs?

(A) Ampicillin and piperacillin
(B) Gentamicin and tobramycin
(C) Trimethoprim and pyrimethamine
(D) Erythromycin and clindamycin
(E) Cefazolin and ceftizoxime

16. R_1 is important in determining a drug's

(A) spectrum of antibacterial activity
(B) spectrum of antiviral activity
(C) spectrum of antitumor activity
(D) pharmacologic properties
(E) mechanism of action

17. R_2 is important in determining a drug's

(A) spectrum of antibacterial activity
(B) spectrum of antiviral activity
(C) spectrum of antitumor activity
(D) pharmacologic properties
(E) mechanism of action

18. Adequate therapy of both erythrocytic and exoerythrocytic forms of malaria would be provided by combination chemotherapy with

(A) chloroquine and metronidazole
(B) primaquine and chloroquine
(C) clotrimazole and niclosamide
(D) primaquine and piperazine
(E) sulfisoxazole and trimethoprim

19. The mechanism of action of pyrimethamine involves

(A) muscle paralysis
(B) inhibition of glucose absorption
(C) interference with folate metabolism
(D) inhibition of glycolysis
(E) enhanced immune function

20. The mechanism of action of miconazole is best described as

(A) binding to 80S ribosomes
(B) inhibition of sterol synthesis
(C) blockade of tetrahydrofolate reductase
(D) DNA intercalation
(E) inhibition of ribonucleotide reductase

21. Which group of topical agents would be used to treat fungal infections?

(A) Ketoconazole, amphotericin B, and clotrimazole
(B) Moxalactam, miconazole, and mebendazole
(C) Flucytosine, nystatin, and ketoconazole
(D) Nystatin, clotrimazole, and tolnaftate

22. An appropriate use of doxycycline would be therapy of an infection caused by

(A) *Plasmodium vivax*
(B) *Schistosoma mansoni*
(C) *Rickettsiae*
(D) *Histoplasma capsulatum*
(E) Herpes simplex type II

23. A major step in the excretion of chloramphenicol involves

(A) peroxidation
(B) acetylation
(C) glucuronide formation
(D) accumulation in the bile
(E) deamination

24. Each of the following agents inhibits bacterial cell wall synthesis EXCEPT

(A) vidarabine
(B) nafcillin
(C) cycloserine
(D) bacitracin
(E) cefotaxime

25. Metronidazole would provide appropriate therapy of infections with which one of the following pairs of organisms?

(A) *Enterobius* and *Necator*
(B) *Microsporum* and *Trichophyton*
(C) *Entamoeba histolytica* and *Giardia lamblia*
(D) *Cryptococcus neoformans* and *Histoplasma capsulatum*
(E) *Plasmodium vivax* and *Leishmania donovanii*

26. Which of the following drugs produces its action by inducing flaccid paralysis of nematode muscle?

(A) Niclosamide
(B) Piperazine
(C) Nifurtimox
(D) Metronidazole
(E) Pyrimethamine

Directions: Each group of items in this section consists of lettered options followed by a set of numbered items. For each item, select the **one** lettered option that is most closely associated with it. Each lettered option may be selected once, more than once, or not at all.

Questions 27–30

Match each of the following drugs with the adverse effect most closely related to it.

(A) Red-orange body secretions
(B) Discoloration of teeth
(C) Gray baby syndrome
(D) Parkinsonian-like effect
(E) Nephrotoxicity

27. Chloramphenicol

28. Rifampin

29. Tetracycline

30. Amphotericin B

Questions 31–33

Match each of the following descriptions of mechanisms of action with the appropriate drug.

(A) Griseofulvin
(B) Flucytosine
(C) Isoniazid
(D) Acyclovir
(E) Cephalexin

31. Inhibits peptidoglycan crosslinking

32. Used in therapy of tuberculosis

33. Used for herpesvirus infections

Questions 34–36

Match each of the following descriptions of mechanisms of action with the appropriate drug.

(A) Acyclovir
(B) Rifampin
(C) Streptomycin
(D) Moxalactam
(E) *Para*-aminosalicylic acid

34. Binds to 30S ribosomal subunit

35. Inhibits cell wall synthesis

36. Binds to DNA-dependent RNA polymerase

Questions 37–40

Match each of the following drugs with the adverse effect most closely related to it.

(A) Ototoxicity and nephrotoxicity
(B) Hypersensitivity reactions
(C) Aplastic anemia
(D) Cinchonism

37. Chloramphenicol

38. Gentamicin

39. Quinine

40. Penicillin G

Answers and Explanations

1–A. The combination drug trimethoprim/sulfamethoxazole is one of the few that inhibits the growth of *Pneumocystis*. *Leishmania* and *Ascaris* species and viral infections are not effectively controlled with this drug.

2–C. Clavulanic acid is administered in combination with penicillins because of its activity against β-lactamases. It has little antibiotic activity and is not structurally related to folic acid. It has no effect on transpeptidase activity.

3–C. The extended-spectrum penicillins such as ticarcillin are susceptible to β-lactamases (penicillinases). Methicillin and oxacillin are β-lactamase–resistant penicillin derivatives. Vancomycin and bacitracin are not structurally related to penicillins and are not susceptible to β-lactamase action.

4–D. Because of the high incidence of preexisting resistant mycobacteria, single-agent therapy is not recommended for *Mycobacterium tuberculosis*. Both isoniazid and rifampin are effective antitubercular agents.

5–B. Erythromycin binds to the 50S component of ribosomes and is effective against pneumonia caused by *Mycoplasma* and *Legionella*. The drug is excreted via the biliary route. Serious adverse effects are rare.

6–E. Many antiviral agents exert their effects by incorporation into viral DNA.

7–E. Dapsone, sulfamethoxazole, and *para*-aminosalicylic acid are structural analogs of *para*-aminobenzoic acid and inhibit dihydropteroate synthesis. Trimethoprim inhibits dihydrofolate reductase, another enzyme in the folic acid synthesis pathway.

8–A. Nafcillin is penicillinase-resistant.

9–D. Vancomycin is used to treat methicillin-resistant staphylococcal infections and in patients allergic to penicillins and cephalosporins. Amantadine and isoniazid are not antibacterials; piperacillin is penicillinase-sensitive.

10–C. Third-generation cephalosporins, such as cefotaxime, are effective treatments for *H. influenzae*. First-generation drugs, such as cephalexin, and penicillinase-resistant penicillins (methicillin) have little activity against *H. influenzae*. Interferon is an antiviral agent.

11–D. Probenecid inhibits the elimination of weak organic acids, such as penicillin, excreted by the kidney. Rifampin and erythromycin are excreted via the biliary route; gentamicin is eliminated by glomerular filtration; doxycycline is eliminated by the fecal route.

12–A. Mebendazole is recommended for treatment of nematode (roundworm) infections. Niclosamide and praziquantel are used in the treatment of cestode (tapeworm) and trematode (fluke) infections. Mefloquine is useful for chloroquine-resistant malaria, and suramin is used for African trypanosomiasis (sleeping sickness).

13–D. Stibogluconate is used to treat leishmaniasis. It is not used for trypanosomiasis and is contraindicated in the presence of cardiovascular and renal disease. It has no effect on tooth color.

14–D. Suramin, a treatment for African trypanosomiasis (sleeping sickness), has no effect on viruses and does not penetrate mammalian cells. It must be administered intravenously.

15–E. The structure is the cephalosporin nucleus of cefazolin and ceftizoxime.

16–A. Modifications in R_1 generally affect the spectrum of antibacterial activity for a given cephalosporin.

17–D. R_2 modifications generally affect the pharmacologic properties of a cephalosporin.

18–B. Primaquine is effective only against exoerythrocytic stages of malaria, and chloroquine is only active against erythrocytic forms. Metronidazole is an antiamebic agent; niclosamide is used for tapeworm infections. Trimethoprim possesses slight antimalarial activity restricted to the schizonts.

19–C. Pyrimethamine inhibits parasitic dihydrofolate reductase.

20–B. Miconazole inhibits the synthesis of ergosterol.

21–D. Nystatin, clotrimazole, and tolnaftate are all effective topically.

22–C. Tetracyclines such as doxycycline are the preferred drugs to treat rickettsial infections. They are ineffective against *Plasmodium vivax, Schistosoma mansoni,* and *Histoplasma capsulatum.*

23–C. The lack of adequate chloramphenicol glucuronidation in neonates (because their glucuronidation systems are not sufficiently developed) contributes to the development of gray baby syndrome; they fail to eliminate the drug, and toxic concentrations accumulate.

24–A. Vidarabine, or *ara*-A, is an antiviral agent that inhibits DNA polymerase and ribonucleotide reductase.

25–C. Metronidazole [Flagyl] is an effective antiamebic agent and also possesses activity against *Giardia* infections.

26–B. Piperazine blocks the action of ACh at the myoneural junction and causes flaccid paralysis of nematode muscle.

27–C. Neonates lack adequate glucuronidation systems, and so toxic levels of chloramphenicol can accumulate.

28–A. Orange-colored rifampin often produces red-orange saliva, tears, and other body secretions.

29–B. When administered to children with growing teeth, tetracycline may cause discoloration.

30–E. Amphotericin B is highly nephrotoxic.

31–E. β-Lactam antibiotics inhibit crosslinking of bacterial cell wall peptidoglycans.

32–C. Isoniazid is a first-line drug in the treatment of *Mycobacterium tuberculosis.*

33–D. Acyclovir is a very effective antiherpetic agent.

34–C. Streptomycin is the prototypical inhibitor of bacterial protein synthesis. It acts by binding to the 30S ribosomal subunit and freezing the initiation complex.

35–D. Moxalactam, a third-generation cephalosporin, inhibits cell wall synthesis by preventing crosslinking of peptidoglycans.

36–B. Rifampin inhibits bacterial growth by binding to the bacterial DNA-dependent RNA polymerase.

37–C. Although it occurs rarely, the aplastic anemia caused by chloramphenicol may be fatal.

38–A. Gentamicin can be both ototoxic and nephrotoxic.

39–D. Quinine, a chinchona alkaloid, may cause cinchonism, a syndrome associated with visual and auditory disturbances.

40–B. The most common adverse effect of penicillin is hypersensitivity.

11

Cancer Chemotherapy

I. Principles of Cancer Chemotherapy

A. Therapeutic effect of anticancer agents

–may require **total cell kill,** elimination of all neoplastic cells.

–often involves drugs that have a narrow therapeutic index; may require combinations of several drugs with different mechanisms of action, dose-limiting toxicities, or cross-resistance to minimize adverse effects on non-neoplastic cells (Table 11.1).

–is usually achieved by killing growing cells, which are most sensitive to this class of agents. Most adverse effects are seen in normally dividing non-neoplastic cells, such as hair follicles and bone marrow.

–may involve the use of agents that act only at specific stages in the cell cycle.

B. Resistance

1. Primary resistance

–is seen in tumor cells that do not respond to initial therapy using currently available drugs.

–is related to the **frequency of spontaneous mutation** (10^{-5}–10^{-10}). There is less likelihood that a small tumor burden has resistant cells. The probability that any tumor population has primary resistance to two non–cross-resistant drugs is even less likely (approximately the product of the two individual probabilities).

2. Acquired resistance

–develops or appears **during therapy**.

–can result from amplification of target genes (e.g., the gene for dihydrofolate reductase, which is the target for **methotrexate**). Gene amplification also occurs in the **multidrug resistance phenotype**. In this case, cells overproduce proteins that apparently transport bulky, natural product agents out of cells. As a result, the cell fails to accumulate toxic concentrations of several different types of drugs.

–can also occur via changes in the cellular targets of the drugs (e.g., in their affinity for drugs) or changes in transport or "activating" enzymes.

279

Table 11.1. Properties of Some Cancer Chemotherapeutic Drugs

Class of Drug	Examples	Dose-limiting Toxicity, Distinguishing Adverse Effects	Mechanism of Action
Alkylating agents	Nitrogen mustards: mechlorethamine, cyclophosphamide, ifosfamide, melphalan, chlorambucil	Myelosuppression, tissue damage at injection site; hemorrhagic cystitis and sterility (with cyclophosphamide and ifosfamide)	Alkylation of target molecules, often *N*-7 of guanine in DNA
	Nitrosoureas: carmustine, lomustine, semustine	Myelosuppression, tissue damage at injection site	
	Others: busulfan, streptozocin, dacarbazine	Myelosuppression, tissue damage at injection site	
Antimetabolites	Methotrexate	Myelosuppression, hepatotoxicity, mucositis	Inhibition of dihydrofolate reductase and subsequent thymidylate synthesis by depletion of required tetrahydrofolate cofactor
	Fluorouracil, floxuridine	Myelosuppression	Inhibition of thymidylate synthetase by forming ternary complex between enzyme and F-dUMP
	Cytarabine (cytosine arabinoside)	Myelosuppression	Triphosphate analog inhibits DNA polymerase, and, when incorporated into DNA, causes mispairing
	Mercaptopurine, thioguanine	Myelosuppression	Nucleotide analogs inhibit nucleotide metabolism; also incorporated into DNA and may cause aberrant base pairing
Natural products	Vinca alkaloids: vincristine, vinblastine	Myelosuppression (vinblastine > vincristine), neurotoxicity (vincristine > vinblastine)	Disrupt microtubule apparatus
	Epipodophyllotoxins: etoposide, teniposide	Myelosuppression	Inhibit DNA topoisomerase II
Antibiotics	Actinomycin D (dactinomycin)	Myelosuppression	DNA intercalating agent; inhibits RNA and DNA synthesis
	Doxorubicin, daunorubicin	Cardiomyopathy	DNA intercalating agents; inhibit DNA and RNA synthesis

Bleomycin	Pulmonary toxicity	Complexes with DNA and produces strand scission
Others		
Cisplatin	Renal toxicity	Crosslinks DNA
Procarbazine	Myelosuppression	Produces chromosomal breaks; inhibits DNA, RNA synthesis
L-Asparaginase	Antibodies to enzyme; anaphylaxis	Reduces level of L-asparagine, a required amino acid for some tumors
Steroids and antagonists: estrogen, tamoxifen, leuprolide	Adverse effects relating to hormone, antagonist properties	Antagonize or lower concentrations of normally occurring hormones in hormone-dependent tumors

II. Alkylating Agents

A. Structure and mechanism

—contain **strong electrophilic center**. Clinically useful drugs have a **nitrosourea,** *bis*-**(chloroethyl) amine,** or **ethylenimine** moiety. The electrophilic center becomes covalently linked to nucleophilic centers of target molecules, often via a carbonium ion intermediate. The end result is transfer of an alkyl moiety from the drug to the target. Nitrosoureas can also cause **carbamylation**.

—target nitrogens (especially the *N*-7 of guanine) and oxygens of purines and pyrimidines in DNA. May lead to abnormal base pairing, depurination (followed by DNA chain scission), ring cleavage, and DNA strand crosslinks.

—also target other biological moities, which become alkylated, including carboxyl, imidazole, amino, sulfhydryl, and phosphate groups.

—can act at all stages of the cell cycle.

—**resistance** can involve increases in DNA repair processes, reduction in cellular permeability to the drug, and production of molecules containing thiols that react with and neutralize the alkylating agents.

—are **direct vesicants;** except for cyclophosphamide, most can damage tissue at the injection site.

—dose-limiting toxicity is **bone marrow suppression**. Most also cause nausea and vomiting that can be minimized by pretreatment with **phenothiazines** or **cannabinoids**. Most can cause sterility. Some (**cyclophosphamide** and **ifosfamide**) may result in hemorrhagic cystitis.

B. Nitrogen mustards: bifunctional alkylating agents

1. Mechlorethamine [Mustargen]

—is extremely hygroscopic and unstable. The active drug is present only for minutes.

—is administered intravenously (IV); causes severe local reactions.

—is used primarily in the treatment of **Hodgkin's disease** and other lymphomas; it is included in the **MOPP** regimen (*m*echlorethamine, *v*incristine [Oncovin], *p*rocarbazine, and *p*rednisone).

—**leukopenia** and **thrombocytopenia** are dose-limiting toxicities; repeat courses of treatment are given only after marrow function has recovered. Nausea and vomiting generally occur.

2. Cyclophosphamide [Cytoxan] and ifosfamide [Ifex]

a. Cyclophosphamide may be administered orally, intravenously, or intramuscularly. It needs to be metabolically activated to 4-hydroxycyclophosphamide by the mixed-function oxidase system of the liver. **Phosphoramide mustard** and **acrolein,** active drugs, are produced by nonenzymatic cleavage of 4-hydroxycyclophosphamide.

—is used to treat **Hodgkin's disease** and other lymphomas. In combination with other agents, it has been shown to be effective against **Burkitt's lymphoma** and **acute lymphoblastic leukemia of childhood**.

—is frequently used for adjuvant therapy after **surgery for breast cancer** in combination with **methotrexate** and **fluorouracil**. Is also used in combinations to treat **small-cell lung cancer, retinoblastoma,** and **adult soft-tissue sarcomas**.

–has less incidence of thrombocytopenia than **mechlorethamine,** but **immunosuppression** is still the most important toxic effect. Reversible alopecia often occurs; nausea and vomiting are common.

b. Ifosfamide
   –is a **cyclophosphamide** analog with less potential to cause hemorrhagic cystitis.
   –appears to be effective (in combination with other agents) in the treatment of **germ-cell testicular cancer, carcinomas of the cervix,** and **Hodgkin's and non-Hodgkin's lymphomas**. It is administered with **mesna** to detoxify its harmful urinary metabolites.

3. Melphalan [Alkeran] and chlorambucil [Leukeran]
   –are derivatives of **nitrogen mustard** containing phenylalanine and an aromatic ring, respectively.
   –can be administered orally. Therapeutic use and adverse effects are similar to those of other nitrogen mustards.

   a. Chlorambucil is the slowest-acting nitrogen mustard and is the agent of choice in the treatment of **chronic lymphocytic leukemia** and **Waldenström's macroglobulinemia**. It produces less severe marrow suppression than other nitrogen mustards.

   b. Melphalan is often used to treat **multiple myeloma, malignant melanoma,** and **carcinoma of the ovary and breast**.

4. Busulfan [Myleran]
   –is an alkyl sulfonate that is selectively myelosuppressive, inhibiting granulocytopoiesis.
   –is administered orally to treat **chronic granulocytic leukemia** and other myeloproliferative disorders.
   –produces adverse effects related to myelosuppression. It rarely produces nausea and vomiting.
   –is administered concurrently with **allopurinol** to reduce renal precipitation of urates resulting from cellular destruction. (Allopurinol is frequently used for this purpose with highly toxic agents.)

5. Nitrosoureas
   –include **carmustine** (BCNU) [BiCNU], **lomustine** (CCNU) [CeeNU], and **semustine** (methyl-CCNU).
   –are highly lipophilic; cross the blood–brain barrier.
   –are given orally except for **carmustine,** which is administered intravenously.
   –are useful in **Hodgkin's disease** and other lymphomas as well as **meningeal leukemia** and **tumors of the brain**.
   –are markedly **myelosuppressive** (delayed effect, possibly up to 6 weeks). May also result in renal failure.

6. Streptozocin [Zanosar]
   –is a natural antibiotic that is comprised of methylnitrosourea linked to the 2-carbon of glucose.
   –has an affinity for beta cells of islets of Langerhans and is diabetogenic in animals. It is useful for the treatment of **pancreatic islet cell carcinoma** and other malignant carcinomas.

—is not myelosuppressive. Nausea and vomiting almost always occur. **Renal toxicity** is dose-limiting.

7. Dacarbazine (dimethyltriazenoimidazolecarboxamide) [DTIC-Dome]

—is activated in the liver by oxidative *N*-demethylation. The active compound is **diazomethane**.

—is administered intravenously primarily to treat **malignant melanoma** and in combination with **doxorubicin** in **Hodgkin's disease** and some soft-tissue sarcomas.

—is moderately myelosuppressive. Nausea and vomiting occur in 90% of patients.

III. Antimetabolites

A. Methotrexate [Folex, Mexate]

1. Mechanism of action

—is a **folic acid analog** that inhibits dihydrofolate reductase. This reduces the pool of tetrahydrofolate and, consequently, *N*-5,10-methylene tetrahydrofolate is not formed. Hence, transfer of the methyl group from this cofactor to 2'-deoxyuridylate by thymidylate synthetase to form thymidylate cannot occur. Net result is **indirect inhibition of DNA synthesis**.

—also inhibits dihydrofolate reductase by the intracellular formation of polyglutamates.

—is actively taken up into cells by folate carrier. The most common resistance results from transport defects. Resistance can also result from amplification or alterations in gene for dihydrofolate reductase.

2. Pharmacologic properties

—is administered orally, intrathecally, intravenously, or intramuscularly.

—is excreted by glomerular filtration and tubular secretion.

—is poorly transported across the blood–brain barrier. Therapeutic concentrations in the central nervous system (CNS) occur only with high-dose therapy (combined with **leucovorin rescue**).

3. Therapeutic uses

—is an important agent in the **maintenance of remission,** especially in **childhood acute lymphoblastic leukemia,** choriocarcinoma, and other trophoblastic tumors in women.

—is also useful in combination with other drugs in the treatment of **Burkitt's lymphoma and other non-Hodgkin's lymphomas, osteogenic sarcoma,** and various carcinomas.

—can be used for treatment of **severe psoriasis** and has been used for immunosuppression following transplantation or in the management of a variety of immune disorders.

4. Adverse effects

—is **myelosuppressive,** producing severe leukopenia, bone marrow aplasia, and thrombocytopenia. Dose monitoring and **leucovorin** treatment are important adjuncts to successful therapy.

—may produce severe gastrointestinal disturbances. Other adverse effects can occur in most body systems; hepatotoxicity and mucositis are common.

5. Adjunct agents

a. Leucovorin (folinic acid, *N*-5-formyltetrahydrofolic acid, citrovorum factor) is a form of folate that can function directly without need for reduction by dihydrofolate reductase. Administration of **leucovorin** can "rescue" an individual from **methotrexate toxicity**.

b. Thymidine, which can be converted to thymidylate by thymidine kinase, can also relieve **methotrexate** inhibition by eliminating the need for conversion of deoxyuridylate to thymidylate.

B. Cytarabine (cytosine arabinoside, 1-β-D-arabinofuranosylcytosine, ara-C) [Cytosar-U]

1. Structure and mechanism of action

—is an analog of 2′-deoxycytidine. It is converted intracellularly to the monophosphate (AraCMP), diphosphate (AraCDP), and triphosphate nucleotides (AraCTP), sequentially. Accumulation of the triphosphate analog inhibits activity of DNA polymerases and, if incorporated into DNA, results in altered function of newly replicated DNA.

—is most active in the S phase of the cell cycle.

2. Resistance

—can occur via changes in any of the enzymes required for conversion of the nucleoside to the various phosphorylated forms. Deoxycytidine kinase, which produces AraCMP, is one target since it is rate-limiting in the phosphorylation pathway.

—might also involve increased concentrations of the normal substrate dCTP, reduced affinity of DNA polymerases for AraCTP, decreased uptake of ara-C, or increased deoxycytidine deaminase.

3. Pharmacologic properties

—is administered intravenously or intrathecally because absorption after oral administration is poor and unpredictable. Therapeutic concentrations in cerebrospinal fluid (CSF) are achieved after continuous infusion or intrathecal injection.

4. Therapeutic uses

—is useful for induction of remission in **acute leukemia,** especially adult myelocytic leukemia. It is generally used in combination, often with **thioguanine** and **daunorubicin**.

—is beneficial in the treatment of **Hodgkin's disease** and other lymphomas; it is seldom used for carcinomas.

5. Adverse effects

—is highly **myelosuppressive** and can produce severe leukopenia, thrombocytopenia, and anemia.

—also produces many other **toxic effects,** most frequently involving gastrointestinal disturbances.

C. Fluorouracil (5-FU) [Adrucil] and floxuridine (fluorodeoxyuridine) [FUDR]

1. Mechanism of action

—need to be converted to deoxynucleotide monophosphate, F-dUMP, which inhibits thymidylate synthetase by forming a ternary complex between itself, N-5,10-methylene tetrahydrofolate, and the enzyme. The pathway for synthesis of F-dUMP occurs in many ways.

   a. Fluorouracil is converted to fluorouridine (by uridine phosphorylase) and then to F-UMP (by uridine kinase); synthesis can also occur by formation of F-UMP by phosphoribosyl transferase and 5-phosphoribosyl-1-pyrophosphate (PRPP). F-UMP can then be converted to the diphosphate and reduced by ribonucleotide reductase to form F-dUMP.

   b. When **floxuridine** is used, formation of F-dUMP occurs directly since this analog is a substrate for thymidine kinase. Floxuridine can also be degraded to fluorouracil. The triphosphate forms of the analog can also be found in cells, and incorporation into DNA and ribonucleic acid (RNA) occurs with resulting deleterious effects.

2. Pharmacologic properties
   −are administered parenterally and penetrate the CSF well.
   −are metabolized in liver to inactive compounds.

3. Therapeutic uses
   −are useful in certain types of carcinoma; major use is in the treatment of **metastatic colon carcinoma** by infusion into the hepatic artery.
   −applied topically, **fluorouracil** is used to treat **premalignant keratoses, superficial basal cell carcinomas,** and **severe psoriasis**.

4. Adverse effects
   −are markedly **myelosuppressive**.
   −produce gastrointestinal disturbances, alopecia, and neurologic manifestations, along with other toxic effects.

D. Purine analogs: mercaptopurine and thioguanine

1. Structure and mechanism of action
   −are analogs of the natural purines hypoxanthine and guanine, respectively. Must be converted to ribonucleotides by hypoxanthine-guanine phosphoribosyltransferase (HGPRT) to produce 6-thioguanosine-5′-phosphate (6-thioGMP) and 6-thioinosine-5′-phosphate (T-IMP).

   a. 6-thioGMP can be further phosphorylated and is incorporated into DNA. This appears to be its major site of action, although the precise mechanism of cytotoxicity is unknown.

   b. T-IMP accumulates and inhibits nucleotide metabolism at several steps. It can be converted into **thioguanine** derivatives and can also be incorporated into DNA.

2. Mercaptopurine [Purinethol]
   −can be administered orally. Desulfuration can occur; it is also metabolized by xanthine oxidase. (This led to the development of **allopurinol,** which inhibits xanthine oxidase and decreases metabolism of **mercaptopurine**.) Although allopurinol increases the antineoplastic action of mercaptopurine, it does not improve the therapeutic index. Dose reduction necessary when administered with allopurinol.
   −is useful in maintenance therapy of children with **acute leukemia**.
   −**bone marrow depression** is dose-limiting toxicity. Gastrointestinal disturbances occur, including anorexia, nausea, and vomiting.

3. Thioguanine
—is administered orally, although absorption is incomplete.

—is used to treat **acute leukemia** and, in combination with **cytarabine,** for induction of remission in **acute granulocytic leukemia.**

—**bone marrow depression** is dose-limiting toxicity. Gastrointestinal disturbances are less severe than with **mercaptopurine**.

IV. Natural Products

A. Vinca alkaloids

1. Mechanism of action
—are derived from periwinkle plants. They bind to tubulin and disrupt microtubule apparatus, resulting in **metaphase arrest**.

—are most active during mitosis.

2. Selected drugs

a. Vinblastine [Velban]
—is administered intravenously. **Marrow suppression** is dose-limiting toxicity; other adverse effects, including neurologic toxicity, are also observed.

—is used in combination with **bleomycin** and **cisplatin** for **metastatic testicular tumors**. It also is used for various lymphomas and several solid tumors.

b. Vincristine [Oncovin]
—is administered intravenously; it is less toxic to marrow than **vinblastine**. **Neurologic manifestations** may limit dose.

—is used in combination with corticosteroids to induce remissions in **childhood leukemia**. It is used in several important combinations (e.g., MOPP regimen for advanced Hodgkin's disease). It is not cross-resistant with **vinblastine**.

B. Epipodophyllotoxins

1. Structure and mechanism of action
—are bulky multiringed structures derived from the mayapple plant. They block cells at boundary of S phase and prevent entry into G_2 phase.

—most probably act through inhibition of DNA topoisomerase II.

2. Selected drugs

a. Etoposide [VePesid]
—is administered intravenously or orally. **Leukopenia** is dose-limiting toxicity.

—is used for recalcitrant **testicular tumors,** in combination with **bleomycin** and **cisplatin** for **small-cell lung carcinoma, carcinoma of the breast,** and **Kaposi's sarcoma**.

b. Teniposide
—has mechanism similar to **etoposide**.

—is administered intravenously; it is used investigationally.

C. Antibiotics

1. Dactinomycin (actinomycin D) [Cosmegen]

a. Structure and mechanism of action

- −is a chromophore containing peptides isolated from *Streptomyces*. It is one of the most potent cytotoxic agents.
- −intercalates between adjacent guanosine–cytosine base pairs of DNA double helix.
- −strongly impairs RNA synthesis and to a lesser extent DNA synthesis.

b. Pharmacologic properties

- −is administered by intravenous infusion; does not enter the CSF.

c. Therapeutic uses

- −is used to treat **rhabdomyosarcoma and Wilms' tumor in children**. Activity has been observed in Ewing's tumor, Kaposi's sarcoma and other sarcomas, and **methotrexate-resistant choriocarcinoma**.
- −has been used in combination with **vincristine** and **cyclophosphamide** for solid tumors in children.

d. Adverse effects

- −causes bone marrow suppression and gastrointestinal disturbances.

2. Doxorubicin [Adriamycin] and daunorubicin [Cerubidine]

a. Pharmacologic properties

- −are tetracycline rings with the sugar daunosamine. Thus are DNA intercalating agents; affect DNA function.
- −also can produce superoxide anion radicals.
- −are primarily toxic during S phase.
- −are administered intravenously.
- −produce both reversible acute and **irreversible chronic cardiomyopathies;** chronic type is related to cumulative dose of drug and is dose-limiting.

b. Daunorubicin (daunomycin)

- −is used in the treatment of **acute lymphocytic and granulocytic leukemias,** often in combination with **cytarabine**.
- −is also used in some solid tumors of children (but not adults).

c. Doxorubicin

- −is one of the most useful anticancer agents.
- −is extensively cleared via hepatic route, and dose reduction is recommended in presence of hepatic dysfunction. Is myelosuppressive.
- −is employed to treat **acute leukemias,** lymphoma, and a number of solid tumors. One combination regimen (BACOP: *b*leomycin, *A*driamycin [doxorubicin], *c*yclophosphamide, *O*ncovin [vincristine], *p*rednisone) is useful for **non-Hodgkin's lymphomas,** and another combination regimen (ABVD: *A*driamycin [doxorubicin], *b*leomycin, *v*inblastine, *d*acarbazine) is effective in **Hodgkin's disease**.
- −is also used in combination with **cyclophosphamide** and **cisplatin** in treatment of **carcinoma of the ovary** and in combinations with other drugs to treat various carcinomas, sarcomas, and metastatic adenosarcomas.

3. Bleomycin [Blenoxane]

a. Structure and mechanism of action

—is a mixture of copper-chelating glycopeptides produced by *Streptomyces verticillus*. It causes DNA chain scission and fragmentation. Cells with chromosomal aberrations accumulate in the G_2 phase of cell cycle.

—is inactivated by bleomycin hydrolase.

b. Pharmacologic properties

—is administered parenterally. Does not enter the CSF. High drug concentrations are found in the lungs and skin.

—is excreted predominantly by glomerular filtration, and dose reduction is required in the presence of renal impairment.

c. Therapeutic uses

—is used to treat **testicular carcinoma** (usually in combination with **vinblastine** and **cisplatin**) and **squamous cell carcinomas**.

d. Adverse effects

—only minimally myelosuppressive. Most serious adverse effect is **pulmonary toxicity**.

4. Other antibiotics

a. Plicamycin (mithramycin) [Mithracin]

—is a highly **toxic antibiotic** whose use is primarily limited to treatment of **advanced embryonal testicular tumors**.

—lowers plasma calcium concentrations via action on osteoclasts.

b. Mitomycin [Mutamycin]

—is a **natural antibiotic** that is activated to a bifunctional alkylating agent. Results in the impairment of DNA function.

—is used in palliative treatment of **gastric adenocarcinoma,** other carcinomas, and melanoma.

—is **myelosuppressive**.

V. Miscellaneous Agents

A. Cisplatin (*cis*-diamminedichloroplatinum [II]) [Platinol]

1. Structure and mechanism of action

—is a small platinum coordination complex that enters cells by diffusion and acts by complexing with DNA to form crosslinks. Adjacent guanines are most frequently crosslinked.

—also reacts with other nucleophils.

2. Pharmacologic properties

—is administered intravenously. Poor penetration into the CNS.

3. Therapeutic uses

—is employed to treat **testicular tumor** (usually with **bleomycin** and **vinblastine**) or **ovarian carcinoma** (with **doxorubicin**). Also used for several other carcinomas and childhood lymphomas.

4. Adverse effects

−dose-limiting toxicity is **cumulative damage to renal tubules** (may be irreversible following high or repeated doses). Also ototoxic.

−almost always produces nausea and vomiting. Only moderately immunosuppressive.

B. Procarbazine [Matulane]

1. Structure and mechanism of action

−is a substituted hydrazine that needs to be activated metabolically.

−produces chromosomal breaks and inhibits DNA, RNA, and protein synthesis.

2. Pharmacologic properties

−is administered orally and is lipophilic. It enters most cells by diffusion, and is found in the CSF.

3. Therapeutic uses

−is particularly useful in the treatment of **Hodgkin's disease** as part of the MOPP regimen; it is also active against non-Hodgkin's lymphoma, small-cell carcinoma of the lung, melanoma, and brain tumors.

−has no cross-resistance with other anticancer drugs.

4. Adverse effects

−most commonly produces **leukopenia** and **thrombocytopenia,** along with gastrointestinal disturbances. Myelosuppression is dose-dependent.

−augments the effects of sedatives (most probably by competing for drug-metabolizing enzymes in the liver).

−is a monoamine oxidase inhibitor, and some adverse effects related to this inhibition occur.

C. Hydroxyurea [Hydrea]

−inhibits ribonucleoside diphosphate reductase.

−is primarily used in the management of **chronic granulocytic leukemia** and other myeloproliferative disorders.

−produces **hematopoietic depression,** the major adverse effect.

D. Amsacrine (m-AMSA) [Amsidyl]

−intercalates and inhibits DNA synthesis, most probably by inhibiting DNA topoisomerase II.

−produces dose-limiting **leukopenia**.

−is used for induction of remission in **refractory adult leukemia** in combination with **cytarabine**.

E. L-Asparaginase [Elspar]

−is an enzyme that reduces levels of L-asparagine, an amino acid not synthesized by some tumors.

−is synergistic with **methotrexate** when the folic acid analog is administered prior to L-asparaginase.

−is administered intravenously or intramuscularly.

−is used in **lymphoblastic leukemia** and for the induction of remission in **acute lymphocytic leukemia** (with **vincristine** and **prednisone**).

–is minimally marrow suppressive. Toxicity to several body organs, particularly liver and pancreas, occurs; **antibodies to the protein** may develop.

F. Biological response modifiers

–are naturally occurring compounds that influence how an individual responds to the presence of a neoplasm; a number are being tested for efficacy as cancer therapeutics, alone or in combination.

–many have been produced using recombinant DNA technology, including **tumor necrosis factor,** the **interferons,** the **interleukins,** and **epoietin alfa,** among others.

–**alpha-interferons** have been approved for treatment of **hairy cell leukemia** and **Kaposi's sarcoma**. The clinical place of the other agents in cancer chemotherapy remains to be established.

VI. Steroid Hormones and Antagonists

A. Use in neoplasia

–is predicated on the presence of steroid hormone receptors in certain cells and on the ability of the hormone to stimulate or inhibit cell growth. In the former case, hormonal antagonists are used; in the latter, hormonal agonists are employed.

B. Adrenocorticosteroids

–are lymphocytic and antimitotic agents.

–can be administered orally. They are useful in **acute leukemia** in children and **malignant lymphoma**. They are commonly used in combination with **vincristine** to induce remissions; sometimes useful in breast carcinomas; and are also helpful in reducing radiation edema.

C. Aminoglutethimide [Cytadren]

–inhibits synthesis of adrenocorticosteroids.

–when administered with **hydrocortisone,** can effectively reduce estradiol levels.

–is useful in **advanced carcinoma of the breast** when tumor contains estrogen receptors (receptor–positive tumors).

D. Mitotane (*o,p'*-DDD) [Lysodren]

–selectively attacks adrenocortical cells by unknown mechanism.

–is used in palliative treatment of **inoperable adrenocortical carcinoma**.

–produces dose-limiting **CNS depression**.

E. Progestins

–are useful in management of **endometrial carcinoma**.

F. Estrogens

–are used to treat **prostatic carcinoma**. Androgen dependence of prostatic carcinoma renders it an attractive target for estrogen therapy because estrogens can competitively block the effects of androgens.

–are more effective when combined with orchiectomy. Carcinoma of the male breast can also be controlled by orchiectomy and estrogen therapy.

–at high doses, are of some use in **carcinoma of the breast** in postmenopausal women.

G. Estramustine [Emcyt]

–is a **nitrogen mustard** linked to estradiol.

–acts by unknown mechanism; adverse effects are related to estrogenic component.

–is used in palliative treatment of **advanced prostatic carcinoma**.

H. Androgens

–are used to treat **carcinoma of the breast** in both premenopausal and postmenopausal women.

I. Tamoxifen [Nolvadex]

–is an antiestrogenic drug that competes with estrogen for binding to receptors.

–is most effective in **carcinoma of the breast** in women who have estrogen receptor–positive tumors.

J. Gonadotropin-releasing hormone analog: leuprolide [Lupron]

–reduces circulating levels of gonadotropins and testosterone.

–is effective in **prostatic carcinoma**.

Review Test

Directions: Each of the numbered items or incomplete statements in this section is followed by answers or by completions of the statement. Select the **one** lettered answer or completion that is **best** in each case.

1. Which one of the following statements is characteristic of any given cytotoxic antitumor agent?

(A) The dose–response curve is shallow
(B) The cell kill is a function of drug concentration and time of exposure to the drug
(C) The therapeutic index (TI) is wide
(D) The cytotoxic drugs will kill a constant number rather than a constant fraction of the tumor cell population
(E) A set of drugs is chosen for combination chemotherapy because the dose-limiting toxicity of each drug is the same

2. The combination of vinblastine, bleomycin, and cisplatin is a curative regimen for metastatic testicular tumors. This combination is desirable because

(A) the three agents have the same mechanism of action
(B) at least one of the three drugs can be given orally
(C) two agents are natural products and the third is a synthetic chemical
(D) the three agents have different dose-limiting toxicities

3. Which one of the following statements regarding characteristics of cytotoxic antitumor agents is incorrect?

(A) The curves of the dose–response relationships are steep
(B) The chemotherapeutic indices are small
(C) The agents kill a constant fraction of the tumor cell population
(D) Drug-resistant cells are less likely to be present when the tumor burden is large
(E) The agents are more active toward dividing cancer cells

4. Citrovorum factor is used to reverse toxicity of which one of the following anticancer agents?

(A) Mercaptopurine
(B) Bleomycin
(C) Doxorubicin
(D) Methotrexate
(E) Etoposide

5. Which one of the following agents can produce hearing loss and renal impairment?

(A) Cisplatin
(B) Nitrogen mustard
(C) Melphalan
(D) Mercaptopurine
(E) Vinblastine

6. Which one of the following statements concerning cancer chemotherapeutic agents characterized as natural products is true?

(A) Vincristine and vinblastine have the same mechanism of action and the same dose-limiting toxicities
(B) Actinomycin D produces severe cardiomyopathy as a dose-limiting toxicity
(C) Bleomycin may produce pulmonary fibrosis but is considered to have low bone marrow toxicity
(D) Doxorubicin and daunomycin have different mechanisms of action and are used clinically for the same neoplastic diseases

7. Which of the following cancer chemotherapeutic agents is least likely to exhibit cross-resistance with other agents listed?

(A) Actinomycin D
(B) Doxorubicin
(C) 6-Mercaptopurine
(D) Vincristine
(E) Bleomycin

8. Which of the following biochemical reactions is influenced by both fluorouracil and methotrexate?

(A) The synthesis of DNA from RNA by reverse transcriptase
(B) The conversion of thymidine to thymidylic acid (dTMP) by thymidine kinase
(C) The conversion of hypoxanthine to inosinic acid (IMP) by hypoxanthine-guanine phosphoribosyltransferase (HGPRT)
(D) The conversion of deoxycytidine to deoxycytidylic acid (dCMP) by deoxycytidine kinase
(E) The conversion of deoxyuridylic acid (dUMP) to thymidylic acid (dTMP) by thymidylate synthetase

9. Assuming that there are no drug-resistant tumor cells, which one of the following is a consequence of the log cell kill concept?

(A) Antitumor agents will be rapidly distributed and eliminated in the host
(B) A different dose of antitumor agent will be required for cure if the tumor burden is small rather than large
(C) The same dose of antitumor agent will be required for cure if the tumor burden is small rather than large
(D) Metabolism of the drug is a function of its plasma concentration
(E) Endogenous metabolites will always interfere with antitumor drug activity

Directions: Each group of items in this section consists of lettered options followed by a set of numbered items. For each item, select the **one** lettered option that is most closely associated with it. Each lettered option may be selected once, more than once, or not at all.

Questions 10–13

Match each of the agents listed below with the most likely mechanism for expression of drug resistance.

(A) Increased levels of dihydrofolate reductase
(B) Increased levels of nonspecific phosphatases
(C) Development of antibodies
(D) Increased DNA repair processes
(E) Reduced intestinal drug absorption

10. Methotrexate

11. L-Asparaginase

12. Cytosine arabinoside

13. Cisplatin

Questions 14–16

Match the drugs listed below with the phase of the cell cycle in which the drugs would be active.

(A) G_1
(B) G_2
(C) M
(D) S
(E) All of the above

14. Cytosine arabinoside

15. Nitrogen mustard

16. Vincristine

Questions 17–21

Match the drug listed below with its most likely mechanism of action.

(A) Inhibits ribonucleoside diphosphate reductase
(B) Alkylates DNA
(C) Intercalates DNA
(D) Inhibits DNA topoisomerase II
(E) Has antiestrogenic effects

17. Cyclophosphamide

18. Actinomycin D

19. Hydroxyurea

20. Tamoxifen

21. Etoposide

Answers and Explanations

1–B. Cell kill is a function of drug concentration and time of exposure. The dose–response curve is usually steep and the TI is narrow. If the TI is wide, the dose required for significant tumor cell kill is seldom toxic to the host. Antitumor agents kill a constant fraction of the tumor cell population. Drugs are often chosen for use in combination because they have different dose-limiting toxicities.

2–D. Vinblastine, bleomycin, and cisplatin all have different dose-limiting toxicities. Although vinblastine and bleomycin are natural products and cisplatin is a synthetic chemical, this has no relationship to the rationale for the combinations.

3–D. Because the number of cells present with a large tumor burden is high, there is an increased probability of resistant cells.

4–D. Citrovorum factor, or leucovorin, is a form of folate that can function without need for reduction by dihydrofolate reductase and, therefore, is used to rescue individuals from methotrexate toxicity. Methotrexate is a folic acid analog that inhibits dihydrofolate reductase.

5–A. An ototoxic agent, cisplatin also produces cumulative damage to renal tubules. Leukopenia and thrombocytopenia are dose-limiting for nitrogen mustard and phenylalanine mustard (melphalan). Bone marrow depression is dose-limiting for mercaptopurine and vinblastine.

6–C. Vincristine and vinblastine are both vinca alkaloids and have the same mechanisms of action; the dose-limiting toxicity for vincristine is related to neurologic effects while the dose-limiting toxicity for vinblastine is related to bone marrow suppression. The dose-limiting adverse effect of actinomycin D (dactinomycin) is bone marrow suppression. Doxorubicin and daunorubicin (daunomycin) have the same mechanism of action.

7–C. 6-Mercaptopurine is a small molecule. Actinomycin D, doxorubicin, vincristine, and bleomycin are all large, bulky, natural products that are transported out of the cells, and the multidrug resistance phenotype can confer cross-resistance to these agents

8–E. Fluorouracil is converted to F-dUMP, which inhibits thymidylate synthesis by forming a ternary complex with thymidylate synthetase. Methotrexate reduces the pool of tetrahydrofolate and subsequently N-5,10-methylenetetrahydrofolate, which is a required cofactor for thymidylate synthetase.

9–C. The same dose of antitumor agent will be required for cure if the tumor burden is small (i.e., 10^6 cells) rather than large (i.e., 10^{10} cells). This is a major consequence of the total cell kill concept; that is, that a constant fraction of cells are killed by antitumor agents.

10–A. Although the most common cause of drug resistance to methotrexate is transport defects, resistance can also result from amplification or alteration in the gene for dihydrofolate reductase.

11–C. L-Asparaginase is an enzyme; antibodies to the protein may develop.

12–B. Resistance to cytarabine (cytosine arabinoside) can occur via changes in any of the enzymes required for conversion of the nucleoside to various phosphorylated forms.

13–D. Cisplatin causes DNA crosslinks, which then induce DNA repair processes.

14–D. Cytosine arabinoside, or cytarabine, is converted to the triphosphate form. This analog inhibits DNA synthesis, which takes place in the S phase of the cell cycle.

15–E. Nitrogen mustards, which are alkylating agents, can act at all stages of the cell cycle.

16–C. Vincristine disrupts microtubules and inhibits metaphase.

17–B. Cyclophosphamide is activated in the liver; the resultant phosphoramide mustard alkylates DNA.

18–C. Actinomycin D, or dactinomycin, intercalates between adjacent guanine–cytosine base pairs.

19–A. Hydroxyurea inhibits ribonucleoside diphosphate reductase.

20–E. Tamoxifen is structurally related to estrogen and can bind to, but not activate, estrogen receptors.

21–D. Etoposide inhibits DNA topoisomerase II.

12

Toxicology

I. Principles and Terminology

A. **Toxicology** is concerned with the deleterious effects of physical and chemical agents (including drugs) in humans (see Table 12.1). **Toxicity** refers to the ability of an agent to cause injury; **hazard** refers to the likelihood of injury.

    1. **Occupational toxicology** is concerned with chemicals encountered in the workplace. For many of these agents, **threshold limit values** (TLV) are defined in either parts per million (ppm) or milligrams per cubic meter (mg/m^3). These limits are either time-weighted averages (TLV-TWA; i.e., concentrations for a workday or workweek); short-term exposure limits (TLV-STEL), which reflect the maximum concentration that should not be exceeded in a 15-minute interval; or ceilings (TLV-C).

    2. **Environmental toxicology** deals not only with humans but with all living organisms and their surroundings (air, water, soil); some chemicals that enter the food chain are defined in terms of their **acceptable daily intake,** the level at which they are considered safe even if taken daily.

B. **Dose–response relationship** implies that higher doses in an individual result in a graded response and that higher doses in a population result in a larger percentage of individuals responding to the agent (**quantal dose–response**). It is used for determination of LD_{50} (**mean lethal dose**).

C. **Risk** is defined as the expected frequency of occurrence of unwanted effects. Ratios of benefits to risks influence the acceptability of compounds.

D. **Duration of exposure** is used to classify toxic response.

    1. **Acute exposure** resulting in a toxic reaction represents a single exposure or multiple exposures over 1–2 days.

    2. **Chronic exposure** resulting in a toxic reaction represents multiple exposures over longer periods of time.

    3. **Delayed toxicity** represents the appearance of a toxic effect after a delayed interval.

Table 12.1. Acute and Evident Changes in the Poisoned Patient and Possible Causes

Changes	Causes
Cardiorespiratory abnormalities	
Hypertension, tachycardia	Amphetamines, cocaine, phencyclidine (PCP), nicotine, antimuscarinic drugs
Hypotension, bradycardia	Narcotics, clonidine, β-receptor blocking agents, sedatives, hypnotics
Hypotension, tachycardia	Tricyclic antidepressants, phenothiazines, theophylline
Rapid respiration	Sympathomimetics (including amphetamines, salicylates), carbon monoxide, any toxin that produces metabolic acidosis (including alcohol)
Hyperthermia	Sympathomimetics, salicylates, antimuscarinics, most drugs that induce seizures or rigidity
Hypothermia	Narcotics, phenothiazines, sedatives
Central nervous system effects	
Nystagmus, dysarthria, ataxia	Phenytoin, alcohol, sedatives
Rigidity, muscular hypertension	Methaqualone, phencyclidine, haloperidol, sympathomimetics
Seizures	Tricyclic antidepressants, theophylline, isoniazid, phenothiazines
Flaccid coma	Narcotics and sedative–hypnotics
Hallucinations	LSD, poisonous plants (nightshade, jimsonweed)
Gastrointestinal changes	
Ileus	Antimuscarinics, narcotics, sedatives
Cramping, diarrhea, increased bowel sounds	Organophosphates, arsenic, iron, theophylline, *Amanita phalloides*
Nausea, vomiting	*Amanita phalloides*
Visual disturbances	
Miosis (constriction)	Clonidine, narcotics, phenothiazines, cholinesterase inhibitors (including organophosphate insecticides)
Mydriasis (dilation)	Amphetamines, cocaine, LSD, antimuscarinics (including atropine)
Horizontal nystagmus	Phenytoin, alcohol, sedatives (including barbiturates)
Horizontal and vertical nystagmus	Phencyclidine
Ptosis, ophthalmoplegia	Botulism
Changes in skin	
Flushed, hot, dry skin	Antimuscarinics (including atropine)
Excessive sweating	Nicotine, sympathomimetics, organophosphates
Cyanosis	Drugs that induce hypoxemia or methemoglobinemia
Icterus	Hepatic damage from acetaminophen or *Amanita phalloides*
Mouth and taste alterations	
Burns	Caustic substances, soot
Odors	Garlicky breath: arsenic, organophosphates Bitter almond breath: cyanide Rotten egg odor: hydrogen sulfide Pear-like odor: chloral hydrate Chemical smell: Alcohol, hydrocarbon solvents, paraldehyde, gasoline, ammonia
Green tongue	Vanadium
Metallic taste	Lead, cadmium

II. Air Pollutants

—enter the body primarily through inhalation and are either absorbed into the blood (e.g., gases) or eliminated by the lungs (e.g., particulates).

—are characterized as either **reducing types** (sulfuroxides) or **oxidizing types** (nitrogen oxides, hydrocarbons, photochemical oxidants).

A. Carbon monoxide (CO)

1. Properties and mechanism of action

—is a colorless, odorless, nonirritating gas produced from incomplete combustion of organic matter.

—competes for and **combines with the oxygen-binding site of hemoglobin** to form carboxyhemoglobin. Its binding affinity for hemoglobin is 220 times higher than oxygen itself.

—binds to cellular respiratory cytochromes.

—CO concentrations of 0.1% in air will result in 50% carboxyhemoglobinemia. **Smokers** may routinely exceed normal carboxyhemoglobin levels of 1% by up to 10 times.

2. Poisoning and treatment

—CO intoxication (> 15% carboxyhemoglobin) results in **progressive hypoxia**. Symptoms include headache, dizziness, nausea, vomiting, syncope, seizures, and coma.

—chronic low-level exposure may be harmful to the cardiovascular system and to a developing fetus.

—**treatment** includes removal from the source of CO, maintenance of respiration, and administration of oxygen. Hyperbaric oxygen may be required in severe poisonings.

B. Sulfur dioxide (SO_2)

1. Properties and mechanism of action

—is a colorless, irritant gas produced by the combustion of sulfur-containing fuels.

—forms **sulfuric acid** on contact with moisture.

2. Poisoning and treatment

—at low levels (5 ppm), SO_2 has severe irritant effects on exposed membranes (eyes, mucous membranes, skin, and upper respiratory tract with bronchoconstriction). **Delayed pulmonary edema** may be observed after severe exposure.

—is treated by therapeutic maneuvers that reduce irritation of the respiratory tract.

C. Nitrogen dioxide (NO_2)

1. Properties and mechanism of action

—is an irritant brown gas produced in fires and from decaying silage. It also is produced from a reaction of nitrogen oxide (from auto exhaust) with O_2.

—causes **degeneration of alveolar type I cells** with rupture of alveolar capillary endothelium.

2. Poisoning and treatment

—acute symptoms include irritation of eyes and nose, coughing, dyspnea, and chest pain.

–produces **pulmonary edema;** severe exposure may result in delayed pulmonary edema. Chronic low-level exposure also may result in pulmonary edema.

–is treated with therapeutic maneuvers that reduce pulmonary irritation and edema.

D. Ozone (O_3)

1. Properties and mechanism of action

–is an irritating naturally occurring bluish gas found in high levels in polluted air and around high-voltage equipment.

–is formed by a complex series of reactions involving NO_2 absorption of ultraviolet light with generation of free oxygen.

–causes degeneration of **alveolar type I cells** with rupture of the alveolar capillary endothelium (similar to NO_2). Toxicity may result from free radical formation.

2. Poisoning and treatment

–irritates mucous membranes and can cause bronchoconstriction and pulmonary edema. Chronic exposure may cause decreased respiratory reserve, bronchitis, and pulmonary fibrosis.

–is treated with maneuvers similar to those used in NO_2 poisoning.

E. Hydrocarbons

–are oxidized by sunlight and by incomplete combustion to short-lived aldehydes such as **formaldehyde** and **acrolein;** aldehydes are also found in and can be released from certain construction materials.

–irritate mucous membranes of the respiratory tract and eyes, producing a response similar to that seen with SO_2 exposure.

F. Particulates

–inhalation can lead to **pneumoconiosis,** most commonly caused by **silicates (silicosis)** or **asbestos (asbestosis).** Bronchial cancer and mesothelioma are associated with asbestos exposure, particularly in conjunction with cigarette smoking.

–adsorb other toxins, such as polycyclic aromatic hydrocarbons, and deliver them to the respiratory tract.

–increase susceptibility to pulmonary dysfunction and disease. May yield fibrotic masses in the lungs that develop over years of exposure.

III. Solvents

A. Aliphatic and halogenated aliphatic hydrocarbons

–include fuels and industrial solvents such as ***n*-hexane, gasoline, kerosene, carbon tetrachloride, chloroform** and **methylchloroform, trichloroethylene,** and **tetrachloroethylene.**

–are central nervous system (CNS) depressants and cause neurologic, liver, and kidney damage. Cardiotoxicity is also possible.

–**polyneuropathy** predominates with ***n*-hexane** poisoning; CNS effects predominate with **chloroform** and **tetrachloroethylene** exposure.

–**hepatotoxicity** (delayed) and **renal toxicity** are common with **carbon tetrachloride** poisoning; may be mediated by free radical interaction with cellular lipids and proteins.

−aspiration with chemical pneumonitis and pulmonary edema is common.

−**treatment** is primarily supportive and oriented to the organ systems involved.

B. Aromatic hydrocarbons

−of this class of solvents, **benzene** poisoning is most common; **CNS depression** is the major acute effect. Chronic exposure can result in **severe bone marrow depression,** resulting in aplastic anemia. Low-level benzene exposure has been linked to leukemia. No specific treatment is available for benzene poisoning.

C. Aliphatic alcohols and glycols

−**methanol, isopropanol,** and **ethylene glycol** are CNS depressants that are **substrates for alcohol dehydrogenase;** resultant metabolites are generally toxic. Ethanol is used to compete for alcohol dehydrogenase and reduce toxic effects. Hemodialysis may be necessary to remove alcohol and metabolites; sodium bicarbonate is used to correct metabolic acidosis.

D. Polychlorinated biphenyls (PCBs)

−are stable, highly lipophilic agents used industrially before 1977 but still persist in the environment.

−dermatologic disorders, reproductive dysfunction, and carcinogenic effects linked to PCBs may be largely due to other contaminating polychlorinated agents.

IV. Insecticides and Herbicides

A. Organophosphorus insecticides

1. Properties and mechanism of action

−include **parathion, malathion,** and **diazinon**.

−are preferred over chlorinated hydrocarbons because they do not persist in the environment. However, the potential for acute toxicity is higher.

−are characterized by their ability to **phosphorylate the active site of acetylcholinesterase (AChE).** Toxic effects result from acetylcholine (ACh) accumulation.

−are well absorbed through the skin and via the respiratory and gastrointestinal tracts.

−some compounds also phosphorylate a "neurotoxic esterase," which results in a **delayed neurotoxicity** with sensory and motor disturbances of the limbs.

2. Treatment of poisoning

−assisted respiration and decontamination are needed as soon as possible to prevent irreversible inhibition ("aging") of AChE, which involves strengthening of the phosphorus–enzyme bond.

−**atropine** reverses all muscarinic effects but does not reverse neuromuscular activation or paralysis.

−**pralidoxime** (2-PAM) [Protopam] reactivates AChE, particularly at the neuromuscular junction. It often is used as an adjunct to **atropine** (may reverse some toxic effects); however, it is most effective in **parathion** poisoning.

B. Carbamate insecticides

—include **carbaryl, carbofuran, isolan,** and **pyramat**.

—are characterized by their ability to **inhibit AChE by carbamoylation**.

—produce toxic effects similar to those of the phosphorus-containing insecticides. Generally the toxic effects of carbamate compounds are less severe than those of the organophosphorus agents since carbamoylation is rapidly reversible.

—**pralidoxime** therapy is contraindicated in poisoning with these agents.

C. Chlorinated hydrocarbons

—include **chlorophenothane (DDT)** and its derivatives, **benzene hexa-chlorides,** cyclodienes such as **dieldrin** and **chlordane,** and **toxaphenes**.

—are absorbed through the skin, lungs, and gastrointestinal tract to varying degrees.

—persist in the environment after application. Use of chlorinated hydrocarbons is curtailed in many countries.

—**inactivate the sodium channel of excitable membranes,** resulting in repetitive neuronal firing with tremor or seizures. No specific treatment for poisoning with chlorinated hydrocarbons exists.

D. Botanical insecticides

1. Nicotine stimulates nicotine receptors and results in membrane depolarization. Poisoning is characterized by salivation, vomiting, muscle weakness, seizures and respiratory arrest; can be treated with anticonvulsants and agents for symptomatic relief.

2. Pyrethrum, a common household insecticide, is toxic only at high levels. Allergic manifestations are the most common adverse effect.

3. Rotenone poisoning is rare in humans and generally results in gastrointestinal disturbances.

E. Herbicides

1. Paraquat

—causes **acute gastrointestinal irritation** followed by delayed respiratory distress and development of **congestive hemorrhagic pulmonary edema,** which is thought to be caused by superoxide radical formation and subsequent **cell membrane lipid peroxidation**. Death may ensue several weeks after ingestion.

—treatment consists of prompt gastric lavage, administration of cathartics and adsorbents, and hemodialysis or hemoperfusion.

2. 2,4-Dichlorophenoxyacetic acid (2,4-D) and related compounds

—cause neuromuscular paralysis and coma. Long-term toxic effects are rare. Dioxin contaminants may be responsible for some of the toxic effects that have been observed.

V. Fumigants and Rodenticides

A. Cyanide

1. Commercial uses

—fumigants for ships and soil
—metal cleaners (silver polish)

—insecticides and rodenticides

—may be released on combustion of nitrogen-containing plastics

2. Mechanism

—possesses a high affinity for ferric iron; **reacts with iron and cytochrome oxidase** in mitochondria to inhibit cellular respiration, thereby blocking oxygen utilization.

3. Poisoning and treatment

—causes transient CNS stimulation followed by **hypoxic seizures** and death.

—is signalled by bright red venous blood and a characteristic **odor of bitter almonds**.

—treatment must be immediate.

   a. Elevate pool of ferric iron to compete for cyanide by administering **amyl or sodium nitrite,** which oxidizes hemoglobin and produces methemoglobin (effectively competes for cyanide ion).

   b. Accelerate conversion of cyanide to nontoxic thiocyanate by mitochondrial rhodanase (transsulfurase) with administration of **sodium thiosulfate**.

B. Warfarin

—is one of the most frequently used rodenticides; it also is used as an anticoagulant.

—induces bleeding and hemorrhagic conditions on repeated ingestion of high doses; can be reversed with **phytonadione (vitamin K$_1$)**.

C. Methyl bromide

—major toxicity is referrable to the CNS and includes headache, visual disturbances, and seizures. Pulmonary edema is possible after respiratory exposure.

—treatment includes supportive therapy, possibly with sulfhydryl agents. **Chloropicrin,** a stimulant of lacrimation, is added to methyl bromide products as a precaution.

D. Strychnine

—competitively **blocks postjunctional glycine inhibition of neuronal activity,** resulting in CNS excitation and seizures, including dramatic and violent contractions of voluntary muscle. Death is by **respiratory paralysis**.

—poisoning must be treated immediately; treatment includes support of respiration and **diazepam** administration to prevent seizures.

E. Thallium

—acute poisoning results in gastrointestinal irritation, motor paralysis, and respiratory arrest.

—chronic exposure results in hair loss (alopecia) and reddening of the skin. Liver, kidney, and brain damage with prominent neurologic symptoms and encephalopathy can occur.

—treatment includes administration of oral **ferric ferrocyanide (Prussian blue),** which binds thallium in the gastrointestinal tract and increases its fecal excretion. Hemodialysis and forced diuresis are also used.

VI. Heavy Metal Poisoning and Management

A. Lead

1. General properties and toxicity

—inorganic metallic lead oxides and salts are slowly absorbed through all routes except the skin. Organic lead compounds are also well absorbed across the skin. The gastrointestinal route is the most common route of exposure in nonindustrial settings; the respiratory route is more common for industrial exposure.

—binds to erythrocytes and then distributes to soft tissues such as the brain and kidney. It later accumulates in bone, where its elimination $t_{1/2}$ is 20–30 years.

—chronic exposure results in **inhibition of δ-aminolevulinic acid dehydratase** and a block in the conversion of δ-aminolevulinic acid to porphobilinogen. This leads to anemia and also to the **excretion of δ-aminolevulinic acid in urine,** a diagnostic sign of lead ingestion. Ferrochelatase is also inhibited, resulting in the **accumulation of protoporphyrin IX.**

—**CNS effects** are common after chronic exposure to lead; wristdrop is a common sign of **peripheral neuropathy**. Childhood encephalopathy with seizures and high mortality may be an acute sign of the ingestion of lead-based paint.

—kidney and reproductive functions may be affected after chronic exposure to lead. Gastrointestinal upset, including epigastric distress, is also seen.

2. Inorganic lead poisoning and treatment

a. Acute lead poisoning

—occurs rarely in industrial settings or from ingestion of lead-based paints.

—symptoms include severe gastrointestinal distress followed by CNS abnormalities and anemia.

b. Chronic lead exposure

—occurs more often than acute poisoning.

—is characterized by weakness, anorexia or weight loss, nervousness, headache, and gastrointestinal distress.

—**wristdrop** often signals exposure. Findings of lead in the blood and metabolic abnormalities related to disturbed porphyrin metabolism confirm the diagnosis.

c. Treatment

—requires termination of exposure.

—**chelation therapy**: severe exposures are generally treated with **calcium disodium EDTA** (ethylenediamine tetraacetic acid versenate) or **dimercaprol** [BAL]; less severe cases may be treated with **penicillamine** [Cuprimine, Depen].

3. Organic lead poisoning and treatment

—is often caused by tetraethyl or tetramethyl lead (antiknock components in gasoline), which are highly volatile and are absorbed through the skin and respiratory tract.

—occurs in commercial settings and from sniffing gasoline.

—**acute CNS abnormalities** (hallucinations, headaches, insomnia) are generally seen.

—treatment involves decontamination and elimination of the lead source.

B. Arsenic

1. Inorganic arsenic

a. Properties and mechanism of action

—can be found in coal and metal ores, ocean water, and seafood.

—is absorbed through the gastrointestinal tract and lungs.

—trivalent forms (arsenites) are more toxic than the pentavalent forms (arsenates).

—**arsenites inhibit sulfhydryl enzymes** (pyruvate dehydrogenase/glycolysis is especially sensitive), resulting in damage to the epithelial lining of the gastrointestinal and respiratory tracts and damage to tissues of the nervous system, liver, bone marrow, and skin.

—**arsenates uncouple mitochondrial oxidative phosphorylation.**

b. Acute poisoning and treatment

—symptoms include severe nausea, vomiting, abdominal pain, laryngitis, and bronchitis; capillary damage with dehydration and shock may occur. Diarrhea is characterized as **"rice-water stools."** There is often a garlicky breath odor.

—initial episodes may be fatal; if the individual survives, bone marrow depression, severe neuropathy, and encephalopathy may occur.

—treatment is primarily supportive and involves emesis, gastric lavage, rehydration, and restoration of electrolyte imbalance. Chelation therapy with **dimercaprol** for up to 2 weeks is indicated in severe cases.

c. Chronic poisoning

—may result in weight loss due to gastrointestinal irritation, perforation of the nasal septum, hair loss, sensory neuropathy, depression of bone marrow function, and kidney and liver damage. The skin often appears pale and milky ("milk and roses" complexion) due to anemia and vasodilation. Skin pigmentation, hyperkeratosis of the palms and soles, and white lines over the nails may be observed after prolonged exposure.

—inorganic arsenicals have been implicated in cancers of the respiratory system.

2. Organic arsenicals

—are excreted more readily and are less toxic than inorganic forms; poisoning is rare.

—**arsine gas** (AsH_3) poisoning may occur in industrial settings; effects are **severe hemolysis** and subsequent renal failure. Symptoms include jaundice, dark urine, and severe abdominal pain.

—treatment includes **transfusion** and **hemodialysis** for renal failure. Chelation therapy is ineffective.

C. Mercury

1. Inorganic mercury

a. Properties and mechanism of action

—occurs as a potential hazard in dental laboratory materials, wood preservatives, herbicides and insecticides, thermometers, batteries, and other products.

(1) Elemental mercury (Hg) is poorly absorbed by the gastrointestinal tract but is volatile and can be absorbed by the lungs. Hg itself causes CNS effects; the ionized form, Hg^{2+}, accumulates in the kidneys and causes damage in the proximal tubules by combining with sulfhydryl enzymes.

(2) Mercuric chloride ($HgCl_2$) is well absorbed by the gastrointestinal tract and is toxic.

(3) Mercurous chloride (HgCl) is also absorbed by the gastrointestinal tract but is less toxic than $HgCl_2$.

b. Acute poisoning and treatment

(1) Mercury vapor

—produces chest pain, shortness of breath, nausea, vomiting, and a metallic taste. **Severe kidney impairment,** gingivitis, and gastroenteritis follow. Muscle tremor and psychopathology can develop.

—treatment involves removal from exposure and chelation therapy with **dimercaprol** or **penicillamine**. Hemodialysis may be required.

(2) Inorganic mercury salts

—cause precipitation of mucous membrane proteins in the mouth and gastrointestinal tract, producing intense pain and vomiting. Hypovolemic shock may also occur.

—**renal tubular necrosis** is the most prevalent and serious systemic toxicity. Metallic taste and gingivitis may also result from systemic toxicity.

—treatment involves supportive therapy to restore electrolyte and hematologic balance. Emesis or gastric lavage is used to remove mercury, and a cathartic or activated charcoal is used to limit absorption.

c. Chronic poisoning

(1) Mercury vapor

—neurologic effects predominate and include a syndrome referred to as the **asthenic vegetative syndrome** (neurasthenic symptoms accompanied by such other abnormalities as goiter, tachycardia, gingivitis, labile pulse, and mercury in urine).

—may lead to tremor, depression, irritability, confusion, and vasomotor disturbances. Excessive salivation and gingivitis are often present.

(2) Inorganic mercury salts

—renal injury predominates. Erythema of extremities (**acrodynia**) is often coupled with anorexia, tachycardia, and gastrointestinal disturbances.

2. Organic mercurials
  —are found in seed dressings and fungicides.
  —can be absorbed from the gastrointestinal tract and often distribute to the CNS, where they exert their toxic effects. **Visual disturbances** often predominate.
  —treatment is primarily supportive.

D. Cadmium
  —may be found in **tobacco smoke** and **contaminated food,** especially shellfish, liver, and kidney. **Industrial exposure** may occur in smelting and refining operations.
  —acute inhalation poisoning from cadmium dusts and fumes causes irritation to the respiratory tract; death can occur as a result of **pulmonary edema**.
  —oral intake of cadmium salts results in local **gastrointestinal irritation**.
  —chronic exposure produces changes in the lungs as well as **renal** effects. Dyspnea, emphysema, and fibrosis are the most frequent **pulmonary** effects. Proteinuria, glycosuria, and aminoaciduria from tubule injury are the most frequent renal effects.
  —chelating agents are used in treatment but with limited success.

E. Metal chelating agents
1. General properties
  —usually contain two or more electronegative groups that form stable coordinate–covalent complexes with cationic metals that can then be excreted from the body. The complex is referred to as monodentate, bidentate, or polydentate, depending on the number of metal-ligand bonds. The greater the number of metal-ligand bonds, the more stable the complex and the greater the efficiency of the chelator.
  —contain functional groups such as $-OH$, $-SH$, and $-NH$, which compete for metal binding with similar groups on cell proteins.
  —may also bond with essential metals important for body function. Adverse effects can be circumvented by coadministration of the essential metal with the chelating agent.

2. EDTA (ethylenediaminetetraacetic acid)
  —is an efficient chelator of many transition metals. Because it can also chelate body calcium, **EDTA** is administered intramuscularly or by intravenous (IV) infusion as the **disodium salt of calcium**.
  —is excreted by glomerular filtration.
  —is used primarily in treatment of **lead poisoning**.
  —is nephrotoxic, particularly of renal tubules, at high doses.

3. Dimercaprol [BAL]
  —is an oily, foul-smelling liquid administered intramuscularly as a 10% solution in peanut oil.
  —interacts with metals and reactivates or prevents their inactivation of cellular sulfhydryl-containing enzymes. **Dimercaprol** is most effective if administered immediately following exposure.
  —is useful in **arsenic, mercury, and lead poisoning**.
  —adverse effects include tachycardia, hypertension, gastric irritation, and pain.

4. Penicillamine [Cuprimine, Depen]

   –is related to **penicillin**.

   –is well absorbed from the gastrointestinal tract.

   –**allergic reactions** and rare **bone marrow toxicity** and **renal toxicity** are the major adverse effects.

   –is used primarily to chelate excess copper in individuals with **Wilson's disease**.

   –is also used for **copper and mercury poisoning** and as an adjunct for the treatment of lead and arsenic poisoning.

5. Deferoxamine [Desferal]

   –is a specific **iron-chelating agent** that binds with ferric ions to form ferrioxamine; it also binds to ferrous ions. **Deferoxamine** can also remove iron from ferritin and hemosiderin outside of bone marrow, but does not capture iron from hemoglobin, cytochromes, or myoglobin.

   –rapid IV infusion may result in hypotensive shock due to release of histamine. It may also be administered intramuscularly.

   –is metabolized by plasma enzymes and excreted by the kidney, turning urine red.

   –may cause allergic reactions and rare **neurotoxicity** or **renal toxicity**. **Deferoxamine** therapy is contraindicated in patients with renal disease or renal failure.

6. Trientine [Cuprid]

   –is a **copper-chelating agent**.

   –therapy is restricted to treatment of **Wilson's disease** in individual's who cannot tolerate **penicillamine**.

VII. Drug Poisoning

A. General management of the poisoned patient (see Table 12.1)

1. Observe vital signs.

2. Obtain history.

3. Perform toxicologically oriented physical examination.

B. Symptoms

   –most poisonings occur in children younger than age 3.

   –the symptoms of most drug and chemical poisonings are extensions of their pharmacologic properties. Common causes of death include CNS depression with respiratory arrest, seizures, cardiovascular abnormalities with severe hypotension and arrhythmias, cellular hypoxia, and hypothermia.

C. Treatment

   –measures to support vital functions, slow drug absorption, and promote excretion are generally sufficient for treatment. If available, specific antidotes can also be used.

1. Vital function support

   –in the presence of severe CNS depression, it is important to clear the airway and maintain adequate ventilation. Comatose patients may die as a result of airway obstruction, respiratory arrest, or aspiration of gastric contents into the tracheobronchial tube.

–other important supportive measures include maintaining electrolyte balance and maintaining vascular fluid volume with IV **dextrose infusion**.

2. Drug absorption

–may be slowed or prevented by decontamination of the skin and induction of **emesis** with **ipecac** orally or with **apomorphine** parenterally.

–emesis is **contraindicated** if corrosives have been ingested (reflux may perforate the stomach or esophagus), petroleum distillates have been ingested (may induce chemical pneumonia if aspirated), the patient is comatose or delirious and may aspirate gastric contents, or CNS stimulants have been ingested (may induce seizure activity with stimulation of emesis).

a. Gastric lavage

–is performed only when the airway is protected by an endotracheal tube.

–is generally not useful in children.

b. Chemical adsorption with activated charcoal

–activated charcoal will bind many toxins and drugs, including **salicylates, acetaminophen,** and antidepressants.

–can be used in combination with gastric lavage or catharsis but not simultaneously with **ipecac**.

c. Cathartics

–are used occasionally to speed removal of toxins from the gastrointestinal tract. **Sorbitol** is a recommended agent in the absence of heart failure. **Magnesium sulfate** can be used in the absence of renal failure.

3. Promotion of elimination may be achieved by the following:

a. Chemically enhancing urinary excretion with agents such as **ammonium chloride,** which reduces urinary pH and decreases tubular reabsorption of some organic bases such as **amphetamine,** and **sodium bicarbonate,** which raises urinary pH and decreases renal reabsorption of certain organic acids such as **aspirin** and **phenobarbital**.

b. Hemodialysis

–is an efficient way to remove certain toxins and restore electrolyte balance. **Salicylate, methanol, ethylene glycol, paraquat,** and **lithium** poisonings are effectively treated this way; hemoperfusion may enhance whole-body clearance of some agents. Drugs and poisons with large volumes of distribution are not effectively removed by dialysis.

4. Antidotes

–are available for some poisons and should be used when a specific toxin is identified.

a. Naloxone [Narcan] and naltrexone [Trexan]

–are opioid-receptor antagonists that competitively block opioid action.

—are drugs of choice for reversal of respiratory depression due to opioid overdose. Lack of response indicates that opioids are not the source of poisoning or that other agents are also involved.

—are also effective in treating neonates who have depressed respiration due to administration of morphine-like compounds to the mother during delivery.

—may precipitate withdrawal symptoms in opioid-dependent patients.

—are also used to maintain an opioid-free state in abusers.

b. Acetylcysteine [Mucomyst]

—is used for severe **acetaminophen poisoning,** which depletes endogenous glutathione levels.

—provides sulfhydryl groups for hydrolysis to cysteine and protects the liver from reactive acetaminophen metabolites.

c. Physostigmine salicylate [Antilirium]

—inhibits AChE peripherally and in the CNS.

—is useful for **atropine** and **scopolamine** poisoning.

—use is limited to serious poisonings due to potentially severe adverse effects.

d. Other antidotes include metal chelators for metal poisoning, antivenins for snake bites, **atropine** and **pralidoxime** (2-PAM) for poisoning with AChE inhibitors and organophosphates, and **ethanol** to reverse **methanol** poisoning.

Review Test

Directions: Each of the numbered items or incomplete statements in this section is followed by answers or by completions of the statement. Select the **one** lettered answer or completion that is **best** in each case.

1. Sensitive indicators of lead toxicity include which of the following?

(A) Wristdrop
(B) Inhibition of δ-aminolevulinic acid dehydratase
(C) Childhood encephalopathy
(D) Anemia
(E) All of the above

2. CNS disturbances and depression are a major toxic effect of

(A) ionic mercury (Hg^{2+})
(B) trivalent arsenic
(C) pentavalent arsenic
(D) elemental mercury

3. Which of the following toxic agents would pose a problem with dermal exposure?

(A) Inorganic arsenic
(B) Organophosphate insecticides
(C) Inorganic lead
(D) Cadmium

4. Which of the following is the most common result of benzene poisoning?

(A) CNS depression
(B) Stimulation of red blood cell production
(C) Delayed hepatotoxicity
(D) Cardiotoxicity

5. Which of the following toxic agents inhibits sulfhydryl enzymes?

(A) Cyanide
(B) Pentavalent arsenic
(C) Inorganic lead
(D) Trivalent arsenic

6. Atropine can be used effectively as an antidote to poisoning by which toxic agent?

(A) Parathion
(B) Carbaryl
(C) Methanol
(D) Chlorophenothane (DDT)

7. Ipecac has which of the following characteristics or uses?

(A) Induces catharsis
(B) Should be used in combination with activated charcoal
(C) Is an important metal chelator
(D) Is contraindicated in the absence of a gag reflex

Directions: Each group of items in this section consists of lettered options followed by a set of numbered items. For each item, select the **one** lettered option that is most closely associated with it. Each lettered option may be selected once, more than once, or not at all.

Questions 8–17

Match each of these treatments for poisoning with the most appropriate drug or chemical.

(A) Mercury
(B) Heroin
(C) Lead
(D) Acetaminophen
(E) Atropine
(F) Copper
(G) Iron
(H) Carbon monoxide
(I) Cyanide
(J) Thallium

8. Naloxone

9. Calcium disodium edetate (EDTA)

10. Oxygen

11. Acetylcysteine

12. Dimercaprol (BAL)

13. Deferoxamine

14. Physostigmine

15. Penicillamine

16. Sodium nitrite

17. Ferric ferrocyanide (Prussian blue)

Questions 18–24

For each clinical characteristic, select the toxin most closely associated with it.

(A) Nitrite
(B) Arsenic
(C) Thallium
(D) Carbon monoxide
(E) Nitrogen dioxide
(F) Cyanide
(G) Benzene
(H) Carbon tetrachloride

18. Cytochrome oxidase

19. Liver damage

20. Carboxyhemoglobin

21. Bone marrow depression or aplastic anemia

22. Peripheral neuritis and hair loss

23. Delayed pulmonary edema

24. Rice-water stools

Answers and Explanations

1–E. Lead poisoning predominantly affects the hematopoietic system as a result of inhibition of δ-aminolevulinic acid dehydratase (and ferrochelatase). The most common neurologic manifestation is wristdrop. In children, lead poisoning may be manifested by encephalopathy.

2–D. The CNS is the major target organ for elemental mercury. Ionic Hg^{2+} predominantly affects the renal system.

3–B. Inorganic forms of arsenic, lead, and cadmium are poorly absorbed through the skin, in contrast to the organophosphate insecticides.

4–A. The major acute effect of benzene poisoning is CNS depression. Chronic exposure may lead to bone marrow depression.

5–D. Trivalent arsenic inhibits sulfhydryl enzymes. The pentavalent form is minimally toxic.

6–A. If administered early in poisoning, atropine reverses the muscarinic cholinoceptor effects of organophosphate insecticides such as parathion, which inhibit AChE. Inhibition of AChE by carbamate insecticides such as carbaryl is reversed spontaneously. The toxicity of methanol and DDT is unrelated to acetylcholine action.

7–D. Ipecac is an emetic that has a local action on the gastrointestinal tract and the chemoreceptor trigger zone. Its use is contraindicated if there is no gag reflex to prevent aspiration of vomitus. Charcoal can adsorb ipecac and reduce its effectiveness.

8–B. Naloxone is an opioid-receptor antagonist that competitively blocks opioid action and would be used as an antidote to heroin.

9–C. Severe exposure to lead requires chelation therapy with either calcium disodium EDTA or dimercaprol.

10–H. Treatment of carbon monoxide (CO) poisoning includes removal from the source of CO, maintenance of respiration, and administration of oxygen.

11–D. Acetylcysteine protects the liver from reactive acetaminophen metabolites.

12–A. Treatment of poisoning with mercury vapor includes removal from exposure and chelation therapy with dimercaprol or penicillamine.

13–G. Deferoxamine is a specific iron-chelating agent.

14–E. Physostigmine, which inhibits AChE both peripherally and in the CNS, is useful as an antidote for atropine and scopolamine poisoning.

15–F. Penicillamine is used primarily to chelate excess copper in individuals with Wilson's disease.

16–I. Sodium nitrate is used to treat cyanide poisoning because it oxidizes hemoglobin and produces methemoglobin; elevates pool of ferric iron, which effectively competes for cyanide ion.

17–J. Oral ferric ferrocyanide binds thallium in the gastrointestinal tract and increases its fecal excretion.

18–F. Cyanide reacts with iron of cytochrome oxidase in mitochondria to inhibit cellular respiration, thereby blocking oxygen utilization.

19–H. Hepatotoxicity and renal toxicity are common with carbon tetrachloride poisoning and may be mediated by free radical interaction with cellular lipids and proteins.

20–D. Carbon monoxide competes for and combines with the oxygen-binding site of hemoglobin to form carboxyhemoglobin.

21–G. Chronic exposure to benzene can result in severe bone marrow depression, leading to aplastic anemia. Acute benzene exposure produces CNS depression.

22–C. Chronic exposure to thallium results in alopecia and reddening of the skin, along with liver, kidney, and brain damage. Neurologic symptoms are prominent.

23–E. Severe exposure to nitrogen dioxide results in delayed pulmonary edema.

24–B. Symptoms of acute arsenic poisoning include gastrointestinal symptoms such as severe nausea, vomiting, abdominal pain, and characteristic diarrhea known as rice-water stools.

Comprehensive Examination

Directions: Each of the numbered items or incomplete statements in this section is followed by answers or by completions of the statement. Select the **one** lettered answer or completion that is **best** in each case.

1. A 35-year-old premenopausal woman with estrogen-receptor–negative breast cancer undergoes a radical mastectomy and is started on adjuvant chemotherapy. The regimen consists of 5-fluorouracil, cyclophosphamide, and methotrexate. One week into therapy the following laboratory values were obtained:

RBC: $2.9 \times 10^3/\mu l$ (norm: $3.5–5.0 \times 10^3/\mu l$)
WBC: $2.5 \times 10^3/\mu l$ (norm: $3.2–9.8 \times 10^3/\mu l$)
Platelets: 45,000   (norm: $130–400 \times 10^3$)

Which of the following agents is most likely responsible for these abnormalities?

(A) 5-Fluorouracil
(B) Cyclophosphamide
(C) Methotrexate
(D) None of the above

2. Which of the following statements concerning the mechanism of action of levodopa is correct?

(A) It prevents uptake of dopamine into presynaptic vesicles
(B) It increases release of endogenous dopamine into the central nervous system (CNS)
(C) It directly activates postjunctional dopamine receptors
(D) It is decarboxylated to dopamine in the CNS

3. A 68-year-old man is placed under general anesthesia for an operative procedure. On completion of the operation, the anesthesiologist cannot safely extubate the patient because he remains paralyzed. The patient suffered a similar episode years earlier, which was diagnosed as arising from a cholinesterase deficiency. Which of the following agents is responsible for the patient's current condition?

(A) Halothane
(B) Midazolam
(C) Succinylcholine
(D) Morphine

4. A 63-year-old man with metastatic lung cancer complains of nausea, vomiting, increased confusion, increasing lethargy, and weakness of 1 week's duration. Physical examination shows him to be cachectic, with dry mucous membranes and tenting of his skin, and the following vital signs: BP 90/60 mm Hg, heart rate 106 beats/minute, respiratory rate 16 breaths/minute. The patient has the following laboratory values on admission:

Na^+	137 mEq/L	K^+	4.2 mEq/L
BUN	30 mg/dL	Cr	0.9 mg/dL
Ca^+	22 mg/dL	PO_4	4.1 mg/dL
Alb	2.1 gm/dL		

His electrocardiogram showed a decreased QT_c. All of the following agents can be used to decrease the serum calcium level in this patient EXCEPT

(A) plicamycin
(B) calcitonin
(C) cholecalciferol
(D) hydrochlorothiazide

5. A 32-year-old man presents with a 6-month history of palpitations, anxiety, heat intolerance, insomnia, and weight loss. A physical examination reveals mild tremors bilaterally, a diffusely enlarged thyroid, and the following vital signs: BP 170/85 mm Hg, heart rate 120 beats/minute. Laboratory values are as follows:

T_3RU	20%	(norm: 25%–35%)
T_3	250 ng/dL	(norm: 75–220 ng/dL)
Free T_4	0.6 ng/dL	(norm: 0.8–2.8 ng/dL)
TSH	0.5 μU/mL	(norm: 2–11 μU/mL)

All of the following drugs can be used in the primary treatment of thyrotoxicosis in this patient EXCEPT

(A) levothyroxine
(B) methimazole
(C) propranolol
(D) radioactive iodine
(E) propylthiouracil

315

6. Which of the following adverse effects is commonly seen with benzodiazepines?

(A) Hypertension
(B) Daytime drowsiness
(C) Diarrhea
(D) Retrograde amnesia
(E) All of the above

7. Which of the following drugs has been used with success in the treatment of Fanconi's anemia?

(A) Danazol
(B) Spironolactone
(C) Nandrolone
(D) Flutamide

8. Which of the following statements describes the mechanism of action of androgens that is responsible for their stimulation of erythropoiesis?

(A) Antagonizes the binding of endogenous androgens at specific extracellular receptors
(B) Binds with specific intracellular receptors to activate specific genes
(C) Binds with specific extracellular receptors to activate specific genes
(D) None of the above

9. Which of the following agents is usually administered with levodopa to minimize its peripheral decarboxylation?

(A) Carbidopa
(B) Bromocriptine
(C) Benztropine
(D) Amantadine
(E) None of the above

10. Which of the following statements concerning the mechanism of action of carbon monoxide (CO) is correct?

(A) Disrupts the association of the α and β chains of the hemoglobin molecule
(B) Binds to the oxygen-binding site on hemoglobin to form carboxyhemoglobin
(C) Causes a dissociation of iron from the hemoglobin molecule
(D) Binds to oxygen-binding sites on hemoglobin to form methemoglobin
(E) None of the above

11. A 63-year-old woman being treated with a diuretic for mild hypertension presents complaining of weakness. Inverted T waves and U waves are seen on her electrocardiogram. The patient also has a K^+ level of 2.0 mEq/dL (norm: 3.5–5.0 mEq/dL). Which of the following diuretics could be responsible for these findings?

(A) Bumetanide
(B) Amiloride
(C) Triamterene
(D) Spironolactone
(E) None of the above

12. A 25-year-old woman presents with sneezing, rhinorrhea, and nasal stuffiness. She has tried many over-the-counter (OTC) products for allergies without relief; these agents also make her tired. Which of the following antihistamines is least likely to cause sedation?

(A) Diphenhydramine
(B) Cyproheptadine
(C) Terfenadine
(D) Promethazine
(E) Meclizine

13. Adverse effects of loop diuretics include which of the following?

(A) Ototoxicity
(B) Hyperkalemia
(C) Acidosis
(D) All of the above

14. A 24-year-old man comes to the psychiatric service with elevated mood and rapid and pressured speech, and reports an inability to sleep for the past several days. He is easily distracted during the interview. He claims to be a celebrity with many famous friends. He also says that he writes books and has been on television. Acute mania is diagnosed and treatment is begun with lithium. All of the following statements about lithium therapy are true EXCEPT

(A) the onset of lithium's therapeutic effect takes 2–3 days
(B) lithium is usually administered with an antipsychotic drug to control agitation
(C) plasma levels need to be monitored continuously to prevent toxicity
(D) all of the above

15. A 5-year-old girl is seen by her pediatrician after she has complained of headache, dizziness, tinnitus, sweating, and hyperventilation for 3 days. She was recently diagnosed with juvenile rheumatoid arthritis. Which of the following drugs may be associated with these adverse effects?

(A) Naproxen sodium
(B) Acetaminophen
(C) Aspirin
(D) Tolmetin
(E) None of the above

16. Which of the following interventions is used in the treatment of CO poisoning?

(A) Removal from the source
(B) Maintenance of respirations
(C) Administration of supplemental oxygen
(D) All of the above

17. A 3-year-old girl is brought to the emergency department after she was found consuming cyanide-based silver polish that she found in a kitchen cabinet. The patient is expected to present with all of the following signs EXCEPT

(A) bright red venous blood
(B) an increased respiratory rate
(C) an odor of bitter almonds on her breath
(D) pinpoint pupils
(E) transient CNS stimulation

18. A 32-year-old man with no previous psychiatric history presents complaining of an inability to relax, increased tension, and gastrointestinal disturbances. Results of his mental status examination are consistent with a diagnosis of anxiety disorder. Treatment is initiated with diazepam 5 mg orally 3 times/day (tid). Which of the following statements describes the mechanism of action of benzodiazepines?

(A) Antagonize postjunctional dopamine D_2 receptors
(B) Decrease reuptake of norepinephrine into prejunctional vesicles
(C) Potentiate GABA-receptor–mediated inhibition of neuronal activity
(D) Inhibit activity of monoamine oxidase
(E) None of the above

19. Which of the following pharmacologic properties is characteristic of phenobarbital?

(A) Low lipid solubility
(B) Extensive binding to plasma proteins
(C) Weakly basic (low pH)
(D) All of the above

20. Barbiturates act through which of the following mechanisms of action?

(A) Interact with receptors associated with chloride channels to potentiate the inhibitory effects of GABA
(B) Directly increase CNS activity, particularly the activity of the reticular activating system
(C) Directly stimulate inhibitory GABA receptors
(D) All of the above

21. The main limiting adverse effect of androgen treatment is

(A) hepatotoxicity
(B) edema
(C) decreased testicular function
(D) all of the above

22. A 3-year-old girl at risk for generalized tonic–clonic seizures has been receiving prophylactic anticonvulsant therapy with phenobarbital (5 mg/kg/day) for 1 year. Without reviewing the patient's history, an intern abruptly discontinues the medication. Which of the following symptoms will been seen in the withdrawal syndrome?

(A) Minimal anxiety
(B) Somnolence
(C) Tremor
(D) All of the above

23. All of the following interventions are used to treat cyanide toxicity EXCEPT

(A) administer amyl nitrite to increase the pool of ferric iron
(B) delay treatment in order to determine the toxic effects of cyanide poisoning
(C) administer sodium thiosulfate 25% to remove the cyanide in the form of nontoxic thiocyanate
(D) all of the above

24. A patient receiving digoxin for the treatment of congestive heart failure is found on routine screening to have elevated serum cholesterol. A fasting serum cholesterol level obtained several weeks later is also elevated. Which of the following cholesterol-reducing agents should not be prescribed for this patient?

(A) Niacin
(B) Clofibrate
(C) Cholestyramine
(D) Lovastatin

25. Which of the following statements regarding loop diuretics is true?

(A) Can be used synergistically with thiazide diuretics
(B) Can be used in the treatment of acute hypercalcemia
(C) Can be used to treat patients with hypertension
(D) All of the above

Questions 26–28

A 31-year-old man is seen in the outpatient psychiatric clinic. He appears well groomed and can sit in a chair. He makes minimal eye contact, his affect is extremely flat, and his mood neutral. He claims that he is being followed by ninjas who are trying to hurt him. He also hears them speak in his mind. He presents for treatment for schizophrenia, paranoid type.

26. Which of the following drugs can be used in the treatment of this patient?

(A) Chlorpromazine
(B) Thioridazine
(C) Haloperidol
(D) All of the above

27. Antipsychotic agents have the most benefit for which type of symptoms?

(A) Mainly the positive symptoms of psychosis
(B) Mainly the negative symptoms of psychosis
(C) Both the positive and negative symptoms
(D) Neither the positive nor negative symptoms

28. Major adverse effects associated with the use of phenothiazines include which of the following?

(A) Acute dystonia
(B) Gynecomastia
(C) Sedation
(D) Loss of libido
(E) All of the above

Questions 29–30

A 78-year-old man presents with a swollen, painful first metatarsophalangeal joint that is warm to the touch. His serum uric acid level is 12 mg/dL (norm: 2–7 mg/dL). Under the polarized light microscope, an aspirate from the joint is seen to contain needle-shaped negative birefringent crystals consistent with monosodium urate crystals. A diagnosis of gout is made.

29. Which of the following agents can be used to treat gout?

(A) Phenylbutazone
(B) Indomethacin
(C) Allopurinol
(D) All of the above

30. Adverse effects associated with the use of colchicine include all of the following EXCEPT

(A) nausea and vomiting
(B) abdominal pain
(C) liver damage
(D) dermatitis

Questions 31 and 32

A 31-year-old woman is brought to the emergency department after an attempted suicide. This is her second suicide attempt and fourth episode of major depression within the past year. The patient is restarted on the tricyclic antidepressant amitriptyline and is admitted to the hospital.

31. Tricyclic antidepressants act by which of the following mechanisms?

(A) Reduce the active uptake of norepinephrine or serotonin into prejunctional nerve endings
(B) Directly stimulate postsynaptic adrenergic or serotonin (5HT) receptors
(C) Inhibit the metabolism of norepinephrine or serotonin in the synapse
(D) None of the above

32. The patient is clinically less depressed, and she is discharged from the hospital with a prescription for amitriptyline. During an outpatient follow-up visit, she expresses concern that she may be experiencing adverse effects from the amitriptyline. Which of the following adverse effects is possible?

(A) Sedation
(B) Constipation
(C) Dry mouth
(D) Blurred vision
(E) All of the above

33. Which of the following statements correctly describes the mechanism of action of digitalis glycosides?

(A) Stimulate β_1-adrenoceptors to directly increase myocardial contractility
(B) Inhibit phosphodiesterase to increase cyclic AMP (cAMP), which results in an increase in intracellular calcium
(C) Inhibits the Na^+,K^+-ATPase pump, leading to an increase in intracellular calcium level
(D) None of the above

34. A 63-year-old man with a long history of major depression presents to the emergency department with a severe depressive episode. The patient has failed treatment with all available antidepressant medications, and a decision is made to try electroconvulsive therapy. As preparation for the procedure, the anesthesiologist administers tubocurarine to prevent fractures during the induced seizure. Which of the following statements describes the mechanism of action of tubocurarine?

(A) Directly stimulates receptors on motor end-plate in skeletal muscles to produce persistent depolarization of the motor end-plate
(B) Blocks acetylcholine (ACh) receptors and therefore the effect of ACh at the motor end-plate
(C) Blocks the effect of acetylcholinesterase, which results in an excess amount of ACh in the synapse, to produce persistent depolarization of the motor end-plate
(D) All of the above

Questions 35–37

A 17-year-old boy experiences a tonic–clonic seizure at school. The seizure continues as he is being transported to the emergency department, and the boy does not regain consciousness. Shortly after arriving at the hospital, the patient experiences another seizure.

35. Which of the following is the drug of choice for treatment of this patient?

(A) Ethosuximide
(B) Diazepam
(C) Carbamazepine
(D) Valproic acid

36. After the patient's seizure was brought under control and he regained consciousness, he was admitted to the hospital for evaluation; chronic therapy with anticonvulsant medication was initiated. Which of the following medications is indicated for the treatment of generalized tonic–clonic seizures?

(A) Carbamazepine
(B) Valproic acid
(C) Phenobarbital
(D) All of the above

37. The patient received a loading dose of 1260 mg phenytoin followed by 300 mg daily and is discharged several days later. Chronic use of this medication is associated with which of the following adverse effects?

(A) Tremor
(B) Sedation
(C) Nystagmus
(D) Hair loss
(E) All of the above

Questions 38 and 39

38. A 39-year-old male drug addict with suspected morphine overdose presents at the emergency department with all of the following signs and symptoms EXCEPT

(A) mydriasis
(B) respiratory depression
(C) sedation
(D) nausea and vomiting

39. The patient was given naloxone while at the emergency department. Naloxone acts by

(A) binding noncompetitively to opiate receptors, shifting the dose–response curve of the agonist to the right
(B) binding competitively to the opiate receptor and decreasing the maximum response compared to that of the agonist alone
(C) binding competitively to opiate receptors, shifting the dose–response curve of the agonist to the right
(D) none of the above

40. Which of the following statements correctly describes the effect of digitalis glycoside preparations on the failing heart?

(A) They increase the force of contraction
(B) They decrease stroke volume
(C) They decrease cardiac output
(D) None of the above

41. What is the mechanism by which hypokalemia can potentiate digitalis toxicity?

(A) It results in less intracellular Ca^{2+}, causing enhanced effects
(B) It allows more digitalis glycoside to bind to the Na^+,K^+-ATPase complex, resulting in enhanced effects
(C) It results in higher serum concentrations of the digitalis glycoside, resulting in enhanced effects
(D) It results in higher intracellular concentrations of the digitalis glycoside, resulting in enhanced effects

42. A 41-year-old businessman with a Type A personality, history of stable angina, and evidence of a reversible septal defect on his exercise stress test is admitted for cardiac catheterization. His cholesterol level is 375 mg/dL (norm: <200 mg/dL). He begins therapy with lovastatin. Which of the following adverse effects can be expected?

(A) Constipation
(B) Hepatotoxicity
(C) Leukopenia
(D) Flushing

43. The mechanism of action of nicotinic acid includes which one of the following?

(A) Increased activity of lipoprotein lipase
(B) Slightly decreased hepatic cholesterol synthesis
(C) Inhibited lipolysis in adipose tissue
(D) All of the above

44. Which one of the following describes the mechanism of action of nitroglycerin?

(A) Interferes with adenosine uptake, causing coronary vasodilation
(B) Potentiates the effects of PGI_2 to promote coronary vasodilation
(C) Activates guanylate cyclase to dilate all vessels
(D) Increase cAMP, causing dilation of all vessels

45. Which of the following statements correctly describes the mechanism of action of loop diuretics?

(A) Inhibit active sodium reabsorption in the thick descending loop of Henle
(B) Inhibit active sodium reabsorption in the distal and collecting tubules
(C) Inhibit active reabsorption of sodium in the ascending loop of Henle and the early distal tubule
(D) Inhibit active reabsorption of sodium in the thick ascending limb of the loop of Henle

46. Which of the following adverse effects is associated with the use of levodopa?

(A) Mydriasis
(B) Hallucinations
(C) Peripheral edema
(D) Livedo reticularis
(E) None of the above

47. A 75-year-old woman is seen by her family doctor and is found to have a fasting cholesterol level of 322 mg/dL (norm: <200 mg/dL) and triglyceride level of 1210 mg/dL (norm: <160 mg/dL). Nicotinic acid therapy is begun at 100 mg four times daily (qid), which is increased to 800 mg/day. At that dosage, it produces significant adverse effects. Which of the following adverse effects is most likely to cause the patient to discontinue the nicotinic acid?

(A) Flushing and itching of skin
(B) Leukopenia
(C) Myalgia
(D) All of the above

48. Which of the following is an electrophysiologic effect of quinidine at therapeutic levels?

(A) Enhancement of pacemaker rate
(B) Depressed electrical conduction
(C) Enhanced electrical excitability
(D) All of the above

49. A 54-year-old man is brought to the hospital after having chest pain at work. Approximately 30 minutes later, the patient is found to be in ventricular fibrillation, without a pulse or blood pressure. The ACLS protocol is initiated. After he is given a lidocaine bolus (1 mg/kg) followed by a constant infusion of 2 mg/minute, the patient is defibrillated with 360 joules and is successfully converted to normal sinus rhythm. What changes will lidocaine have on the electrophysiology of the heart?

(A) Acts on both activated and inactivated sodium channels
(B) Slows myocardial conduction
(C) Acts on potassium channels
(D) Accelerates myocardial conduction

50. A 12-year-old girl with acute lymphocytic leukemia is being treated with high-dose methotrexate. Which of the following agents can be given to prevent the adverse effects of methotrexate?

(A) Erythromycin
(B) Leucovorin
(C) Clavulanic acid
(D) Cyclophosphamide

51. Which of the following effects does nifedipine have on the cardiovascular system?

(A) Lowers peripheral vascular resistance
(B) Decreases myocardial contractile force
(C) Increases afterload (vascular tone)
(D) All of the above

52. A 68-year-old man being treated with warfarin (5 mg/day) for deep-vein thrombosis presents with midepigastric pain that generally worsens after a meal. An upper endoscopy is performed and reveals an active gastric ulcer. The patient is placed on cimetidine (300 mg/day), which is known to competitively inhibit the cytochrome P-450 mixed-function oxidase system. Which of the following adjustments needs to be made in the patient's warfarin dose to prevent bleeding complications?

(A) Needs to be increased due to the prolongation of its half-life
(B) Needs to be reduced due to the prolongation of its half-life
(C) Needs to be increased due to its shortened half-life
(D) No changes; these drugs can be taken safely together

53. What is the advantage of administering nitroglycerin sublingually rather than by the oral route?

(A) The sublingual route bypasses the liver, resulting in increased serum nitroglycerin levels
(B) The sublingual route allows more predictable absorption, resulting in increased serum levels
(C) The sublingual route minimizes systemic adverse effects
(D) All of the above

54. A 6-year-old girl with otitis media was treated empirically with amoxicillin for 10 days without improvement. Culture results identify penicillinase-producing *Haemophilus influenzae* as the causative agent. Which of the following drugs can be added to the amoxicillin regimen to treat the infection?

(A) Gentamicin
(B) Penicillin G
(C) Clavulanic acid
(D) Tetracycline

55. All of the following agents can be administered by inhalation to produce bronchodilation and relieve the symptoms of upper respiratory tract infection EXCEPT

(A) metaproterenol
(B) propranolol
(C) terbutaline
(D) albuterol

56. A 2-year-old girl is found to have ingested heart medication. The regional poison control center instructs the parents to give the girl syrup of ipecac and bring her to the local emergency department. Ipecac can be expected to produce all of the following actions EXCEPT

(A) stimulation of the chemoreceptor trigger zone
(B) gastrointestinal irritation
(C) rapid action, working within 20 minutes
(D) removal of all toxins from the gastrointestinal tract

57. A family physician suspects myasthenia gravis in a 32-year-old woman and orders a Tensilon (edrophonium) test to confirm the diagnosis. Improvement in her muscle strength indicates a positive test. Which of the following describes the mechanism of action of edrophonium?

(A) Inhibits reuptake of ACh into presynaptic vesicles, thereby increasing the concentration of ACh in the synapse
(B) Directly stimulates nicotinic ACh receptors at the motor end-plate to cause contraction of the muscle
(C) Inhibits acetylcholinesterase to increase the amount of ACh in the synapse and stimulate postsynaptic muscle receptors
(D) None of the above

58. An 82-year-old woman presents to her ophthalmologist with increasing pain in her left eye, nausea, and visual changes. Examination reveals a red, tearing eye with marked corneal edema and a mid-dilated pupil. The eye is firm to palpation; intraocular pressure is 45 mm Hg (norm: 5–21 mm Hg). Acute angle-closure glaucoma is supected. Which of the following intraocular agents is contraindicated in this patient?

(A) Atropine
(B) Physostigmine
(C) Pilocarpine
(D) Timolol
(E) None of the above

59. Which of the following is a dose-limiting toxicity associated with the use of vinblastine?

(A) Pulmonary toxicity
(B) Bone marrow suppression
(C) Ototoxicity
(D) All of the above

60. What is the mechanism of action of ondansetron?

(A) Serotonin-receptor antagonist
(B) Dopamine-receptor antagonist
(C) Histamine-receptor antagonist
(D) None of the above

Questions 61 and 62

A 6-year-old boy is brought to the hospital because he is wheezing; he had an upper respiratory tract infection in the recent past. He has had similar wheezing attacks in the past. Physical examination reveals a respiratory rate of 22 breaths/minute, use of accessory muscles for respiration, and slightly blue-tinged lips. As long-term treatment to prevent recurrent asthma attacks, a loading dose of theophylline followed by a maintenance regimen is administered.

61. Which of the following statements describes the most probable mechanism of action of theophylline?

(A) Stabilizes mast cells to prevent the release of histamine and ultimately prevent bronchospasm
(B) Stimulates β_2-receptors to relax bronchial smooth muscle and cause bronchodilation
(C) Blocks adenosine receptors in the bronchial smooth muscle to prevent bronchospasm
(D) None of the above

62. On a 3-week follow-up visit, the patient's serum theophylline level is markedly elevated. Adverse effects that may be seen with high blood levels of theophylline include which of the following?

(A) Seizures
(B) Arrhythmias
(C) Nervousness
(D) Nausea and vomiting
(E) All of the above

Directions: Each group of items in this section consists of lettered options followed by a set of numbered items. For each item, select the **one** lettered option that is most closely associated with it. Each lettered option may be selected once, more than once, or not at all.

Questions 63–65

Match the clinical scenario with the most appropriate drug.

(A) Erythromycin
(B) Penicillin G
(C) Metronidazole
(D) Gentamicin
(E) Clavulanic acid
(F) Chloramphenicol
(G) Tetracycline
(H) Leucovorin

63. A healthy 24-year-old man presents acutely with slightly productive blood-tinged sputum, a temperature of 37°C, and a chest X-ray consistent with bilateral basilar patchy infiltrate. A diagnosis of *Mycoplasma* pneumonia is made.

64. A 58-year-old man placed on antibiotic therapy for a *Pseudomonas aeruginosa* infection is found to have a rising serum creatinine level beginning on day 8 of treatment.

65. A 2-year-old child with *H. influenzae* meningitis has a platelet count of 12,000 after several days of drug treatment.

Questions 66–72

For each patient scenario, choose the most appropriate causative agent.

(A) Clomiphene
(B) Glyburide
(C) Levothyroxine
(D) Medroxyprogesterone
(E) Chlorpropamide
(F) Thiocyanate
(G) Flutamide
(H) Prednisone
(I) Nandrolone
(J) Oxytocin
(K) Vasopressin
(L) Diethylstilbestrol

66. A 62-year-old male alcoholic being treated for non-insulin dependent diabetes mellitus comes to the emergency department with a 1-hour history of nausea, vomiting, headache, hypotension, and profuse sweating.

67. An 81-year-old man with a history of coronary artery disease and a recent diagnosis of hypothyroidism presents to the emergency department with an acute myocardial infarction.

68. A 32-year-old woman being treated for an acute exacerbation of lupus erythromatosus complains of pain on eating.

69. A 31-year-old woman with chronic anemia presents with a deepening of her voice and a decrease in breast size.

70. A 26-year-old woman with primary infertility presents with hot flashes, nausea, and a palpable adnexal mass.

71. A 31-year-old woman has lower abdominal pain and hypertension after undergoing a cesarean section.

72. A 68-year-old postmenopausal woman presents with acute shortness of breath.

Questions 73–79

Match the scenario with the most appropriate treatment.

(A) Pralidoxime
(B) Calcium disodium EDTA
(C) Dimercaprol
(D) Flumazenil
(E) Penicillamine
(F) Ethanol
(G) Acetylcysteine
(H) Deferoxamine
(I) Vitamin K
(J) Naloxone

73. A 17-year-old boy is brought to the emergency department by a friend after he is discovered to have consumed antifreeze. He has metabolic acidosis, is stuporous, and has decreased urine output.

74. A 38-year-old farmer is found unresponsive after exposure to parathion from a crop duster spraying.

75. A 4-year-old boy presents to the emergency department secondary to bleeding that will not stop. He is found to have eaten rat poison that he found under the bathroom sink.

76. A 3-year-old girl was found ingesting paint chips in the hallway of her apartment building. She presents to the emergency department with signs and symptoms of encephalopathy.

77. A 2-year-old boy is brought to the emergency department with midepigastric pain. Laboratory studies show a pH of 7.15 and elevated liver enzymes. The patient presents with abdominal pain, diarrhea, and vomiting, and appears slightly cyanotic and tachypneic. His baby sitter says that he swallowed an entire bottle of iron pills.

78. A 62-year-old man with metastatic prostate cancer who takes meperidine for pain is brought to the emergency department unresponsive and with a respiratory rate of 4 breaths/minute.

79. An 18-year-old woman is brought to the emergency department after she confesses that she has ingested several hundred acetaminophen tablets. Laboratory values are consistent with acute acetaminophen toxicity.

Questions 80–84

Match each of the characteristics or uses with the agent it best describes.

(A) Mannitol
(B) Furosemide
(C) Metolazone
(D) Acetazolamide
(E) Spironolactone

80. Inhibits carbonic anhydrase and can be used to treat glaucoma

81. Used in patients with closed head injuries to decrease intracranial pressure

82. Contraindicated in patients who have undergone adrenalectomy and require diuretic therapy for moderate peripheral edema

83. Potentially results in the development of a serum potassium level of 2.6 mEq/L in a patient receiving therapy for mild hypertension

84. An antihypertensive agent that can cause "gout-like" symptoms

Questions 85–90

Match each of the following drugs with the mechanism of action that is most closely associated with it.

(A) Inhibits bacterial protein synthesis by binding to the 30S ribosomal subunit, effectively preventing formation of the initiation complex
(B) Inhibits the synthesis of *para*-aminobenzoic acid by blocking the synthesis of dihydropteroic acid, decreasing folic acid synthesis
(C) Inhibits synthesis of the mycobacterial cell wall
(D) Inhibits protein synthesis by binding to the 50S ribosomal subunit, restricting the length of the peptide under construction
(E) Binds to the microtubules and inhibits spindle formation, effectively stopping cell mitosis
(F) Binds to ergosterol, altering the permeability of cell membranes and leading to osmotic damage in the infecting organism

85. Erythromycin

86. Gentamicin

87. Isoniazid

88. Sulfamethoxazole

89. Amphotericin B

90. Griseofulvin

Questions 91–95

Match each of the agents below with its appropriate mechanism of action.

(A) Inhibits prostaglandin and leukotriene synthesis by inhibiting phospholipase A activity
(B) Stimulates β_1-, β_2-, and α-adrenoceptors to produce bronchodilation
(C) Stabilizes mast cells, thereby inhibiting the release of histamine and other autacoids, to prevent bronchospasm
(D) Antagonizes ACh at muscarinic receptors to inhibit constriction of the bronchial airways
(E) Prevents elastase from destroying lung parenchyma

91. Cromolyn sodium

92. Alpha-1 proteinase inhibitor

93. Epinephrine

94. Ipratropium

95. Triamcinolone

Questions 96–100

Match each of the drugs below with the appropriate mechanism of action.

(A) Coats fecal material to inhibit the reabsorption of water by the large intestine
(B) Causes an increase of water in the gastric lumen by osmosis, resulting in a reflex increase in peristaltic activity
(C) Decreases the absorption of water from the gastric lumen and stimulates intestinal secretions to increase the luminal content, resulting in an increase in peristalsis
(D) Retains water and so causes an increase in luminal mass in the bowel, resulting in stimulation of peristalsis
(E) Facilitates the emulsification of the water and fat content of fecal material to increase luminal mass, resulting in an increase in peristaltic activity

96. Psyllium

97. Magnesium citrate

98. Mineral oil

99. Docusate sodium

100. Bisacodyl

Answers and Explanations

1–A. 5-Fluorouracil causes marked myelosuppression, characterized by a reduction in all bone marrow elements (red blood cells, white blood cells, and platelets). Neither cyclophosphamide nor methotrexate generally result in total bone marrow failure.

2–D. Levodopa is decarboxylated to dopamine in the CNS. The increase in dopamine directly activates the dopamine receptors in the basal ganglia. Amantadine causes an increase in dopamine release into the CNS.

3–C. Succinylcholine is comprised of two linked molecules of acetylcholine. In patients with a deficiency of plasma cholinesterase, the drug's half-life is markedly increased, thus prolonging its effects. Halothane, midazolam, and morphine are not metabolized by plasma cholinesterase.

4–C. Cholecalciferol (vitamin D_3), when hydroxylated to $1,25\text{-}(OH)_2D_3$, can increase serum calcium levels through increased gastrointestinal absorption, mobilization from bone, and increased renal reabsorption. All the other agents listed can be used to lower plasma calcium levels, either by decreasing bone resorption (plicamycin, calcitonin), antagonizing parathyroid hormone (calcitonin), or increasing renal excretion of calcium (calcitonin, hydrochlorothiazide).

5–A. Levothyroxine, a preparation of thyroid hormone, would exacerbate the patient's condition. The other agents listed are antithyroid drugs that either interfere in the synthesis of endogenous thyroid hormones (methimazole, propylthiouracil), destroy follicular cells with high-energy emissions (radioactive iodine), or block the symptoms of thyrotoxicosis (propranolol).

6–B. Daytime drowsiness, a common adverse effect of benzodiazepines, is seen particularly with long-acting benzodiazepines and may lead the patient to self-discontinuation of the medication. Other adverse effects of benzodiazepines include ataxia, confusion, hypotension, and constipation. Amnesia, if present, is usually anterograde in nature.

7–C. Nandrolone, a synthetic androgen, stimulates the secretion of erythropoietin and hemoglobin synthesis. The other agents do not have any effect on erythropoiesis.

8–B. Androgens form a complex with intracellular receptors to activate genes that stimulate secretion of erythropoietin as well as genes to increase the production of hemoglobin.

9–A. Carbidopa does not cross the blood–brain barrier. It decreases the amount of levodopa decarboxylated in the periphery and increases the amount of levodopa that reaches the CNS and is converted to dopamine in the basal ganglia.

10–B. Carbon monoxide combines with the oxygen-binding sites on hemoglobin to form carboxyhemoglobin. Hemoglobin in this form is unable to carry oxygen, decreasing the amount of oxygen available to tissues. CO has a much greater affinity for these binding sites than does oxygen; therefore, low concentrations of CO can be very dangerous.

11–A. Loop diuretics (bumetanide, furosemide, ethacrynic acid) all can cause hypokalemia, or low serum potassium. This condition results from an increase in the tubular flow rate in the distal nephron. Amiloride, triamterene, and spironolactone are potassium-sparing diuretics that maintain serum potassium levels within the normal range.

12–C. Terfenadine is a nonsedating antihistamine. Sedation following the administration of an antihistamine results from direct CNS depression. Because terfenadine does not cross the blood–brain barrier, it lacks a sedative effect.

13–A. Loop diuretics are associated with dose-related ototoxicity, especially in patients with renal impairment. Caution should be taken when administering other ototoxic drugs with loop diuretics. Loop diuretics are also associated with hypokalemia (unless a supplement is provided) and alkalosis.

14–A. The onset of the therapeutic effect of lithium usually takes 2–3 weeks. Antipsychotic drugs typically are required to control the psychotic symptoms associated with a severe manic episode. The potential for toxic effects (seizures, cardiovascular collapse, coma) exists if plasma lithium levels exceed 2.5 mmol/L; therefore, routine monitoring of plasma levels is indicated.

15–C. All of these effects are seen in mild chronic salicylate toxicity, also known as salicylism. None of the drugs listed except aspirin produce this toxic syndrome.

16–D. All of the listed interventions are indicated in the acute management of CO poisoning. Intubation and artificial ventilation with 100% oxygen may be required.

17–D. Pinpoint pupils are not associated with cyanide poisoning but rather with certain opiate intoxication. The remaining signs listed are all seen due to the inhibition of mitochondrial respiration, which results in the blockage of oxygen utilization.

18–C. Benzodiazepines bind to specific benzodiazepine receptors associated with chloride channels. Stimulation of these receptors leads to an increase in the frequency of the opening of the chloride channels, causing hyperpolarization of the neuron and thereby potentiating the effects of γ-aminobutyric acid (GABA).

19–B. Pharmacologic properties of barbiturates, such as phenobarbital, include lipid solubility, which allows penetration into the CNS and affects the onset and duration of action of the drug. All barbiturates are weak acids that result in 50% un-ionized drug in the serum. In addition, barbiturates are extensively bound to plasma proteins; this also affects the onset of action, duration of action, and metabolism of the individual drug.

20–A. Barbiturates interact with a distinct and separate receptor associated with chloride channels to potentiate the inhibitory effects of GABA. The interaction results in prolongation of the opening time of the chloride channels, leading to a hyperpolarization of the neuron.

21–D. All of the adverse effects listed are associated with the use of androgenic compounds. Long-term steroid use could lead to hepatocellular carcinoma and testicular atrophy.

22–C. Withdrawal symptoms are usually seen when phenobarbital is discontinued after long-term use, and may last up to 1 week. Characteristically, patients experience anxiety, insomnia, and tremor. Seizures, coma, and death may also occur. Withdrawal should be gradual, tapering over a period lasting up to 3 weeks.

23–B. Treatment of cyanide poisoning must be immediate in order to reverse the binding of cyanide with ferric iron.

24–C. Cholestyramine is a binding resin and will bind and eliminate significant amounts of digoxin if given simultaneously or within 2 hours of the digoxin. This interaction will result in a decrease in the amount of digoxin absorbed from the gastrointestinal tract and nontherapeutic blood digoxin levels.

25–D. Loop diuretics act synergistically with thiazide diuretics by providing an increase in tubular flow to the ascending loop of Henle and early distal tubule. They are also first-line agents used in the treatment of acute hypercalcemia because they enhance renal excretion. Diuretics are commonly employed in the treatment of hypertension.

26–D. All of the drugs listed are useful in the treatment of schizophrenia. Haloperidol is available in an intramuscular form and may be useful in noncompliant patients.

27–A. Antipsychotic agents are more useful in treatment of the positive symptoms of paranoia, delusions, and hallucination. There is much less effect on the negative symptoms of mood disturbances.

28–E. Acute dystonia, gynecomastia, sedation, and loss of libido may all be seen in patients being treated with neuroleptic agents. Acute dystonic reactions can be prevented by administering anticholinergic agents such as benztropine mesylate along with phenothiazines.

29–D. All of the agents listed can be used to treat gout. Because indomethacin has a rapid onset of action, it is effective for acute episodes of gout. Phenylbutazone can only be used for a short time because of its toxicity, and allopurinol is the drug of choice for chronic tophaceous gout.

30–D. Except for dermatitis, all of the adverse effects listed are associated with the use of colchicine. A pruritic, erythematous, or maculopapular eruption is commonly seen with allopurinol; it may also be exfoliative, urticarial, or purpuric in nature.

31–A. Tricyclic antidepressants work by increasing levels of norepinephrine or serotonin in the neuronal synapses. The mechanism is by decreasing the reuptake of previously secreted neurotransmitters.

32–E. Sedation, constipation, dry mouth, and blurred vision are common adverse effects seen with tricyclic antidepressants. Sedation is more common with amitriptyline than with other second-generation antidepressants. Autonomic effects generally result in patient noncompliance and require a change in medication.

33–C. Digitalis glycosides bind to the Na^+,K^+-ATPase pump, inhibiting its normal function and increasing the number of intracellular sodium ions. To maintain electroneutrality, the calcium–sodium ion exchanger is enhanced, resulting in increased levels of intracellular Ca^{2+}. Some of the additional calcium ions bind to the actin–myosin complexes to produce an increased force of contraction in cardiac muscle.

34–B. The prototype of nondepolarizing neuromuscular blocking agents, tubocurarine directly blocks the ACh receptors at the motor end-plate, thereby inhibiting the depolarization and contraction of the muscle. The effects of tubocurarine are seen at the autonomic ganglia.

35–B. Intravenous diazepam or lorazepam are the drugs of choice in the treatment of status epilepticus. Ethosuximide, carbamazepine, and valproic acid are useful in the chronic prevention of generalized tonic–clonic seizures.

36–D. All of the agents listed are effective in long-term prevention of generalized tonic–clonic seizures. The actual choice of the appropriate agent must be tailored to the needs of the individual patient.

37–C. Nystagmus is a common adverse effect in patients receiving chronic phenytoin therapy. Other adverse effects include gingival hyperplasia, hirsutism, ataxia, and diplopia.

38–A. Miosis ("pinpoint pupils") rather than mydriasis (pupil dilation) is the classic ocular manifestation of opiate intoxication.

39–C. Naloxone competitively binds to opiate receptors and therefore will precipitate a withdrawal reaction. It is actively metabolized in the liver, requiring repeat administration until the patient clears all of the opiate.

40–A. Digitalis glycosides increase the speed of shortening and the force of contraction of the cardiac muscle because they increase intracellular Ca^{2+}. The net result is positive inotropic activity. They do not have any chronotropic effects.

41–B. Hypokalemia reduces the activity of the normal Na^+,K^+-ATPase mechanism. Higher concentrations of a digitalis glycoside can then bind to the Na^+,K^+-ATPase complex, resulting in further inhibition. As a result, higher concentrations of Ca^{2+} can be exchanged for Na^+ to keep the cells electroneutral. This results in higher levels of intracellular Ca^{2+} and increased force of contractions (enhanced digitalis glycoside activity).

42–B. The major limiting adverse effect of HMG-CoA reductase inhibitors such as lovastatin is hepatotoxicity. Therefore, serum liver enzymes should be monitored for the duration of therapy.

43–D. Nicotinic acid exerts its cholesterol- and triglyceride-lowering effects by all the mechanisms listed.

44–C. Nitroglycerin activates guanylate cyclase, which results in an increase in cyclic guanine phosphate compounds (cGMP) in smooth muscle cells. A cGMP-sensitive protein kinase is activated that phosphorylates many intracellular proteins. This process results in dilation of vascular smooth muscle and decreased vascular resistance.

45–D. Loop diuretics inhibit active reabsorption of sodium in the thick ascending limb of the loop of Henle, resulting in an increase in fluid flow through the tubules. Thiazide diuretics inhibit reabsorption of sodium in the ascending loop of Henle and the early distal tubule.

46–B. Nightmares, vivid dreams, and visual hallucinations are some of the behavioral manifestations of levodopa therapy. Other adverse effects include dyskinesias, akinesias, nausea and vomiting, and orthostatic hypotension.

47–A. The dose-limiting adverse effect commonly encountered when treating a patient with nicotinic acid is flushing and pruritus. This effect is prostaglandin-mediated and can be reduced by premedicating the patient with aspirin. If this adverse effect can be controlled, nicotinic acid is a very effective means of lowering cholesterol and serum triglyceride levels.

48–B. At therapeutic levels, quinidine depresses the pacemaker firing rate as well as electrical conduction and excitability. However, at low doses, quinidine has a vagolytic effect and speeds conduction though the atrioventricular node. This may cause some problems when titrating the dose in patients with an initially rapid ventricular rate.

49–A. Lidocaine acts on both the activated and inactivated sodium channels to decrease the duration of the action potential in ventricular muscle. Therefore, there is no significant slowing of myocardial conduction.

50–B. Leucovorin is a form of folate that can be used by the cell in the absence of dihydrofolate reductase, which is inhibited by methotrexate. Therefore, leucovorin can block the toxic effects of methotrexate in normal cells, allowing DNA synthesis in those cells to continue unaffected.

51–A. Nifedipine blocks the calcium channels of vascular smooth muscle, resulting in a decrease in contraction and dilation of the vessels (lowered peripheral vascular resistance). This effectively reduces afterload, the force that the heart pumps against. Unlike diltiazem and verapamil, nifedipine had little to no effect on the contractile force of the myocardium.

52–B. Inhibition of the cytochrome P-450 mixed-function oxidase system results in an increase in the half-life of drugs whose metabolism relies on that system. If no dosage adjustments were made, the serum warfarin concentration would increase, with resultant adverse effects. Therefore, the dosage of the warfarin must be reduced to maintain therapeutic serum levels.

53–A. Nitroglycerin undergoes significant first-pass metabolism in the liver, which results in a very short half-life. Sublingual administration can bypass enteric absorption and portal circulation, resulting in higher blood levels. Topical preparations are also available; however, they are not effective in treating acute angina attacks because they are absorbed at a slower, controlled rate.

54–C. Clavulanic acid, structurally related to penicillin, irreversibly inhibits β-lactamase, allowing penicillinase-producing bacteria to be exposed to higher, more therapeutic levels of amoxicillin.

55–B. Propranolol is a β-adrenoceptor antagonist that produces bronchoconstriction. Because of this effect, β-adrenoceptor antagonists are contraindicated in patients with underlying asthma or lung disease. The remaining agents listed are β-adrenoceptor agonists that stimulate β_2-receptors to produce bronchodilation.

56–D. Ipecac is useful only for the removal of unabsorbed toxins still in the stomach. Once the ingested material has passed into the duodenum, the efficacy of ipecac is markedly reduced. Due to its purgatory action, ipecac is contraindicated in patients with an altered state of consciousness and in persons who have ingested caustic substances that cause tissue damage (e.g., acids or lye).

57–C. Edrophonium combines with acetylcholinesterase to inhibit hydrolysis of ACh. This results in increased synaptic concentrations of ACh, stimulating the remaining receptors in myasthenia gravis patients.

58–A. Atropine blocks the parasympathetic tone to the eye and results in a dilated pupil. In acute angle-closure glaucoma, this action will lead to further blockage of aqueous humor outflow and a further decrease in intraocular pressure. The other agents listed can lead to a decrease in intraocular pressure in acute angle-closure glaucoma. Physostigmine and pilocarpine cause pupillary constriction, which will aid in aqueous humor outflow; timolol decreases the production of additional aqueous humor.

59–B. The dose-limiting toxicity associated with vinblastine therapy is bone marrow suppression. Pulmonary toxicity is usually associated with the use of bleomycin, and ototoxicity is seen with cisplatin therapy.

60–A. Ondansetron is a specific serotonin-receptor antagonist that acts both in the CNS and in the gastrointestinal tract. It is used specifically to treat the nausea and vomiting associated with cisplatin.

61–C. It is currently thought that theophylline and other methylxanthines produce bronchodilation by acting as adenosine antagonists. These agents will prevent adenosine-mediated histamine release and ultimately produce bronchoconstriction. Theophylline analogs that lack the adenosine antagonist component cause bronchodilation by inhibiting intracellular phosphodiesterase. It is not yet known how this proposed mechanism contributes to the bronchodilating effects of this drug class.

62–E. Theophylline is associated with all of the reactions listed. They usually occur at elevated blood levels, generally accepted as greater than 20 μg/dL. However, adverse drug reactions may occur at any blood level.

63–A. The drug of choice for the treatment of community-acquired *Mycoplasma* pneumonia is erythromycin. Hospitalization is generally not required. It will take several weeks for the chest X-ray to clear, but symptoms will improve within 1 week.

64–D. Aminoglycoside antibiotics such as gentamicin can cause acute reversible tubular necrosis, leading to an increase in serum creatinine and blood urea nitrogen. These results are usually noticeable on laboratory tests within approximately 5 days.

65–F. Chloramphenicol can produce an idiosyncratic reaction resulting in a potentially fatal pancytopenia. Leukopenia, thrombocytopenia, and aplasia of the bone marrow are generally experienced as part of this reaction.

66–E. A disulfiram-like reaction may be seen in non-insulin dependent diabetics treated with chlorpropamide, an oral hypoglycemic, when used in combination with alcohol.

67–C. Elderly patients with subclinical hypothyroidism are at risk for arrhythmias, angina, or myocardial infarction if they have underlying cardiovascular disease when they begin treatment with thyroid hormones such as levothyroxine. These potential adverse effects occur because of increased cardiovascular work load as well as the direct effect of thyroid hormone on the heart.

68–H. Prednisone, a steroid commonly used to treat exacerbations of lupus erythematosus, can cause peptic ulcer disease due to the inhibition of the prostaglandins that normally protect the mucosa.

69–I. Androgens such as nandrolone are used in the treatment of anemia. These agents produce masculinization in female patients.

70–A. Clomiphene, an anti-estrogen used in the treatment of primary infertility, produces adverse effects that include hot flashes, nausea, and ovarian enlargement.

71–J. Oxytocin is commonly used to induce labor. It is also used to contract uterine muscle and so inhibit postpartum bleeding. In women who have undergone a cesarean section, uterine cramping or rupture can occur, resulting in lower abdominal pain. If rupture occurs, hypotension can result from bleeding; however, oxytocin causes hypertension directly.

72–L. The use of postmenopausal estrogens such as diethylstilbestrol can result in an increased risk of thromboembolic disease. Pulmonary embolism may result in shortness of breath, and death can occur. A ventilation and perfusion scan is indicated.

73–F. Ethylene glycol, antifreeze, causes CNS depression that can lead to coma and death. It can also cause acute renal failure. Ethanol is given because it competes for alcohol dehydrogenase, leading to a reduction in toxic metabolites. Treatment includes bicarbonate for the metabolic acidosis. Dialysis may be required until the renal failure resolves.

74–A. Parathion, an insecticide, phosphorylates the active site on acetylcholinesterase, resulting in an increase in acetylcholine in the neuromuscular junction. This causes prolonged depolarization of the motor end-plate, resulting in paralysis. Pralidoxime (administered with atropine) reactivates acetylcholinesterase to promote the degradation of acetylcholine.

75–I. Rodenticides contain warfarin and can cause toxicity and hemorrhage if ingested. Treatment consists of vitamin K administered intravenously for serious hemorrhage or orally for minor bleeding.

76–B. Calcium disodium EDTA is administered to chelate lead when the blood lead concentration is > 50 μg/dL or when the patient is symptomatic. Calcium disodium EDTA is often administered with dimercaprol. Treatment of acute lead poisoning also involves supportive measures, such as seizure prophylaxis, fluid and electrolyte management, and prevention of cerebral edema.

77–H. Deferoxamine is a specific iron-chelating agent that binds ferric iron without removing iron from hemoglobin, myoglobin, or cytochromes. It is indicated when plasma concentrations of iron exceed > 500 μg/dL.

78–J. Naloxone is a competitive opiate-receptor antagonist and can produce an increase in respiratory rate in the presence of opiate overdose within 1–2 minutes. The sedative effects of opiates are reversed, and blood pressure is returned to normal. Due to the relatively short half-life of naloxone, multiple doses may be required.

79–G. Acetylcysteine provides sulfhydryl groups, replenishing hepatic stores of glutathione depleted by acetaminophen overdosage. It is generally well tolerated with minimal adverse effects and should be administered within 24 hours of acetaminophen ingestion.

80–D. Acetazolamide inhibits carbonic anhydrase and is useful as a diuretic. However, it is far more commonly used for glaucoma. It acts by decreasing the formation of aqueous humor and consequently reduces intraocular pressure.

81–A. Mannitol reduces cerebral edema and also acts as an osmotic diuretic. It is easily filtered at the glomerulus and is poorly reabsorbed, pulling water into the tubules to equalize the osmotic gradient.

82–E. Spironolactone acts by inhibiting the effects of naturally occurring aldosterone. In a patient who had undergone total adrenalectomy, serum aldosterone concentrations would be low, rendering this diuretic ineffective in reducing edema.

83–B. Furosemide is a potent loop diuretic that can cause hypokalemia by decreasing reabsorption of sodium and chloride in the distal convoluted tubule and the ascending loop of Henle.

84–C. Metolazone, like other thiazide diuretics, may cause increased reabsorption of uric acid from the kidney and result in elevated serum uric acid. This condition can often precipitate an acute gouty attack or produce "gout-like" symptoms.

85–D. Erythromycin binds to the 50S ribosomal subunit and inhibits protein synthesis. Erythromycin is a bacteriostatic agent: It does not directly kill microorganisms but prevents further growth, allowing the immune system to eradicate the infection.

86–A. Aminoglycoside antibiotics such as gentamicin inhibit the formation of initiation complexes and suppress the synthesis of proteins necessary for survival of the cell.

87–C. Isoniazid inhibits mycobacteria by preventing the synthesis of mycolic acids, important and unique components of the mycobacterial cell wall. Other proposed mechanisms of action for isoniazid include inhibition of nucleic acid biosynthesis and glycolysis.

88–B. Sulfonamides, such as sulfamethoxazole, inhibit the synthesis of *para*-aminobenzoic acid by competing for the bacterial enzyme responsible for incorporating *para*-aminobenzoic acid into dihydropteroic acid. This action diminishes the substrate (dihydropteroic acid) required for folic acid synthesis. Mammalian cells must use preformed folic acid and are therefore not affected by sulfonamides.

89–F. Amphotericin B acts primarily by binding to sterol moieties in the fungal cell wall, primarily ergosterol. This results in the formation of pores or channels within the membrane, which allow for increased cell-wall permeability and leakage of small molecules. However, amphotericin also works on fungi with sterol-free cell walls, suggesting other mechanisms of action.

90–E. Griseofulvin causes a disruption of the mitotic spindle apparatus by interacting with the microtubules, thereby interrupting fungal mitosis.

91–C. Cromolyn sodium, used to prevent asthma attacks, acts by preventing sensitized mast cells from degranulating and releasing histamine and other factors. Cromolyn sodium may block calcium channels within the mast cell membrane and may regulate the intracellular phosphorylation of regulatory proteins as well. Therefore, it must be used prophylactically rather than as treatment for acute attacks.

92–E. Alpha-1 proteinase inhibitor (Prolastin) is used for the treatment of alpha-1 antitrypsin deficiency in genetically predisposed patients. It is given weekly for treatment of hereditary emphysema and acts by preventing elastase from destroying lung parenchyma.

93–B. Epinephrine, available OTC for the treatment of bronchospasm, is a relatively nonselective adrenoceptor agonist that stimulates β_1-, β_2-, and α-receptors. Stimulation of β_2-receptors results in dilation of bronchioles. This product has many adverse effects related to its relative nonselectivity (arrhythmias, tachycardia, tremors, and hypertension).

94–D. Ipratropium bromide, used primarily to treat bronchospasm in patients with underlying lung disease, antagonizes ACh at muscarinic receptors to inhibit bronchoconstriction.

95–A. Triamcinolone acetonide is an inhaled steroid preparation that treats asthma by inhibiting local mediators of inflammation. Current research suggests that inflammation is a major component in the pathogenesis of asthma. Administering steroids by inhalation results in a decrease in systemic effects.

96–D. Psyllium, a bulk-forming laxative, is poorly absorbed from the gastrointestinal tract and retains water, ultimately increasing luminal contents. This increase causes stretching of the bowel wall and stimulates peristalsis. Psyllium should be taken with water.

97–B. Magnesium citrate solution contains ions that are poorly absorbed from the gastrointestinal tract and acts as an osmotic agent. This agent also increases luminal water, stretching the bowel wall and increasing peristalsis.

98–A. Mineral oil is a laxative that forms a waterproof barrier around fecal material, inhibiting the reabsorption of water, increasing fecal mass, and stimulating peristalsis.

99–E. Docusate sodium acts by increasing the mixture of water and fat in the stool, resulting in an increased luminal mass. A stool softener, it provides a gentle laxative effect. Preparations of docusate usually contain gentle cathartic agents that can increase the propulsion of fecal material through the gastrointestinal tract.

100–C. Bisacodyl, an irritant laxative, acts by irritating the mucosal surface, resulting in increased intestinal secretions, direct stimulation of peristalsis, and a decrease in the reabsorption of water secondary to the increased rate of movement through the bowel.

Index

Note: Page numbers in italics indicate figures; those followed by (t) indicate tables; those followed by Q indicate questions; and those followed by E indicate explanations. Generic drug names are followed by tradenames in parentheses; tradenames also appear as individual entries.

333

Anhidrosis, muscarinic-receptor antagonists and, 33
Anhydron, *see* Cyclothiazide
Anisindione (Miradon), 179
Anistreplase (APSAC; Eminase), 181
Anorexigenic(s), 188
Ansaid, *see* Flurbiprofen
Anspor, *see* Cephradine
Antabuse, *see* Disulfiram
Antacid(s)
  aspirin and, 160
  described, 188
  drug interactions with, 189
  renal effects of, 189
  uses of, 196Q, 197E
Antagonist(s)
  adrenergic-receptor, 46–50, 47(t), *49*, *see also* Adrenoceptor antagonist(s)
  adrenocortical, 227
  cholinergic, 186
    described, 190
  competitive
    actions of, 17Q, 20E
    described, 2–3
    graded dose–response curves for, *3*
  defined, 2–3
  dopamine, 186
  histamine₁-receptor, 186, 206Q, 207E
  histamine₂-receptor, 196Q, 197E
    described, 189–190
  muscarinic-receptor, 32–34, *33*
    for asthma, 202–203
  noncompetitive
    described, 3
    graded dose–response curves for, *4*
Antepar, *see* Piperazine
Antiandrogen(s), 222–223
Antianxiety agent(s), prolactin secretion increase due to, 210
Antiarrhythmic agent(s), 73–78
Antibacterial(s), 244–258, *245*, 246(t), 249(t)
  for malaria, 266
Antibiotic(s), *see also specific types*
  cancer and, 280(t), 288–289
  warfarin and, 179
Anticholinergic(s)
  for anesthesia, 129
  for diarrhea, 194
Anticoagulant(s), 177–179
  aspirin and, 160
Antidepressant(s), 104–109, 105(t), *106*
  adverse effects of, 105(t), 107–109
  bicyclic, biochemical activity of, 105(t)
  cardiovascular effects of, 108
  classification of, 104, 105(t), *106*
  CNS effects of, 107–108
  contraindications for, 107–109
  cyclic, biochemical activity of, 105(t)
  drug interactions with, 109
  mechanism of action of, 105(t), *106*
  morphine and, 115
  overdose of, 109
  pharmacologic properties of, 106–107
  prolactin secretion increase due to, 210
  second-generation, mechanism of action of, 105(t), *106*
  structure of, 104, 106, *106*
  tetracyclic, biochemical activity of, 105(t)
  toxicity of, 109
  tricyclic
    adverse effects of, 45
    biochemical activity of, 105(t)
    described, 104, *106*
    drug interactions with, 109
    levodopa and, 119
    mechanism of action of, 105(t), *106*, 318Q, 328E
    narrow-angle glaucoma due to, 141Q, 144E
  uses of, 107
Antidiarrheal(s), 194–195
Antidiuretic hormone (ADH, vasopressin)
  adverse effects of, 323Q, 330E
  agents influencing, 61–62

described, 214
for diabetes mellitus, 89Q, 93E
increased release of
  morphine and, 115
  opioids and, 115
Antidiuretic hormone (ADH) antagonists, 62
Antidote(s), for poisonings, 309–310
Antiemetic(s), 185–187
  levodopa and, 119
Antiepileptic drug(s), 120–124
Antiestrogen(s), described, 220–221
Antifungal agent(s), 259(t), 262–264
Antihistamine(s), 148–150, 149(t)
  for rhinitis, 204
Antihypertensive(s), 80–87, 82(t)-83(t)
  vertigo due to, 185
Anti-inflammatory drug(s)
  nonsteroidal (NSAIDs), 157–164
    analgesic effect of, 158
    anti-inflammatory effect of, 147–158
    antipyretic effect of, 158
    described, 157, 161
    mechanism of action of, 147–158, 169Q, 170E
    types of, 158–163
    uses of, 158
  penicillamine, 162–163
Antilirium, *see* Physostigmine
Antimalarial(s), 264–266
Antimetabolite(s), 280(t), 284–287
Antiminth, *see* Pyrantel pamoate
Antimycobacterial agent(s), 258–262, 259(t)
  for leprosy, 261–262
  for tuberculosis, 258–261, 259(t)
Antiparasitic agent(s), 264–270
Antiparkinsonian drug(s), *see* Parkinsonian disorders, drugs for
Antipsychotic(s), 99–104, 100(t), *101*
  adverse effects of, 102–104
  autonomic nervous system effects of, 103
  classification of, 99–100, 100(t)
  clonidine and, 104
  CNS effects of, 102–103
  contraindications for, 102–104
  drug interactions with, 104
  endocrine and metabolic effects of, 103
  guanethidine and, 104
  levodopa and, 104, 119
  mechanism of action of, 101
  α-methyldopa and, 104
  morphine and, 115
  overdose of, 104
  prolactin secretion increase due to, 210
  structure of, 99–100, *101*
  uses of, 101–102
Antipyresis, NSAIDs for, 158
Antipyretic(s), nonopioid, 163–164
Antithrombotic agent(s), 180–181
Antithyroid agent(s), described, 229
Antitumor agent(s), features of, 293Q, 295E
Antitussive agent(s), for cough, 205
Antivert, *see* Medizine
Anturane, *see* Sulfinpyrazone
  actions of, 180
  for gout, 164–165
  warfarin and, 179
Anxiety
  benzodiazepines for, 95, 97
  buspirone for, 97
  morphine for, 113–114, 113(t)
  propranolol for, 50
Aortic aneurysm, acute dissecting
  ganglionic-blocking drugs for, 35
  trimethaphan for, 86
A.P.L., *see* Human chorionic gonadotropin
Apnea
  in preterm infants, methylxanthines for, 202
  prolonged, nondepolarizing neuromuscular junction-blocking drugs and, 37
Apomorphine
  described, 187
  for poisonings, 309
Appetite suppressant(s), 188

histamine (H₁)-receptor antagonists for, 150
Aprazone, *see* Sulfinpyrazone
Apresoline, *see* Hydralazine
Aprindine (Fibocil), for tachyarrhythmias, 76
Aprotinin (Trasylol), 154
APSAC, *see* Anistreplase
Aqueous humor, decreased formation of, timolol and, 53Q, 55E
ara-A, *see* Vidarabine
ara-C, *see* Cytarabine
Arachidonic acid, formation of, 154
Aralen, *see* Chloroquine
Aramine, *see* Metaraminol
Arfonad, *see* Trimethalphan
Arildone, for viruses, 271
Aristocort, *see* Triamcinolone
  administration of, 225
  described, 203
  mechanism of action of, 325Q, 332E
  properties of, 224(t)
  for skin disorders, 240Q, 242E
Armour Thyroid, *see* Thyroid USP
Arrhythmia(s)
  α-adrenoceptor antagonists for, 48
  β-adrenoceptor antagonists for, 50
  antidepressants and, 108
  antipsychotics and, 103–104
  cardiac glycosides and, 71
  cardiac glycosides for, 69
  causes of, 73
  potassium for, 71
  quinidine and, 89Q, 93E
  theophylline and, 322Q, 330E
  treatment of, goal of, 73
  ventricular
    bepridil and, 80
    disopyramide for, 75
    life-threatening, moricizine for, 76
Arsenic
  described, 312Q, 313E
  inorganic, poisoning by, 305
  mechanism of action of, 305
  organic, 305
    poisoning by, 305
  properties of, 305
  trivalent, described, 311Q, 312E
Arsine gas, poisoning by, 305
Arsobal, *see* Melarsoprol
Artane, *see* Trihexyphenidyl
Arteritis, necrotizing, amphetamine and, 138
Arthritis
  juvenile, aspirin for, 159
  rheumatoid
    aspirin for, 159
    azathioprine for, 166
    cyclophosphamide for, 167
Asacol, *see* Mesalamine
Asbestosis, particulate poisoning and, 300
Ascariasis, piperazine citrate for, 270
Asendin, *see* Amoxapine
L-Asparaginase (Elspar), 280(t), 290–291
  drug resistance to, 294Q, 295E
Aspirin, 158–161
  actions of, 180
  adverse effects of, 159–160, 317Q, 327E
  characteristics of, 182Q, 183E
  contraindications for, 160, 168Q, 170E
  drug interactions with, 160
  inhibition of eicosanoid synthesis by, 157
  pharmacologic properties of, 159
  during pregnancy, 160
  toxicity of, 160–161
  uses of, 159
  warfarin and, 179
Astemizole (Hismanal), 149, 149(t)
  described, 169Q, 170E
Asthenic vegetative syndrome, 306
Asthma
  described, 199
  drugs for, 200–203, 206Q, 207E
    cromolyn, 150

HydroDIURIL, *see* Hydrochlorothiazide
   hypokalemia due to, 91Q, 94E
Hydromorphone (Dilaudid), 116
   for analgesia, 113–114, 113(t)
   for cough, 205
Hydroperoxyeicosatetraenoic acids
   (HPETEs), *see* HPETEs
Hydroxocobalamin (AlphaRedisol), 175
Hydroxyamphetamine (Paredrine)
   effects of, 43–44
   uses of, 45
Hydroxychloroquine (Plaquenil), 163
Hydroxyeicosatetraenoic acids (HETEs), *see*
   HETEs
5-Hydroxyindoleacetic acid (5-HIAA), 150
Hydroxylation, aromatic, reaction for, 12
Hydroxyprogesterone caproate (Delalutin),
   218
5-Hydroxytryptamine, *see* Serotonin
Hydroxyurea (Hydrea)
   described, 290
   mechanism of action of, 294Q, 296E
Hygroton, *see* Chlorthalidone
Hylorel, *see* Guanadrel sulfate
Hyperaldosteronism, trilostane for, 227
Hypercalcemia
   acute, loop diuretics for, 59
   calcitonin for, 236
   cardiac glycosides and, 71
   furosemide for, 239Q, 241E
Hypercalciuria, idiopathic, thiazide diuretics for, 58, 237
Hypercholesterolemia(s), drugs for, 68
Hyperglycemia
   drugs for, 232(t), 234–235
   glucocorticoids and, 227
   thiazide diuretics and, 58
Hyperglycemic(s), 232(t), 234–235
Hyperkalemia
   potassium-sparing diuretics and, 60
   succinylcholine and, 38
Hyperlipidemia(s), drugs for, 65–69
   clofibrate for, 66
   gemfibrozil for, 67
Hyperlipoproteinemia(s), 64
Hyperparathyroidism, β-adrenoceptor antagonists for, 240Q, 242E
Hyperplasia
   adrenal, congenital, aminoglutethimide
      for, 227
   adrenocortical, glucocorticoids for, 226
   gingival, cyclosporine and, 166
Hyperprolactinemia, ergots for, 153
Hyperreflexia, autonomic, ganglionic-
   blocking drugs for, 35
Hypersensitivity (intolerance), aspirin and,
   159–160
Hypersensitivity reaction(s)
   cephalosporins and, 250
   chloramphenicol and, 255
   heparin and, 178
   insulin and, 233
   loop diuretics and, 59
Hyperstat, *see* Diazoxide
Hypertension
   ACE inhibitors for, 63, 83(t), 84
   adrenergic neuronal blocking agents for,
      83(t), 85–86
   adrenoceptor antagonists for, 46, 47t, 48,
      50, 81, 82(t)-83(t), 84
   calcium channel blockers for, 83(t), 84–85
   catecholamine synthesis blockers for, 86
   congestive, 57
   cyclosporine and, 166
   diuretics for, 81, 82(t)
   drugs for, 81–87, 82(t)-83(t)
      amiloride, 60
      captopril, 63
      chlorothiazide, 91Q, 94E
      enalapril, 64
      propranolol, 49
      trimethaphan, 86
   ganglionic-blocking drugs for, 35
   glucocorticoids and, 227

loop diuretics for, 59
MAO inhibitors and, 109
oral contraceptives and, 241Q, 242E
pheochromocytoma-induced
   labetalol for, 84
   metyrosine for, 86
pulmonary, of the newborn, tolazoline
   for, 87
sympathomimetic agents for, 45, 83(t), 85
thiazide diuretics for, 58
vasodilators for, 83(t), 86–87
Hypertensive crisis
   α-adrenoceptor antagonists for, 47(t),
      48
   MAO inhibitors and, 143Q, 145E
Hyperthermia
   aspirin and, 161
   malignant
      dantrolene for, 51Q, 54E
      succinylcholine and, 38
   MAO inhibitors and, 109
Hyperthyroidism
   arrhythmias and, propranolol for, 90Q,
      93E
   oral cholecystographic agents for, 230
   radioactive iodine for, 230
   thioamides for, 229
Hypertrophy, insulin and, 233
Hyperventilation, aspirin and, 160
Hypnosis, defined, 95
Hypoadrenalism, drugs for, 213
Hypocalcemia
   acute, calcium supplements for, 238
   vitamin D for, 237, 239Q, 241E
Hypocalcemic tetany, calcium supplements
   for, 238
Hypoglycemia
   aspirin and, 161
   insulin and, 232
   leucine-sensitive, diazoxide for, 235
   tolbutamide and, 233
Hypoglycemic agent(s)
   diazoxide, 235
   oral, 233–234
      mechanism of action of, 233
      pharmacologic properties of, 233–234
      structure of, 233
      uses of, 234
Hypoglycemic crisis, glucagon for, 234
Hypogonadism
   estrogens for, 217
   hypogonadotropic, pituitary function as-
      sessment in, GnRH for, 210
   nandrolone for, 239Q, 241E
   prepubertal and postpubertal, androgens
      for, 222
Hypokalemia
   cardiac glycosides and, 71
   described, 320Q, 328E
   drugs causing, 91Q, 94E
Hypoparathyroidism
   dihydrotachysterol for, 240Q, 242E
   parathyroid hormone for, 235
Hypotension
   α-adrenoceptor antagonists for, 48
   bretylium and, 77
   local anesthetics and, 132
   morphine and, 115
   nondepolarizing neuromuscular junction-
      blocking drugs and, 37
   opioids and, 115
   orthostatic
      antidepressants and, 108
      antipsychotics and, 103
      drugs causing, 142Q, 145E
   sympathomimetic drugs for, 44
Hypothalamus, drug effects on, 209–211
Hypothrombinemia of newborn, vitamin K
   for, 179
Hypothyroidism
   levothyroxine and, 323Q, 330E
   radioactive iodine for, 230
   thyroid hormones for, 229

Hypoxia, carbon monoxide poisoning and,
   299
Hytakerol, *see* Dihydrotachysterol
Hytrin, *see* Terazosin

I

Ibuprofen (Advil, Motrin), 161
Idiopathic nephrosis, of children, glucocorticoids for, 226
Idoxuridine (IDU, iododeoxyuridine)
   actions of, 274Q, 277E
   viral synthesis inhibited by, 271
IDU, *see* Idoxuridine
Ifex, *see* Ifosfamide
Ifosfamide (Ifex), described, 280(t), 283
Imipenem/cilastatin (Primaxin)
   described, 251
   pharmacologic properties of, 249(t)
Imipramine (Janimine, Tofranil)
   biochemical activity of, 105(t)
   mechanism of action of, 143Q, 146E
   orthostatic hypotension due to, 142Q,
      145E
   prolactin secretion increase due to, 210
Immune disorder(s), insulin and, 233
Immune response, inhibition of, drugs for,
   165–167
Immunosuppression, glucocorticoids for,
   226, 241Q, 242E
Immunosuppressive agent(s), 165–167
   types of, 166–167
   uses of, 165–166
Imodium, *see* Loperamide
Impotence
   antipsychotics and, 103
   ganglionic-blocking drugs and, 35
Impromidine, 148
Imuran, *see* Azothiaprine
Inapsine, *see* Droperidol
Indanedione derivative(s), 179
Indapamide (Lozol, Lozide), 58
   hypokalemia due to, 91Q, 94E
Inderal, *see* Propranolol
Indocin, *see* Indomethacin
Indoline, 58
Indomethacin (Indocin), 162
   ADH effects of, 62
   features of, 169Q, 171E
   for gout, 164, 169Q, 170E, 318Q,
      327E
Inert ingredients, drug absorption affected
   by, 7
Infalyate, for diarrhea, 195
Infant(s)
   preterm, apnea in, 202
   vomiting in, Emetrol for, 187
Infantile spasm(s), drugs for, 124
Infection(s)
   cestode, drugs for, 270
   dermatophyte, tolnaftate for, 264
   fluke, drugs for, 270, 275Q, 278E
   fungal, drugs for, 275Q, 278E
   gastrointestinal, trimethoprim/
      sulfamethoxazole for, 257
   gram-negative, amikacin for, 252
   Haemophilus influenzae, cefotaxime for,
      274Q, 277E
   herpes zoster virus, interferons for, 273
   herpetic
      acyclovir for, 272, 276Q, 278E
      of the eye, vidarabine for, 271
      in neonates, vidarabine for, 271
      mucocutaneous, acyclovir for, 272
   HIV, didanosine for, 272
   metazoan, drugs for, 269–270
   mycobacterial
      cycloserine for, 251
      streptomycin for, 252
   Mycobacterium leprae, drugs for,
      261–262
   nematode, drugs for, 269–270, 275Q,
      278E
   protozoal, drugs for, 264–269